European F

Endorsements

The European Pain Federation has contributed to a greater understanding of health challenges across the EU with this book. Policymakers in the European Union and nationally will benefit from this expertise and more fully understand their political responsibility.

Heinz K. Becker, Member of the European Parliament

It has been said that 'an unexamined life is not worth living'. Yet examination requires both insight and courage. *European Pain Management* is an exercise in self-examination that reflects the high value of the pain workforce, as well as those living with the experience of pain. The book reviews with clarity and integrity the current state of pain management in Europe and fearlessly looks ahead to explore strategic possibilities. The European Pain Federation and its members are to be commended for the publication of this outstanding book on the eve of its 25th anniversary.

Chris Hayes, Dean, Faculty of Pain Medicine,
Australian and New Zealand College of Anaesthetists

This book provides a timely and comprehensive overview of pain practice and research from a uniquely European perspective. Featuring chapters by key leaders in the field, it highlights advances as well as challenges for those seeking to understand and manage pain. The book is the only one of its kind to address pain-related issues across 37 countries in the European community. This book has much to teach not only Europeans, but also those in international pain practice and the research community at large. It deserves to be on the shelf of anyone interested in pain-related issues that are of common concern across different countries as well as unique issues that arise in the context of individual countries.

Francis J. Keefe, Editor-in-Chief, PAIN

For many years, pain was studied and addressed in accordance with the body region affected. This practice lead to an under appreciation of how many individuals suffered from pain in aggregate. When studied as a whole, pain emerges as a significant public health problem for which adequate treatments are lacking. The European Pain Federation (EPF) has nicely documented the breadth of this problem in Europe and has identified both similarities across and unique challenges within countries with respect to how practitioners are trained, how the public is educated, how pain is treated, how multidisciplinary care is accessed and delivered, and which gaps in our knowledge should serve as priorities for research. This book can serve as a guide to those wishing to make systemic impact on how pain is recognized and addressed. From the perspective outside of Europe, this book also provides valuable insights into the shared challenges of pain that apply globally. I found this book enlightening and I plan to include it among the top references supporting the need for better education, access, and treatments for pain.

David A. Williams,
President, American Pain Society

European Pain Management

Edited by

Christopher Eccleston
Professor of Medical Psychology, and Director,
Centre for Pain Research, The University of Bath, UK

Christopher Wells
Vice President, European Pain Federation EFIC®, Belgium

Bart Morlion
President, European Pain Federation EFIC® and
Professor and Director, Leuven Centre for Algology and Pain
Management, University of Leuven, Belgium

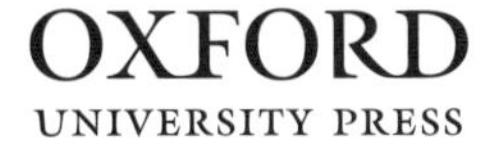

OXFORD
UNIVERSITY PRESS

OXFORD
UNIVERSITY PRESS

Great Clarendon Street, Oxford, OX2 6DP,
United Kingdom

Oxford University Press is a department of the University of Oxford.
It furthers the University's objective of excellence in research, scholarship,
and education by publishing worldwide. Oxford is a registered trade mark of
Oxford University Press in the UK and in certain other countries

First Edition published in 2018

Impression: 1

Published in the United States of America by Oxford University Press
198 Madison Avenue, New York, NY 10016, United States of America

British Library Cataloguing in Publication Data

Data available

Library of Congress Control Number: 2017952074

ISBN 978–0–19–878575–0

Printed in Great Britain by
Bell & Bain Ltd., Glasgow

Acknowledgements

We are grateful for the help and support of all of the councillors of the European Pain Federation and their country authors who worked hard to put this material together. The team in the federation office was also helpful, in particular Christel Geevels who oversaw the contributions. None of it would have been possible without the constant support and encouragement of Caroline Smith, from Oxford University Press, who project-managed, worked with our changing deadlines, and kept the faith in our goal to produce the first summary report of the state of European Pain.

Contents

Contributors *xi*
Abbreviations *xvii*

Section 1 **Foundations**

1.1 Pain in Europe *3*
Christopher Eccleston, Bart Morlion, and Christopher Wells

1.2 Epidemiology of pain: Its importance for clinical management and research *8*
Harald Breivik

Section 2 **National chapter reports**

2.1 Albania *19*
Apostol Vaso

2.2 Austria *22*
Rudolf Likar

2.3 Belgium *27*
Patrice Forget, Susan Broekmans, Lies de Ruddere, Conny Goethals, Koen Lauwers, Bruno Leroy, Marie-Claire Schommer, and Guy Hans

2.4 Bosnia and Herzegovina *31*
Amira Karkin-Tais

2.5 Bulgaria *37*
Atanas Temelkov

2.6 Croatia *41*
Mira Fingler and Ivan Radoš

2.7 Czech Republic *46*
Richard Rokyta and Jiří Kozák

2.8 Denmark *52*
Gitte Handberg and Thorvaldur Skuli Palsson

2.9 Estonia *57*
Maksim Kunevich and Aleksandra Shilova

2.10 Finland *62*
Juha Nevantaus

2.11 France *67*
Didier Bouhassira and Nadine Attal

2.12 Germany *75*
Thomas Tölle, Michael Schäfer, and Thomas Isenberg

2.13 Greece *80*
Emmanouil P. Anastassiou

2.14 Hungary *85*
János Tajti, Délia Szok, and János Szolcsányi

2.15 Ireland *91*
David P. Finn, Brona M. Fullen, Brian E. McGuire, Joanne O'Brien, Laserina O'Connor, Raymond Victory, and Shelagh Wright

2.16 Israel *98*
Elon Eisenberg and Silviu Brill

2.17 Italy *103*
Stefano Coaccioli and Antonella Paladini

2.18 Kosovo *107*
Adem Bytyqi, Agron Bytyqi, and Bashkim Sylaj

2.19 Latvia *111*
Iveta Golubovska, Mihails Arons, Aleksejs Miscuks, and Inara Logina

2.20 Lithuania *117*
Arunas Sciupokas

2.21 Moldova *121*
Adrian Belîi

2.22 Norway *127*
Petter Borchgrevink and Astrid Woodhouse

2.23 Poland *130*
Jan Dobrogowski and Magdalena Kocot-Kępska

2.24 Portugal *136*
Ana Valentim and Pedro Ferreira

2.25 Romania *141*
Adriana Sarah Nica

2.26 Russia *147*
Nikilay N. Yakhno, Michael L. Kukushkin, and Maxim V. Churyukanov

2.27 San Marino *152*
Daniele Battelli

2.28 Serbia *155*
Miroslava Pjevic

2.29 Slovakia *160*
Marta Kulichová

2.30 Slovenia *165*
Marija Cesar Komar, Nevenka Krčevski-Škvarč, and Gorazd Požlep

2.31 Spain *169*
Rafael Galvez Mateos and Juan Perez Cajaraville

2.32 Sweden *174*
Anna Bjarnegård, Carina Carlsson, Eva Gåve, Rolf Karlsten, Malin Lindbäck, Elisabeth Persson, and Malin Ernberg

2.33 Switzerland *181*
André Ljutow and Christine Cedraschi

2.34 The Netherlands *185*
Gertie Filippini, Kris Vissers, and Michiel Reneman

2.35 Turkey *191*
Nuri Süleyman Ozyalcin

2.36 Ukraine *195*
Vladimir Romanenko

2.37 United Kingdom *199*
Ann Taylor

Section 3 **Special issues**

3.1 Pain in later life *207*
Gisèle Pickering

3.2 Pain in children *216*
Julia Wager and Boris Zernikow

3.3 Opioids for pain in Europe: Differing problems and differing solutions *225*
Cathy Stannard

3.4 Specialty pain medicine *243*
Andreas Kopf

3.5 Working at the frontiers of pain management in Europe *249*
Nevenka Krčevski-Škvarč

3.6 European pain policy: Challenges and opportunities *255*
Norbert van Rooij, Joop van Griensven, Mariano Votta, and Bart Morlion

3.7 European pain management: Future directions *267*
Christopher Eccleston, Christopher Wells, and Bart Morlion

Index *275*

Contributors

Emmanouil P. Anastassiou
Head Director of Anaesthesia Department and Pain Clinic, Thriassio General Hospital of Elefsina, Greece

Mihails Arons
Senior Consultant, P. Stradins University Hospital Pain Clinic, Head of the Medical Center D.A.P. Pain clinic, President of Latvian Association for the Study of Pain, Latvia

Nadine Attal
Head of the Pain Center, Ambroise Paré Hospital and member of the INSERM U 987 Research Team Centre d'Evaluation et de Traitement de la Douleur Hôpital Ambroise Paré, Boulogne-Billancourt, France

Daniele Battelli
Consultant, Anesthesia, Intensive Care and Pain Unit, San Marino State Hospital, San Marino Republic

Adrian Belîi
Professor of Anesthesiology and Intensive Care, Chair of Anaesthesiology and Intensive Care 'Valeriu Ghereg', *Nicolae Testemitanu* State University of Medicine and Pharmacy, Chisinau, Republic of Moldova

Anna Bjarnegård
President Swedish Pain Society; and Institute of Neuroscience and Physiology, Department of Health and Rehabilitation/Physiotherapy, University of Gothenburg, Sweden

Petter Borchgrevink
Director, Multidisciplinary Pain Center and National Center for Competence in Complex Symptom Disorders, St. Olav's Hospital, Trondheim, Norway

Didier Bouhassira
Past President of the French Pain Society; and Head of Pathophysiology and Clinical Pharmacology of Pain Research Center (Inserm U987), Centre d'Evaluation et de Traitement de la Douleur Ambroise Paré Hospital, Boulogne-Billancourt, France

Harald Breivik
Professor of Anaesthesiology, Department of Pain Management and Research; and Department of Anaesthesiology, Oslo University Hospital, and The University of Oslo, Norway

Silviu Brill
Past President Israel Pain Association; and Director, Institute of Pain Medicine, Tel Aviv Medical Center, Israel

Susan Broekmans
Clinical Nurse Specialist Pain, Leuven Center for Algology and Pain Management, Nursing Center of Excellence, UZ Leuven, Belgium

Adem Bytyqi
Specialist of Anesthesiology and ICU, General Hospital of Prizren, Kosovo

Agron Bytyqi
Coordinator, Centre for Continuing Professional Education, General Hospital of Prizren, Kosovo

Juan Perez Cajaraville
Clinical Director, Pain Services, HM University Hospitals, Madrid, Spain

Carina Carlsson
Head of Pain Clinic, Department of Anesthesia, Södertälje Hospital, Sweden

Christine Cedraschi
Senior Lecturer, Faculty of Medicine, University of Geneva; and Multidisciplinary Pain Centre, Division of General Medical Rehabilitation; and Clinical Pharmacology and Toxicology, Geneva University Hospitals, Switzerland

Maxim V. Churyukanov
EFIC Councillor; and Assistant Professor, Department of Neurology and Neurosurgery, I.M. Sechenov First MSMU, Neurologist, Pain Clinic of the B.V. Petrovsky Russian National Surgery Center, Moscow, Russia

Stefano Coaccioli
EFIC Italy Advisor; Head and Chief, Department of Internal Medicine, Rheumatology and Medical Pain Therapy, Perugia University School of Medicine; and 'S.Maria' General Hospital, Terni, Italy

Lies de Ruddere
Senior Research Fellow, Ghent Health Psychology Lab, Department of Experimental-Clinical and Health Psychology, Ghent University, Belgium

Jan Dobrogowski
President of Polish Association for the Study of Pain, and Chair of Anaesthesiology and Intensive Therapy, Department for Pain Research and Treatment, Medical College, Jagiellonian University, Krakow, Poland

Christopher Eccleston
Professor of Medical Psychology, and Director Centre for Pain Research, The University of Bath, UK

Elon Eisenberg
Past President Israel Pain Association, Professor of Neurology and Pain Medicine and Director, Pain Research Unit, Institute of Pain Medicine, Rambam Health Care Campus, Haifa, Israel

Malin Ernberg
Professor and Division Head, Oral Diagnostics and Rehabilitation, Department of Dental Medicine, Karolinska Institutet; and Scandinavian Center of Orofacial Neurosciences (SCON), Huddinge, Sweden

Pedro Ferreira
Associate Professor, Health Economics, Faculty of Economics, University of Coimbra; Director, Centre for Health Studies and Research, University of Coimbra, Portugal

Gertie Filippini
Past President Dutch Pain Society; and Consultant Anesthesiologist, Bernhoven, Uden, the Netherlands

Mira Fingler
Specialist in Anesthesiology and Intensive Care; and President of Croatian Pain Society, Osijek, Croatia

David P. Finn
Professor of Pharmacology and Therapeutics; and Co-Director, Centre for Pain Research, Pharmacology and Therapeutics, School of Medicine, National University of Ireland, Galway, Ireland

Patrice Forget
Vice-President of the Belgian Pain Society; Anesthesiology and Perioperative Medicine, Vrije Universiteit Brussels; and Universitair Ziekenhuis Brussels, Belgium

Brona M. Fullen
School of Public Health, Physiotherapy and Sports Science and Director, University College Dublin Centre for Translational Pain Research, University College Dublin, Ireland

Eva Gåve
Department of Women's and Children's Health and Department of Neuroscience, Uppsala University Children's Hospital, Sweden

Conny Goethals
Executive Secretary, Belgian Pain Society, Pellenberg, Belgium

Iveta Golubovska
Head, Anaesthesiology and Intensive Care Department, Hospital of Traumatology and Orthopaedics, Riga, Latvia

Gitte Handberg
Chairman, Danish Pain Society; and Chief physician, Pain Center South, Odense University Hospital, Norway

Guy Hans
President of the Belgian Pain Society; and Multidisciplinair Pijncentrum, Universitair Ziekenhuis Antwerpen, Edegem, Belgium

Thomas Isenberg
Executive Officer, German Pain Society (Deutsche Schmerzgesellschaft e.V), Berlin, Germany

Amira Karkin-Tais
President, Association for Pain Therapy in Bosnia and Herzegovina (APTBandH), Sarajevo, Bosnia and Herzegovina

Rolf Karlsten
Head, Rehabilitation Medicine and Pain Centre, Department of Surgical Sciences/Anaesthesiology and Intensive Care, Uppsala University, Sweden

Magdalena Kocot-Kępska
Secretary of Polish Association for the Study of Pain and Chair, Anaesthesiology and Intensive Therapy, Department for Pain Research and Treatment, Medical College, Krakow, Poland

Marija Cesar Komar
Consultant in Anesthesiology, Head of Pain Unit, General Hospital Slovenj Gradec, Slovenia

Andreas Kopf
Chairman of EFIC Educational Committee; Visiting Professor Department of Medical Physiology University of Nairobi; and Head, Benjamin Franklin Pain Centre, Department of Anaesthesiology and Surgical Intensive Care, Campus Benjamin Franklin, Charité University Medicine Berlin, Germany

Jiří Kozák
Head, Centre for the Study and Treatment of Pain, Charles University; and President of Czech Pain Society, Prague, Czech Republic

Nevenka Krčevski-Škvarč
Founder of Slovenian Association for Pain Management (SZZB), First president; Head, Pain Unit and Palliative Care, University Hospital Maribor, Maribor, Slovenia

Michael L. Kukushkin
Executive Secretary, Russian Association for the Study of Pain; and Professor and Director of Fundamental and Applied Pain Laboratory, General Pathology and Pathophysiology Institute, Moscow, Russia

Marta Kulichová
President of Slovak Society for Study and Treatment of Pain (SSSTP); and Head of Chronic Pain Department, Martin University Hospital, Slovakia

Maksim Kunevich
Senior Anesthesiologist, Pain Management; Deputy Director, Anesthesiology and Intensive Care Department, East-Viru Central Hospital; and Board Member, Estonian Pain Society, Kohtla-Järve, Ida-Viruma, Estonia

Koen Lauwers
Head, Pain Centre, AZ Klina Brasschaat, Antwerp, Belgium

Bruno Leroy
Head of Service, Physical Medicine and Rehabilitation, Eupen Hospital, Belgium

Rudolf Likar
Head, Department of Anaesthesiology and Intensive Care, General Hospital Klagenfurt; and Secretary-General, Austrian Pain Society and EFIC Councillor, Austria

Malin Lindbäck
Psychologist, The Pain Clinic, Pain Center, Anaesthesiology and Intensive Care, Danderyd´s University Hospital, Stockholm, Sweden

André Ljutow
President of Swiss Association for the Study of Pain; and Head, Centre for Pain Medicine, Swiss Paraplegic Centre, Nottwil/Lucerne, Switzerland

Inara Logina
Department of Neurology and Neurosurgery, Riga Stradins University; and Consultant in Pain, Care Unit, Pauls Stradins University Hospital, Riga, Latvia

Rafael Galvez Mateos
Head, Pain Unit, Virgen de la Nieves University Hospital, Granada, Spain

Brian E. McGuire
Professor, Clinical Psychology; and Co-Director, Centre for Pain Research, School of Psychology National University of Ireland, Galway, Ireland

Aleksejs Miscuks
Senior Consultant, Anaesthesiology and Intensive Care Department, Hospital of Traumatology and Orthopaedics; and Assistant Professor, Faculty of Medicine, Latvian University, Riga, Latvia

Bart Morlion
President, European Pain Federation EFIC®; and Professor, and Director, Leuven Centre for Algology and Pain Management, University of Leuven, Belgium

Juha Nevantaus
President, Finnish Association for the Study of Pain; and Specialist in Anaesthesiology and Pain Medicine, Department of Anaesthesiology and Intensive Treatment, Central Hospital of Central Finland, Jyväskylä, Finland

Adriana Sarah Nica
Head, Rehabilitation Department, University of Medicine and Pharmacy 'Carol Davila', Bucharest, Bucharest, Romania

Joanne O'Brien
President-Elect, Irish Pain Society; and Registered Advanced Nurse Practitioner, Department of Pain Medicine, Beaumont Hospital, Dublin, Ireland

Laserina O'Connor
Professor, Clinical Nursing; and Director of Pain Programs, University College Dublin School of Nursing Midwifery and Health Systems, University College Dublin, Belfield, Ireland

Nuri Süleyman Ozyalcin
Pain Specialist, Anesthesiology; and President Turkish Society of Pain, Istanbul, Turkey

Antonella Paladini
Department of Anaesthesiology and Pain Therapy, L'Aquila University School of Medicine, Italy

Thorvaldur Skuli Palsson
Assistant Professor, Department of Health Science and Technology, Aalborg University, Denmark

Elisabeth Persson
Department of Pain Rehabilitation Medicine, Skane University Hospital, Lund, Sweden; Department of Clinical Sciences, Danderyd Hospital, Karolinska Institutet, Stockholm; and National Coordinator and Board Member, Swedish Quality Registry for Pain Rehabilitation, Sweden

Gisèle Pickering
Professor of Medicine and Clinical Pharmacology, Clinical Pharmacology Centre, University Hospital, Laboratory of Fundamental and Clinical Pharmacology of Pain, Medical Faculty, Clermont-Ferrand, France

Miroslava Pjevic
Professor of Anaesthesiology, Faculty of Medicine, University of Novi Sad, Serbia

Gorazd Požlep
Consultant in Anesthesiology, Head of Pain Center, University Clinical Center, Ljubljana, Slovenia

Ivan Radoš
Secretary of Croatian Pain Society, Head of the Institute for Pain Management, University Hospital Osijek, Croatia

Michiel Reneman
Co-chair Dutch Pain Society, and Professor, Rehabilitation Medicine, University Medical Center Groningen, the Netherlands

Richard Rokyta
Head, Department of Normal, Pathological and Clinical Physiology, Third Faculty of Medicine, Charles University; International and Scientific Secretary of Czech Pain Society; and Councilor of EAP-EFIC, Prague, Czech Republic

Vladimir Romanenko
Executive Secretary, Ukrainian Association for the Study of Pain; and Head, Department of Science; Shupik National Medical Academy of Postgraduate Education, Bohomolets National Medical University, Kyiv, Ukraine

Michael Schäfer
Professor and Vice-Chairman, Department of Anaesthesiology and Intensive Care Medicine, Charité University Berlin, Germany

Marie-Claire Schommer
Nurse Pain Coordinator, Paediatric and Adult Services, Centre Hospitalier Chretien, Liège, Belgium

Arunas Sciupokas
Associate Professor of Neurology and Senior Lecturer, Department of Neurology, Lithuanian University of Health Sciences, Kaunas, Lithuania

Aleksandra Shilova
General Surgery Resident, Tartu University Hospital; Surgical Department, East-Viru Central Hospital; and Member of the Estonian Pain Society, Kohtla-Järve, Ida-Viruma, Estonia

Cathy Stannard
Consultant in Complex Pain and Pain Transformation Programme Clinical Lead, NHS Gloucestershire Clinical Commissioning Group, UK

Bashkim Sylaj
Treasurer of PHA and Nurse at the General Hospital of Prizren, Kosovo

Délia Szok
Secretary of the Hungarian Pain Society; and Department of Neurology, University of Szeged, Hungary

János Szolcsányi
EFIC Councilor of the Hungarian Pain Society; and Department of Pharmacology and Pharmacotherapy, University of Pécs, Hungary

János Tajti
President of the Hungarian Pain Society; and Department of Neurology, University of Szeged, Hungary

Ann Taylor
Professor and Post Graduate Taught Director, Cardiff University School of Medicine, Centre for Medical Education, Cardiff University, Wales, UK

Atanas Temelkov
Chief, Clinic of Anesthesiology and Intensive Care, Alexandrovska University Hospital, Sofia, Bulgaria

Thomas Tölle
Head, Interdisciplinary Pain Clinic, Department of Neurology, Technische Universität München, Munich, Germany

Ana Valentim
Consultant in Anaesthesiology, Chronic Pain Unit, Department of Anaesthesiology, Centro Hospitalar e Universitário de Coimbra, Coimbra, Portugal

Joop van Griensven
President, Pain Alliance Europe (PAE), Brussels, Belgium

Norbert van Rooij
Head, Governmental Affairs and Patient Centricity, Europe, Grünenthal GmbH, Aachen, Germany

Apostol Vaso
President, Albanian Pain Society (Shoqata Shqiptare E Dhimbjes); and Consultant Anaesthetist, Department of Anaesthesia, University of Tirana, Albania

Raymond Victory
Consultant in Pain Medicine, St. Vincent's Hospital, Dublin, Ireland

Kris Vissers
Co-chair Dutch Pain Society; and Professor Anesthesiology, Pain and Palliative Medicine, Radboud University Medical Center, Nijmegen, the Netherlands

Mariano Votta
Director, Active Citizenship Network, Responsible European Affairs, Cittadinanzattiva, Rome, Italy

Julia Wager
Scientific Coordinator, German Paediatric Pain Centre, Children's and Adolescents' Hospital Datteln; and Department of Children's Pain Therapy and Paediatric Palliative Care, Witten/Herdecke University, Faculty of Health, School of Medicine, Witten, Germany

Christopher Wells
Vice President of the European Pain Federation EFIC®, Belgium

Astrid Woodhouse
President of the Norwegian Association for the Study of Pain; and Physical Therapist, Multidisciplinary Pain Center; and National Center for Competence in Complex Symptom Disorders, St. Olav's Hospital, Trondheim, Norway

Shelagh Wright
Committee Member, Irish Pain Society and Irish Pain Research Network, Ireland

Nikilay N. Yakhno
Professor and Director of Neurology Science Department, I.M. Sechenov First MSMU Research Center; and President, Russian Association for the Study of Pain, Moscow, Russia

Boris Zernikow
Head, German Paediatric Pain Centre, Children's and Adolescents' Hospital, Datteln; and Chair of Children's Pain Therapy and Paediatric Palliative Care, Witten/Herdecke University, Faculty of Health, School of Medicine, Witten, Germany

Abbreviations

AIM	anaesthesiology and intensive medicine
AISD	Associazione Italiana per lo Studio del Dolore
ANZCA	Australian and New Zealand College of Anaesthetists
APED	Portuguese Association for the Study of Pain
APPEAL	Advancing the Provision of Pain Education and Learning
APS	acute postoperative pain
ARSD	Romanian Association for the Study of Pain
BASTP	Bulgarian Association for the Study and Treatment of Pain
BPS	Belgian Pain Society/British Pain Society
CAM	complementary and alternative medicine
CIDR	Computerized Infectious Disease Reporting
CIHI	Croatian Institute for Health Insurance
CME	continuing medical education
CNS	central nervous system
COEGD	Comité d'organisation des états généraux de la douleur
CP	chronic pain
CPR	Centre for Pain Research
CPS	Czech Pain Society
CRPS	complex regional pain syndrome
CSO	Central Statistics Office
CTPR	Centre for Translational Pain Research
DDD	defined daily dose
DIVS	German Interdisciplinary Pain Association
DPS	Dutch Pain Society
DPT	Prime Ministry State Planning Organization of the Turkish Republic
ECMDDA	European Monitoring Centre for Drugs and Drug Addiction
EDPM	European Diploma of Pain Medicine
EFIC	European Pain Federation
EMLA	eutectic mixture of local anaesthetics
ESRA	European Society of Regional Anaesthesia
EU	European Union
FASP	Finnish Association for the Study of Pain
FED	Spanish Pain Foundation
FEDELAT	Latin American Federation of Pain
FPM	Faculty of Pain Medicine
FPS	Federal Public Service
GDP	gross domestic product
GHO	Global Health Observatory
GNHS	Greek National Health System
HPHC	High Public Health Committee
HPS	Hellenic Pain Society
HSA	Hellenic Society of Algology
HSC	Health and Social Care in Northern Ireland
HUCSK	Hospital and University Clinical Service of Kosovo
IASP	International Association for the Study of Pain
ICD	International Classification of Diseases
IMA	Israeli Medical Association
INCB	International Narcotics Control Board
INE	Instituto Nacional de Estatística

IPA	Israeli Pain Association
IPRN	Irish Pain Research Network
IPVZ	Institute for Postgraduate Medical Education
ISS	Istituto per la Sicurezza Sociale
LASP	Latvian Association for the Study of Pain
MED	morphine equivalent daily
MERRI	Missions d'Enseignement, de Recherche, de Recours et d'Innovation
MIG	Missions d'Intérêt Général
NATO	North Atlantic Treaty Organization
NCRI	National Cancer Registry of Ireland
NDTMS	National Drug Treatment Monitoring System
NHF	National Health Fund
NHIF	National Health Insurance Fund
NHS	National Health Service
NICE	National Institute for Health and Care Excellence
NMC	neuromodulation centre
NPFAP	National Programme for the Fight Against Pain
NPS	Norwegian Pain Society
NRS	numeric rating scale
NSK	National Coordination Group for Knowledge Dissemination
OECD	Organisation for Economic Co-operation and Development
OMC	Open Method of Coordination
OPSS	Observatório Português dos Sistemas de Saúde
ÖSG	Austrian Health Care Structure Plan
PAE	Pain Alliance Europe
PASP	Polish Association for the Study of Pain
PEMI	pain and emergency medicine initiative
PHA	Professional Health Association
PMP	pain management programmes
PNS	peripheral nerve stimulation
PPP	persistent post-surgical pain
PTSD	post-traumatic stress disorder
PwSI	practitioners with special interests
RASP	Russian Association for the Study of Pain
RSG	Regional Health Care Structure Plans
SAMHSA	Substance Abuse and Mental Health Services Administration
SAPRT	Serbian Association of Pain Research and Treatment
SASP	Swiss Association for the Study of Pain/Scandinavian Association for the Study of Pain
SBU	The Swedish Agency for Health Technology Assessment and Assessment of Social Services
SECPAL	Spanish Society of Palliative Care
SED	Spanish Pain Society
SEGG	Spanish Society of Geriatrics and Gerontology
SEOM	Spanish Society of Medical Oncology
SEOR	Spanish Society of Radiotherapy Oncology
SER	Spanish Society of Rheumatology
SHI	statutory health insurance
SIP	Societal Impact on Pain
SPS	Swedish Pain Society
SSAI	Scandinavian Society of Anaesthesiology and Intensive Care
SSSTP	Slovak Society for the Study and Treatment of Pain
SZZB	Slovenian Association for Pain Management (Slovensko združenje za zdravljenje bolečine)

TÜBİTAK	Scientific and Technological Research Council of Turkey
UASP	Ukrainian Association for the Study of Pain
UCD	University College Dublin
UEMS	European Union of Medical Specialists
UK	United Kingdom
US	United States (of America)
USG	ultrasonography
VHI	voluntary health insurance
WHO	World Health Organization
WIP	World Institute of Pain
WSPC	World Society of Pain Clinicians

Section 1

Foundations

Chapter 1.1

Pain in Europe

Christopher Eccleston, Bart Morlion, and Christopher Wells

Introduction

There are 37 countries in the European Pain Federation (EFIC), which is made up of chapters of the International Association for the Study of Pain (IASP). These chapters comprise over 20,000 healthcare providers working in the field of pain management and pain research. Absent from this are Andorra, Armenia, Azerbaijan, Belarus, Georgia, Iceland, Liechtenstein, Luxemburg, Malta, Monaco, and the Vatican City, none of which are presently chapters of the IASP. In those 37 countries, there are approximately 740 million people, most of whom will experience an episode of severe pain at some point in their life. For a significant minority, maybe as many as 20%, that pain is chronic—episodic, persistent, or variable. A smaller number of people, perhaps as many as 2% of the overall population, reports severe pain that is persistent, frequent, highly disabling, and difficult to manage. In other words, we believe that today there are 150 million people experiencing pain they would like medical help for, and 15 million who experience their pain as severely distressing and too difficult to live with. That number is approximately equal to the populations of Germany and France combined. Imagine so much pain.

Living with pain

At the centre of our thinking is the person. Pain affects all aspects of life and has the capacity to destroy all joy, all responsibility, and all motivation. Pain is the primary reason people seek help from healthcare providers. It is the main complaint in general practice, the main complaint in pharmacy practice, the main complaint in the emergency room, and the reason people most commonly give for wanting to be free of a life lived with disease (Breivik *et al.*, 2006; Gibson and Lussier, 2012; King *et al.*, 2011; McAteer *et al.*, 2011). The relief of suffering is at the core of the medical, religious, and humanitarian narratives, and the organization of attempts to relieve pain is often considered a symbol of scientific and social advancement (Lewis, 1940; Scarry, 1985). Indeed, access to pain management is now considered a fundamental human right (Cousins and Lynch, 2011; Declaration of Montreal, 2010). There is nothing more civilized than the collective action by a society to organize itself to reduce the pain and suffering of its population.

There are three areas of pain practice to consider. First, there is the use of analgesic and anaesthetic agents in the reduction or abolition of sensation associated with injury, planned or accidental. Much of what we know about such short-lived or 'acute' pain comes from the deliberate injury caused in surgical practice. Second, there is the management of pain that persists for longer than three months, either continually or episodically, which we call 'chronic' pain. And third, there is the palliative management of pain in later or end of life, pain that is often co-morbid with other debilitating symptoms, and often associated with multimorbidity.

Acute pain management is a significant part of the workload of many pain specialists across Europe. It is often considered an extension of anaesthetic practice. Pain management starts outside of hospitals, so-called 'field management', at first response to injurious accident, on the battlefield, or in the doctor's or dentist's office. There has been tremendous effort to improve the quality of acute pain management associated with operative practice, perioperatively, but principally postoperatively. In a challenging review of the current state of acute pain management, Narinder Rawal reminds us that despite there being many advances, acute pain services in Europe remain suboptimal and in need of support (Rawal, 2016). Specifically, although there has been industry in the production of guidelines at national and local levels, there is often poor compliance with the guidelines. Many European hospitals have no acute pain service, and many have no training programmes or written protocols for postoperative pain assessment. There are advances to be made still in reaching the goal of optimal acute pain management. The starting point is to determine what is meant by quality and standards, what is achievable, and how to plan for sustainable change (Zoëga *et al.*, 2016).

Chronic pain management is a major personal, societal, and economic burden. The definition of chronic pain is a temporal, rather than a qualitative one. It means having pain that lasts longer than three months. But, for most people what is important about the persistence of pain is not time, but loss: loss of function, loss of identity, loss of mental health, and for many a loss of hope (Eccleston, 2011, 2016). Hidden is a huge heterogeneity of presentation. There is no common personality, socioeconomic grouping, specific age, or race it affects. Chronic pain, whether it be from headache, disease, injury, or whether it is idiopathic, is non-discriminatory. Typical in a chronic pain presentation is, however, what was once called a syndrome of concomitant symptoms and notable features. Although the label 'syndrome' is no longer fashionable, it was used to draw attention to the importance of reduced function, anxiety, depression, family dysfunction, sleep loss, work and role loss, medication misuse, and elevated risk of further illness that its sufferers live with. The patient with chronic pain often has complex needs. This is a challenging task for the pain professional and there is multiple guidance stressing the need for shared practice, either organizationally in the structure of a service, or individually with the need for support. It is not uncommon for patients to also present with mental health needs. These needs may be secondary to the pain, intimately associated with the pain, and could be relieved as a consequence of good pain management. However, even though we do not consider them primary, for the pain physician one is still faced with helping someone in chronic distress. Chronic pain management, like acute pain management, should be approached with organizational as well as personal solutions.

Cancer pain management is a major part of European medical practice. For many cancer is now a chronic disease, which provides symptom management challenges from the condition and its treatment. There is a strong evidence base for the efficacy and safety of interventions for cancer pain, and modern practice involves the long-term support of cancer sufferers. For many, however, cancer is life-shortening, and the palliative management of pain at end of life is as important as during life. Some definitions of palliative and supportive care are broad enough to encompass much of the practice of chronic pain management, including the focus on symptom control and behavioural adjustment to living with and beyond disease (e.g. Eccleston *et al.*, 2013; Cramp and Bennett, 2013). End-of-life care, however, presents very specific challenges to the pain and symptom management community. Although this is not a specific focus in this volume, and we have not directed contributors to comment specifically on palliative care practice, it would be remiss of us to ignore what for many contributors and in some countries, is a major part of their practice. The populations of most major European countries are ageing. For many people later life is medically characterized by multimorbidity, polypharmacy, and a new challenge of living in the context of multiple symptoms. In short, we are living longer, but more of life is dominated by pain. Inevitably the pain workforce will be called upon to be part of the available solutions to later life and end-of-life needs, and just as there have been developments in the science and practice of acute and chronic pain management, we foresee an invigorated science of pain and symptom management in palliative care, on an unprecedented scale.

The European Pain Federation: Responding to need

2018 is the 25th anniversary of the European Pain Federation. In the early 1990s, Ulf Lindblom recognized the importance of individual countries establishing strong national pain societies after witnessing the growth of the IASP. He was impressed by the success of an earlier federation of national pain chapters in Northern Europe, the Scandinavian Association for the Study of Pain. He proposed the establishment of a European collective of IASP chapters, and in 1993, at the Paris World Congress of Pain, EFIC was born. Professor Lindblom was its founding president (and we are saddened to note his loss as we complete this text —for his obituary see http://onlinelibrary.wiley.com/doi/10.1002/ejp.1046/epdf). It was clearly the right idea, as EFIC grew rapidly. In 1995 the first European Pain Congress was held in Verona, and the *European Journal of Pain* was launched. EFIC has since gone from strength to strength (Erdine and Kress, 2013). The goals of EFIC remain the same today as they were in 1993: to promote awareness of the needs of people in pain across Europe; to support those working to help people in pain by advocacy, training, and scientific exchange; and to increase policy awareness, engagement, and action across Europe. The most visible activities are the large biennial pain congresses (with Copenhagen 2017 being the 10th), the annual Societal Impact for Pain Campaign in collaboration with the EU Commission (see Chapter 3.6), the development of pain curricula, accreditation, and training (see Chapter 3.4), and the establishment of annual pain schools offering access to training and expertise across Europe, from Liverpool in the United Kingdom to Maribor in Slovenia. Less publically, EFIC strives to promote the gold standard in science, policy, and practice, by supporting member chapters in their national endeavours, and in actively promoting multidisciplinary involvement in pain management whenever the opportunity arises.

What follows next?

We set out in this book to take stock and explore what is happening in the 37 countries of the European Pain Federation, and in part to expose the wealth of creativity, novelty, and endeavour that is so often hidden from view. The book is in three parts. First, Harald Breivik helps us to understand the extent of pain in Europe, how many people there are struggling to make sense of their pain and looking for treatments. In section two, there is the taking stock. We asked leaders in the 37 IASP chapters to tell us about where they live and practice. Specifically, we asked to learn more about each country, including any relevant geography, history, or politics. We were then interested in the structure and function of the healthcare systems, because they are intimately related to how people access pain management, and hence experience their pain and pain management. And last, we asked them to describe how pain management is organized, practically and professionally, and to end with an example of a local innovation that could be shared. In the final section, we invited thought leaders from across Europe who have focused on specific issues relevant to all countries to elaborate on these, including the clinical realities of pain management in children and in later life, and on the non-clinical topics of major importance, such as education and training for specialization, policy and practice, opioid prescribing, and what it is like to work at the frontiers of developing new pain services in low-income economies that are just beginning to consider pain at a population level (O'Brien *et al.*, 2017). We end by summarizing the learning from across these 37 countries. In this final chapter we go beyond the descriptive and ask critical questions of us all as we plan for the future. We end with an invitation for change, an invitation for progress, an invitation to work together in building a new future of European pain management.

References

Breivik, H., Collett, B., Ventafridda, V., Cohen, R., & Gallacher, D. (2006). Survey of chronic pain in Europe: prevalence, impact on daily life, and treatment. *Eur J Pain*, **10**, 287–333.

Cousins, M. J. & Lynch, M. E. (2011). The Declaration Montreal: Access to pain management is a fundamental human right. *Pain*, **152**, 2673–4.

Cramp, F. & Bennett, M. I. (2013). Development of a generic working definition of 'supportive care'. *BMJ Support Palliat Care*, **3**, 53–60.

Declaration of Montreal (2010). *Declaration of Montreal*. Available at: http://www.iasp-pain.org/files/Content/NavigationMenu/Advocacy/DeclarationOfMontreal.pdf (accessed 29 July 2016) [Online].

Eccleston, C. (2011). A normal psychology of pain. *Pain Manag*, **1**, 399–403.

Eccleston, C. (2016). *Embodied: The Psychology of Physical Sensation*. Oxford, UK: Oxford University Press.

Eccleston, C., Morley, S. J., & Williams, A. C. (2013). Psychological approaches to chronic pain management: evidence and challenges. *Br J Anaesth*, **11**, 59–63.

Erdine, S. & Kress, H. G. (2013) *EFIC: The First 20 Years*. Vienna, Austria: B&K.

Gibson, S. J. & Lussier, D. (2012). Prevalence and relevance of pain in older persons. *Pain Med*, **13**, S23–6.

King, S., Chambers, C.T., Huguet, A., *et al.* (2011). The epidemiology of chronic pain in children and adolescents revisited: a systematic review. *Pain*, **152**, 2729–38.

Lewis, C.S. (1940). *The Problem of Pain*. London, UK: Harper Collins.

McAteer, A., Elliott, A. M., & Hannaford, P. C. (2011). Ascertaining the size of the symptom iceberg in a UK-wide community-based survey. *Br J Gen Pract*, **61**, e1–e11.

O'Brien, T., Christrup, L. L., Drewes, A. M., *et al.* (2017) European Pain Federation position paper on appropriate opioid use in chronic pain management. *Eur J Pain*, **21**, 3–19.

Rawal, N. (2016). Current issues in post-operative pain management. *Eur J Anaesthesiol*, **33**, 160–71.

Scarry, E. (1985). *The Body in Pain: The Making and Unmaking of the World*. New York, NY: Oxford University Press.

Zoëga, S., Gunnarsdottir, S., & Wilson, M. E. (2016). Quality pain management in adult hospitalized patients: a concept evaluation. *Nurs Forum*, **51**, 3–12.

Chapter 1.2

Epidemiology of pain: Its importance for clinical management and research

Harald Breivik

Introduction

Our ability to notice and react to acute pain is a fundamental life-protecting system for alarm and defence, the importance of which is dramatically demonstrated by persons born with an abnormal voltage gated sodium channel ($Na_V1.7$) that makes them insensitive to pain. Such people suffer extreme tissue damage from painless injuries and die at an early age from complications and serious diseases without the alarm function of symptoms (e.g. acute appendicitis).

Chronic pain does not have any useful function, whether caused by ongoing pathologies (e.g. rheumatoid arthritis), injuries, and diseases of nervous tissues (e.g. multiple sclerosis, post-herpetic neuralgia, spinal cord injuries), or chronic pain from unknown or uncertain causes (e.g. fibromyalgia, chronic low back pain). Such chronic pain conditions are common, cost the individual patients and society large sums directly from cost of healthcare, and indirectly through the loss of ability to work and early disability retirement. Chronic pain conditions are often difficult to treat; ineffective treatments are expensive and can cause further complications. Epidemiological studies have documented a number of risk factors, and focus on these may enable us to reduce prevalence and cost of chronic pain.

Prevalence of chronic pain

In Europe, around 20% of the adult population suffer from pain that has lasted more than six months and is of severe intensity, above halfway from nil to unbearable or the 'worst pain imaginable' on a numeric rating scale (NRS) from 0 to 10, occurring in frequent episodes, or being present most of the time (Breivik *et al.*, 2006). In a pan-European telephone survey, the prevalence varied from only 12% in Spain to 30% in Norway (Breivik *et al.*, 2006). This variation may in part have been due to subtle differences in the meaning of translated questionnaires, as well as different cultural backgrounds. Similar prevalence data appear in other studies (Landmark *et al.*, 2013; Macfarlane, 2016; Macfarlane *et al.*, 2010; Gunnarsdottir *et al.*, 2010; Breivik, 2010; Fayaz *et al.*, 2016), and in cohort studies that followed selections of persons from the general population. In Ireland, pain conditions lasting at least three months were present in 36% (Raftery *et al.*, 2011, 2012), in Portugal in 37% (Azevedo *et al.*, 2012), and 31% in a recent survey in Norway (Landmark *et al.*, 2013). In the ongoing health surveys in Denmark, chronic pain occurred in 25% (Eriksen *et al.*, 2003). Children are not immune: the occurrence of chronic pain increases after puberty, especially among girls (Macfarlane, 2016). The enigmatic pain condition complex, regional pain syndrome (CRPS) occurs among children aged 7–15 years, and mostly in girls with CRPS of the lower extremities (Ramage-Morin and Gilmour, 2010).

CRPS is not an uncommon pain condition; about 30/100,000 cases per year in Western Europe (de Mos *et al.*, 2007), and in up to 7% four months after a fracture (de Mos *et al.*, 2007; Bruehl, 2015). However, CRPS is not well known outside of pain clinics, it is often not recognized as a syndrome as such, and therefore diagnosis is delayed. Misguided therapy can worsen the condition dramatically (Lunden *et al.*, 2015; Breivik and Stubhaug, 2015). This is especially the case when surgeons are tempted to look for causes that can be removed with the surgeon's knife (Lunden *et al.*, 2015). Unfortunately, surgical interventions for undiagnosed CRPS aggravate pain and make therapy even more difficult (Bruehl, 2015; Lunden *et al.*, 2015; Breivik and Stubhaug, 2015). On the other hand, orthopaedic surgery has its place in helping the increasing numbers of elderly patients with painful osteoarthritis; hip or knee joint replacements can reduce pain and improving function.

Risk factors for chronic pain after an episode of acute pain—and how to reduce risk

Documented risk factors comprise:

- increasing age, female gender, and other genetic predispositions (Macfarlane, 2016; Zorina-Lichtenwalter *et al.*, 2016; Nielsen *et al.*, 2008);
- low socioeconomic or employment status (Løyland, 2016; Thomtén *et al.*, 2012);
- geographical and cultural background (Macfarlane, 2016);
- history of psychosocial stressful events (Macfarlane, 2016);
- tissue injury by accidents or surgery (Macrae and Davies, 1999; Kehlet *et al.*, 2006; Kalso, 2013; Haroutiunian *et al.*, 2013; Johansen *et al.*, 2012; Romundstad *et al.*, 2006; Althaus *et al.*, 2012);
- depressed mood, tendency to anxieties and worries (Linton and Bergbom, 2011; Nicholas, 2011; Vlaeyen *et al.*, 2016);
- lifestyle factors including lack of physical activity, unhealthy diet, and obesity (Macfarlane, 2016);
- patients who already have one chronic pain condition (Bruehl, 2015; Althaus *et al.*, 2012);
- opioid-induced hyperalgesia and endocrinopathies increase pain suffering (Breivik and Stubhaug, 2014).

We cannot change all these risk factors. However, focusing on early optimal management of an episode of pain in persons with one or more risk factors may be the best we can do (Macfarlane, 2016). Therefore, we should take special care of patients with these risk factors when they have to undergo well-indicated, elective surgical procedures. Chronic pain after surgery is one of the most common reasons for referrals to pain clinics (Macrae and Davies, 1999). The risk of developing chronic postoperative pain is about 10% after any surgical operation, the risk being higher in those with two or more of the risk factors above (Kehlet *et al.*, 2006).

Females, elderly patients, patients with a recent history of a major life event (e.g. divorce, loss of close family or friend), and especially in patients who already have one chronic pain condition (e.g. headache, low back pain) are at increased risk of having a new and often difficult to treat pain condition after surgery (Kalso, 2013; Kehlet *et al.*, 2006; Romundstad *et al.*, 2006; Johansen *et al.*, 2012; Haroutiunian *et al.*, 2013). The risk is higher when the surgeon cannot avoid nerve damage during the operation (e.g. during thoracotomy or radical surgery for breast cancer) (Haroutiunian *et al.*, 2013). Only about 1% of surgical patients end up with debilitating pain after surgery, pain that was not there before the operation (Kehlet *et al.*, 2006). It is therefore especially tragic when patients develop chronic postoperative pain after operations that were not medically indicated, (e.g. breast enlargement and other cosmetic operations) (Romundstad *et al.*, 2006).

It now appears that high-quality pain relief immediately after surgery will decrease this risk (Breivik *et al.*, 2007; Breivik and Stubhaug, 2008), but even more important is optimal pain management during the weeks after surgery in patients at high risk of developing chronic pain (Tiippana *et al.*, 2016; Breivik, 2014). In Finland they have taken this evidence seriously and expanded the responsibilities of the acute pain service to focus on patients with unusually severe pain immediately after surgery, and follow them up for as long as necessary, and when needed transferring patients early to the chronic pain clinic for specialist care (Tiippana *et al.*, 2014, 2016; Breivik, 2014; Jensen *et al.*, 2016; Katz *et al.*, 2015).

Whereas depression is a frequent co-morbid condition among chronic pain patients, it is difficult to know which came first: did a chronic pain condition lead to low mood, despair, and depression (Linton and Bergbom, 2011; Nicholas, 2011)? Alternatively, did a depression aggravate a simple pain condition, such as mild–moderate low back pain, so that pain and low mood interfered more with mental health and bodily functions (Gerrits *et al.*, 2012)? A depressed mental state easily leads to loss of energy, fatigue, less physical vigour, and less motivation for physical exercises that may reduce the burden of pain (Gerrits *et al.*, 2012).

When a pain episode co-occurs with anxiety—including catastrophizing thoughts, fear, low self-efficacy, and avoidance of movements—the likelihood for the acute pain to persist is well-documented (Vlaeyen *et al.*, 2016). Cognitive educational and cognitive behavioural therapies started early after onset of subacute pain may have beneficial effects (Eccleston *et al.*, 2013; Morley *et al.*, 2013).

Those still with a positive occupational status, being employed in spite of a pain condition, had better outcomes when treated in a multimodal, multidisciplinary pain clinic in Helsinki, compared with those who already had lost their job and had lower educational status (Heiskanen *et al.*, 2012).

History of sexual abuse in childhood, possibly because of recall bias (Macfarlane, 2016), was falsely established as a serious risk factor for chronic pain in adulthood.

However, appropriate epidemiological studies were conducted by selecting persons from court cases (children who definitely had been exposed to sexual abuse). When they were followed prospectively for 30 years, there was no increased risk of developing chronic pain (Gassman *et al.*, 2017). However, children exposed to traumatic social events (raised in care, death of a parent), and also children who had severe physical injuries (e.g. hospitalized after car accidents), were found to have an increased risk of chronic pain later in life (Macfarlane, 2016; Raphael and Widom, 2011).

Epidemiology of opioid treatment—a sad story

Mismanaged long-term opioid use aggravates suffering from chronic pain (Breivik and Stubhaug, 2014, 2017). The severe adverse effects of opioid analgesic drugs increase the burden of chronic pain and even increase the already high mortality among patients with chronic pain (Breivik and Stubhaug, 2014). Chronic pain patients, too often co-medicated with sedatives and hypnotics, when they develop opioid-induced hyperalgesia, reduced androgen production, fatigue, loss of libido, and quality of life, need to reduce the use of prescribed medicines (Breivik and Stubhaug, 2017). For this to be possible, whether they meet the criteria for 'substance use disorder' or not, they need help from addiction medicine specialists, as well as pain specialists (Lovejoy *et al.*, 2017).

The pendulum of opioid use and its regulations by authorities have been swinging between too liberal and too restrictive regulations, with about five to six decades in each category. Thus, about 100 years ago, unrestricted use of tincture of opium led to epidemics of misuse and addiction. The reaction to this by the authorities resulted in excessively restrictive policies for opioid use in the middle of the twentieth century. An editorial in the *Journal of the American Medical Association (JAMA)* from 1940 stated that morphine should hardly be used, even in terminally ill cancer patients. The pendulum gradually moved towards more accepted use of morphine for cancer pain from the early 1980s, and by the new millennium, uncritical marketing and prescription of opioids also for chronic non-cancer pain led to the present 'epidemic' of prescription opioid overdose deaths in the United States, also appearing in some European countries as well (Ekholm *et al.*, 2014). Now the pendulum is swinging again, rapidly back towards much more restrictive regulations and attitudes towards opioids for chronic non-cancer pain (Breivik and Stubhaug, 2017; Gassman *et al.*, 2017). It appears that this is another illustration of the old saying that 'Those who cannot remember the past are condemned to repeat it' (Santayana's curse, attributed to Professor of Philosophy at Harvard University, George Santayana).

Individual and societal burden of chronic pain

Chronic pain is common, often not well managed, and confers a substantial burden on the individual pain patient, on employers, on healthcare systems, and society in general (Breivik *et al.*, 2013).

For the individual patient with chronic pain, her/his pain interferes with many bodily functions, causing the patient to suffer from increasing physical disabilities (Nielsen, 2013; Valentin *et al.*, 2016). Depressed mood ensues (Linton and Bergbom,

2011; Elliott *et al.*, 2003), and all aspects of quality of life are diminished (Elliott *et al.*, 2003). Estimates indicate that the personal and socioeconomic impact of chronic pain conditions is as great as, and likely greater than, other established health priorities such as cardiac diseases or cancer management (Gaskin and Richard, 2012).

The direct costs are mostly hospitalization and outpatient care, medication, and equipment to improve activities of daily living, and indirect societal costs are dominated by social benefits, unemployment benefits, sick leave, productivity losses and absenteeism, and early disability retirement (Nielsen, 2013; Valentin *et al.*, 2016). In Ireland the cost per chronic pain patient per year was estimated at €5,665, of which direct healthcare was 52% and indirect costs 48%—a total of €34 billion, or 3% of gross domestic product (GDP) (Raftery *et al.*, 2012). Sweden had even more staggering cost of €6,429 per year per patient with a diagnosis related to recurring or persisting pain, a total of €32 billion or about 10% of the GDP in Sweden (Breivik, 2012; Gustavsson *et al.*, 2012). The direct cost was 41%, the indirect costs 59%. Similar values from the national administrative healthcare registries in Denmark of annual expenses for care of patients with a diagnosis related to severe pain amounted to DKK 18 billion, of which 71% was direct healthcare costs (Christensen *et al.*, 2011). In the United States, a Medical Expenditure Panel Survey estimated that $560–635 billion (47% direct healthcare costs, 53% indirect societal costs), was about 4% of the GDP (Gaskin and Richard, 2012). These costs exceeded the sum of costs for heart disease ($309 billion), cancer ($243 billion), and diabetes ($188 billion)—all in 2010 prices (Gaskin and Richard, 2012).

EFIC and national IASP Chapters—decreasing deficiencies in knowledge of chronic pain

Numerous epidemiological studies and meta-analysis from the last three decades have increased our knowledge of risk factors for developing persistent pain after episodes of acute pain. I cite Gary Macfarlane (2016): '*Focussing on early management of these people is likely to optimise cost effectiveness of management approaches . . .*' and '*. . . tools such as the Örebro Screening Questionnaire seek to capture such factors (and wider psychosocial factors) in terms of predicting risk of poor outcome*' (Linton and Boersma, 2003).

Knowledge has been weak among the lay public about how acute pain can continue as recurring or persistent pain, and also how chronic pain is different from the alarm function of our ability to sense, modulate, and respond to acute nociceptive pain impulses. This is often true for healthcare providers and healthcare policymakers as well.

Deficiencies in the education of healthcare professionals (e.g. nurses as well as medical doctors), and deficiencies in access to specialized interdisciplinary pain management and rehabilitation services are factors that continue to impede improvement in the care of chronic pain patients (Breivik *et al.*, 2013). However, major efforts by the national pain societies in Europe, greatly aided by the collaboration organized by EFIC, the European Federation of IASP Chapters, are increasing focus on and decreasing these deficiencies (Breivik *et al.*, 2013).

A better future for patients with chronic pain

Discussions of prioritization of efforts for improving the management of chronic pain patients emphasize the importance of improving knowledge among the lay public, and among all types of healthcare workers (Breivik *et al.*, 2013).

Epidemiological studies will continue to bring more knowledge of risk factors and prognosis of the different types of chronic pain conditions and outcome of therapies. Epidemiological studies should continue to document the magnitude of cost to society of chronic pain, and this will continue to impress healthcare policymakers and those who decide where research resources go.

A continued challenge will be to separate the always present 'non-specific context-influenced effect' from more specific effects of our interventions, be they pharmacological, surgical, psychological, or physical (Breivik, 2017).

Basic neuroscience and molecular bioscience will continue to increase our understanding of normal and pathological mechanisms for our experience of pain (and pleasure), the two most powerful 'teachers' of human behaviour to improve quality of life (Basbaum and Bráz, 2016).

When planning trials of treatment for chronic pain, it is necessary to critically select homogenous groups of pain patients (e.g. those with phenotype descriptions of neuropathic pain in one group with highly sensitized neuropathic pain, and one group where there are mostly negative signs: sensory loss being the most prominent sign) (Finnerup *et al.*, 2015).

There is already evidence that therapies that can help 'irritable/hypersensitive' neuropathic pain will not help somatosensory silenced neuropathic pain patients (Finnerup *et al.*, 2015). Further development in understanding of phenotypical characteristics and pathomechanisms of chronic pain patients are necessary to secure progress in research on therapies of pain (Dickenson and Baron, 2016).

Comparing the knowledge of pain epidemiology, understanding of pain mechanisms, and pain management present in 1974 when we founded IASP, with the enormous amount of knowledge we have gained since then, gives hope that the future for patients with now difficult-to-treat chronic pain is a brighter one. It certainly is more hopeful than it was when the UK pain society in the 1960s was still 'The Intractable Pain Society'.

References

Althaus, A., Hinrichs-Rocker, A., Chapman, R., *et al.* (2012). Development of a risk index for the prediction of chronic post-surgical pain. *Eur J Pain*, **16**, 901–10.

Azevedo, L. F., Costa-Pereira, A., Mendonça, L., Dias, C. C., & Castro-Lopes, J. M. (2012). Epidemiology of chronic pain: a population-based nationwide study on its prevalence, characteristics and associated disability in Portugal. *J Pain*, **13**, 773–83.

Basbaum, A. I. & Bráz, J. M. (2016). Cell transplants to treat the disease of neuropathic pain and itch. *Pain*, **157**, S42–7.

Breivik, H. (2010). Whether the weather influences pain: High prevalence of chronic pain in Iceland and Norway: Common genes? Or lack of sunshine and vitamin D? *Scand J Pain*, **1**, 149–50.

Breivik, H. (2012). A major challenge for a generous welfare system: A heavy socio-economic burden of chronic pain conditions in Sweden—and how to meet this challenge. *Eur J Pain*, **16**, 167–9.

Breivik, H. (2014). Persistent post-surgical pain (PPP) reduced by high-quality management of acute pain extended to sub-acute pain at home. *Scand J Pain*, **5**, 237–9.

Breivik, H. (2017). Re-enforcing therapeutic effects by positive expectations of pain-relief from our interventions. *Scand J Pain*, **14**, 76–7.

Breivik, H. & Stubhaug, A. (2008). Management of acute postoperative pain: still a long way to go! *Pain*, **137**, 233–4.

Breivik, H. & Stubhaug, A. (2014). Burden of disease is often aggravated by opioid treatment of chronic pain patients: Etiology and prevention. *Pain*, **155**, 2441–3.

Breivik, H. & Stubhaug, A. (2015). Importance of early diagnosis of complex regional pain syndrome (CRPS-1 and CRPS-2): Delayed diagnosis of CRPS is a major problem. *Scand J Pain*, **11**, 49–51.

Breivik, H. & Stubhaug, A. (2017). Endocrinopathies in women during opioid therapy cause loss of androgens, fatigue, listlessness, loss of libido and quality of life: stop prescribing opioids or follow the 2016 Centers for Disease Control and Prevention Guideline? *Pain*, **158**, 1–3.

Breivik, H., Collett, B., Ventafridda, V., Cohen, R., & Gallacher, D. (2006). Survey of chronic pain in Europe: Prevalence, impact on daily life, and treatment. *Eur J Pain*, **10**, 287–333.

Breivik, H., Curatolo, M., Niemi, G., *et al.* (2007). How to implement an acute postoperative pain service: an update. In: Breivik, H. & Shipley, M. (eds)., *Pain Best Practice and Research Compendium*, pp. 255–79. London, UK: Elsevier.

Breivik, H., Eisenberg, E. R., & O'Brien, T. (2013). The individual and societal burden of chronic pain in Europe: the case for strategic prioritization and action to improve knowledge and availability of appropriate care. *BMC Public Health*, **13**, 1229.

Bruehl, S. (2015). Complex regional pain syndrome. *BMJ*, **350**, h2730.

Christensen, J., Bilde, L., & Gustavsson, A. (2011). *Socio-economic Consequences of Pain-Intensive Diseases in Denmark.* Copenhagen, Denmark: Danish Institute for Health Services Research.

de Mos, M., de Bruijn, A. G., Huygen, F. J., Dieleman, J. P., Stricker, B. H., & Sturkenboom, M. C. (2007). The incidence of complex regional pain syndrome: a population-based study. *Pain*, **129**, 12–20.

Dickenson, A. H. & Baron, R. (2016). Making sense of sensory profiles. *Pain*, **157**, 1177–8.

Eccleston, C., Morley, S. J., & Williams, A. (2013). Psychological approaches to chronic pain management: evidence and challenges. *Brit J Anaesth*, **111**, 59–63.

Ekholm, O., Kurita, G. P., Højsted, J., Juel, K., & Sjøgren, P. (2014). Chronic pain, opioid prescriptions, and mortality in Denmark: A population-based cohort study. *Pain*, **155**, 2486–90.

Elliott, T. E., Renier, C. M., & Palcher, J. A. (2003). Chronic pain, depression, and quality of life: correlations and predictive value of the SF-36. *Pain Med*, **4**, 331–9.

Eriksen, J., Jensen, M. K., Sjøgren, P., Ekholm, O., & Rasmussen, N. K. (2003). Epidemiology of chronic nonmalignant pain in Denmark. *Pain*, **106**, 221–8.

Fayaz A, Croft P, Langford RM, Donaldson LJ, Jones GT. (2016). Prevalence of chronic pain in the UK: a systematic review and meta-analysis of population studies. *BMJ Open*, **6**, e010364.

Finnerup, N. B., Attal, N., Haroutounian, S., *et al.* (2015). Pharmacotherapy for neuropathic pain in adults: a systematic review and meta-analysis. *Lancet Neurol*, **14**, 162–73.

Gaskin, D. J. & Richard, P. (2012). The economic costs of pain in the United States. *J Pain*, **13**, 715–24.

Gassman, A. L., Nguyen, C. P., & Joffe, H. V. (2017). FDA regulations of prescription drugs. *N Eng J Med*, **376**, 674–82.

Gerrits, M. M., Vogelzangs, N., van Oppen, P., van Marwijk, H. W., van der Horst, H., Penninx, B. W. (2012). Impact of pain on the course of depressive and anxiety disorders. *Pain*, **153**, 429–36.

Gunnarsdottir, S., Sandra, W. E., & Serlin, R. C. (2010). A population based study of the prevalence of pain in Iceland. *Scand J Pain*, **1**, 151–7.

Gustavsson, A., Bjorkman, J., Ljungcrantz, C., *et al.* (2012). Socio-economic burden of patients with a diagnosis related to chronic pain—Register data of 840,000 Swedish patients. *Eur J Pain*, **16**, 289–99.

Haroutiunian, S., Nikolajsen, L., Finnerup, N. B., & Jensen, T. S. (2013). The neuropathic component in persistent postsurgical pain: a systematic literature review. *Pain*, **154**, 95–102.

Heiskanen T, Roine RP, Kalso E. (2012). Multidisciplinary pain treatment—Which patients do benefit? *Scand J Pain*, **3**, 201–7.

Jensen, T. S., Stubhaug, A., & Breivik, H. (2016). Important development: Extended Acute Pain Service for patients at high risk of chronic pain after surgery. *Scand J Pain*, **12**, 58–9.

Johansen, A., Romundstad, L., Nielsen, C. S., Schirmer, H., & Stubhaug, A. (2012). Persistent postsurgical pain in a general population: prevalence and predictors in the Tromsø study. *Pain*, **153**, 1390–6.

Kalso, E. (2013). Persistent post-surgery pain: research agenda for mechanisms, prevention, and treatment. *Br J Anaesth*, **111**, 9–12.

Katz, J., Weinrib, A., Fashler, S. R., *et al.* (2015). The Toronto General Hospital Transitional Pain Service: development and implementation of a multidisciplinary program to prevent chronic postsurgical pain. *J Pain Res*, **8**, 695–702.

Kehlet, H., Jensen, T. S., & Woolf, C. J. (2006). Persistent postsurgical pain: risk factors and prevention. *Lancet*, **367**, 1618–25.

Landmark, T., Romundstad, P., Dale, O., Borchgrevink, P. C., Vatten, L., & Kaasa, S. (2013). Chronic pain: One year prevalence and associated characteristics (the HUNT pain study). *Scand J Pain*, **4**, 182–7.

Linton, S. J. & Bergbom, S. (2011). Understanding the link between depression and pain. *Scand J Pain*, **2**, 47–54.

Linton, S. J. & Boersma, K. (2003). Early identification of patients at risk of developing a persistent back problem: the predictive validity of the Örebro Musculoskeletal Pain Questionnaire. *Clin J Pain*, **19**, 80–6.

Lovejoy, T. I., Morasco, B. J., Demidenko, M. I., *et al.* (2017). Reasons for discontinuation of long-term opioid therapy in patients with and without substance use disorders. *Pain*, **158**, 526–34.

Løyland, B. (2016). The co-occurrence of chronic pain and psychological distress and its associations with salient socio-demographic characteristics among long-term social assistance recipients in Norway. *Scand J Pain*, **11**, 65–72.

Lunden, L. K., Kleggetveit, I. P., & Jørum, E. (2015). Delayed diagnosis and worsening of pain following orthopedic surgery in patients with complex regional pain syndrome (CRPS). *Scan J Pain*, **11**, 27–33.

Macfarlane, G. J. (2016). The epidemiology of chronic pain. *Pain*, **157**, 2158–9.

Macfarlane, T. V., Mcbeth, J., Jones, G. T., Nicholl, B., & Macfarlane, G. J. (2010). Whether the weather influences pain? Results from the EpiFunD study in North West England. *Rheumatology*, **49**, 1513–20.

Macrae, W. A. & Davies, H. T. O. (1999). Chronic postsurgical pain. In: **Crombie, I. K.** (ed), *Epidemiology of Pain*, pp. 125–42. Seattle, WA: IASP Press.

Morley, S., Williams, A., & Eccleston, C. (2013). Examining the evidence about psychological treatments for chronic pain: Time for a paradigm shift? *Pain*, **154**, 1929–31.

Nicholas, M. K. (2011). Depression in people with pain: There is still work to do: Commentary on 'Understanding the link between depression and pain'. *Scand J Pain*, **2**, 45–6.

Nielsen, C. S. (2013). Chronic pain is strongly associated with work disability. *Scand J Pain*, **4**, 180–1.

Nielsen, C., Stubhaug, A., Price, D., Vassend, O., Czajkowski, N., & Harris, J. (2008). Individual differences in pain sensitivity: genetic and environmental contribution. *Pain*, **136**, 21–9.

Raftery, M. N., Sarma, K., Murphy, A. W., De la Harpe, D., Normand, C., & McGuire, B. E. (2011). Chronic pain in the Republic of Ireland–community prevalence, psychosocial profile and predictors of pain-related disability: results from the Prevalence, Impact and Cost of Chronic Pain (PRIME) study, part 1. *Pain*, **152**, 1096–103.

Raftery, M. N., Ryan, P., Normand, C., Murphy, A. W., de la Harpe, D., & McGuire BE. (2012). The economic cost of chronic noncancer pain in Ireland: results from the PRIME study, part 2. *J Pain*, **13**, 139–45.

Ramage-Morin, P. L. & Gilmour, H. (2010). Chronic pain at ages 12 to 44. *Health Rep*, **21**, 53–61.

Raphael, K. G. & Widom, C. S. (2011). Post-traumatic stress disorder moderates the relation between documented childhood victimization and pain 30 years later. *Pain*, **152**, 163–9.

Romundstad, L., Breivik, H., Roald, H., Skolleborg, K., Romundstad, P. R., & Stubhaug, A. (2006). Chronic pain and sensory changes after augmentation mammoplasty: long-term effects of preincisional administration of methylprednisolone. *Pain*, **124**, 92–9.

Thomtén, J., Soares, J. J. F., & Sundin, Ö. (2012). Pain among women: association with socioeconomic factors over time and the mediating role of depressive symptoms. *Scand J Pain*, **3**, 62–7.

Tiippana, E., Nelskylä, K., Nilsson, E., Sihvo, E., Kataja, M., & Kalso, E. (2014). Managing postthoracotomy pain: epidural or systemic analgesia and extended care—a randomized study with an "as usual" control group. *Scand J Pain*, **5**, 240–7.

Tiippana, E., Hamunen, K., Heiskanen, T., Nieminen, T., Kalso, E., & Kontinen, V. K. (2016). New approach for treatment of prolonged postoperative pain: APS Out-Patient Clinic. *Scand J Pain*, **12**, 19–24.

Valentin, G. H., Pilegaard, M. S., Vaegter, H. B., *et al.* (2016). Prognostic factors for disability and sick leave in patients with subacute non-malignant pain: a systematic review of cohort studies. *BMJ Open*, **6**, 007616.

Vlaeyen, J. W., Crombez, G., & Linton, S. J. (2016). The fear-avoidance model of pain. *Pain*, **157**, 1588–9.

Zorina-Lichtenwalter, K., Meloto, C. B., Khoury, S., & Diatchenko, L. B. (2016). Genetic predictors of human chronic pain conditions. *Neuroscience*, **338**, 36–62.

Section 2

National chapter reports

Chapter 2.1

Albania

Apostol Vaso

Background information

Albania was established in November 1912, and has had a parliamentary democracy since April 1991. Geographically it sits in the southeast of Europe on the Adriatic and Mediterranean seas. It is bordered by Kosovo, Macedonia, and Greece. It has a population of approximately three million people whose life expectancy is estimated at 77.8 years (WHO, 2014). Most of its inhabitants consider themselves Albanian, but there are minority populations of Greeks, Macedonians, and Montenegrins, among others. The official language is Albanian, although most Albanians speak more than one language. It is a mixed religion country with both Christian and Islamic religions. However, Albania is not currently a member of the European Union (see Fig. 2.1.1).

Healthcare system

Healthcare in Albania is funded and administered centrally. On average, there are about 260 hospital beds, 236 acute hospital beds, and 21 psychiatric beds per 100,000 people. Besides the hospitals, there are about 76 primary healthcare facilities per 100,000. In Albania, there is a small private expenditure on health, which consists mainly of 'out-of-pocket' expenditure, whereas 'private prepaid insurance plans' are still in the early stage of development. The total expenditure on health in Albania as a share of gross domestic product (GDP) was 6% in 2011. Government expenditure on health as a share of total expenditure on health increased, from about 36% in 2000 to 48% in 2011 and 63% in 2016. Per capita expenditure on health in Albania has increased significantly in the past decade (WHO, 2014). However, the health sector remains largely underfinanced as indicated by the lack of access for certain disadvantaged groups, or waiting lists for several examinations and interventions involving mainly heart disease.

There are major inequalities in the health system. For example, the infant mortality rates in rural areas (24 deaths per 1,000 births) are twice as high as in urban areas (12 deaths per 1,000 births). The same pattern was observed for under-five mortality (28 deaths per 1,000 births in rural areas and 13 deaths per 1,000 births in urban areas). Infants and children under five years in the mountainous region of Albania had the highest mortality rates compared to the national averages (42 vs. 22 per 1,000 live births, respectively). Higher levels of educational attainment are usually associated with lower mortality rates in early childhood, in part because education exposes

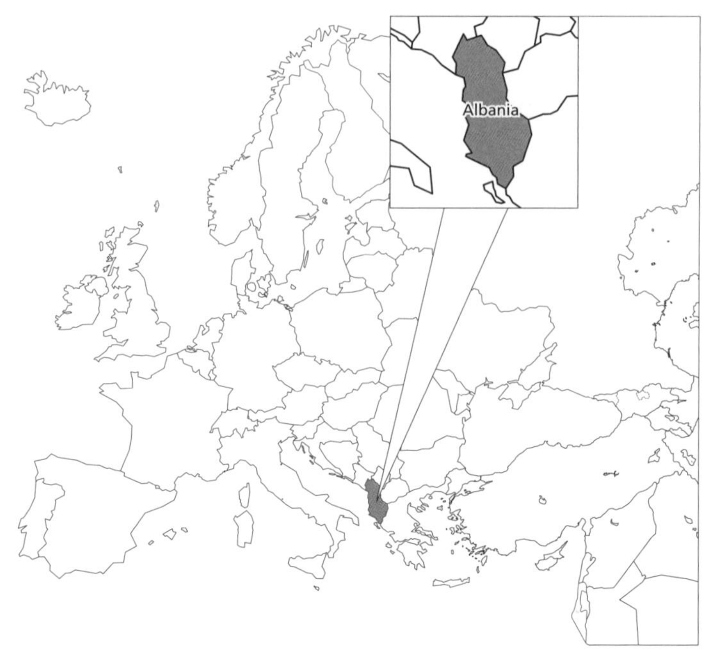

Fig. 2.1.1 Map of Albania.
Copyright © Pyty/Shutterstock.com.

women to information about child feeding practices, child illnesses, and treatment, and the importance of spacing births. In Albania, the differences in the mortality rates by mothers' level of education show that children of mothers with primary education or less are more likely to die before their first or fifth birthday, than children of mothers with secondary education or higher (WHO, 2014).

Albania has no programmes for prenatal or neonatal screening. Recently though, there has been an active screening campaign for breast and cervical cancer in Albanian women. The overall prevalence of unmet need for family planning (consisting mainly of counselling) in Albania was, on average, 13% during 2006–2012. For the same time period, the prevalence of contraceptive use was 69%. The majority of pregnant women (97%) had at least one antenatal care visit during 2006–2013; whereas 67% of women had at least four such visits (WHO, 2014).

The health workforce in Albania includes physicians (general practitioners, family physicians, and specialists), nurses and midwives, as well as other healthcare workers who are together vital for the delivery of high-quality healthcare and preventive services at a population level. Estimates of health personnel densities refer to the active health workforce that is the total manpower participating in the health labour market. According to World Health Organization statistics (GHO 2006–2013), during the period 2006–2013 there were on average 115 physicians and 399 nurses and midwives per 100,000 population in Albania. On average, the number of general practitioners was 50 per 100,000 population during 2006–2012. Furthermore, there were 33 dentists and 43 pharmacists per 100,000 population in 2006 and 2011, respectively.

Current pain workforce

The Albanian Pain Association is the primary professional medical organization which has the objective to promote pain treatment as an essential service, and to improve the quality of life of people through the provision of pain management services. The Association was founded in 2001, and currently has 110 members, of whom most are anaesthetists but there are also neurosurgeons, physical therapists, nurses, and psychologists. Since the Association was founded, it has always had a goal to raise awareness of pain and pain management through education and training. The Albanian Association of Pain has so far successfully organized eight annual national conferences (2001, 2002, 2003, 2004, 2007, 2009, 2010, 2012) and two workshops, a seminar, and an international scientific symposium, whose targets are general best practice and other elements of primary care. Besides the development of the National Conference, the Albanian Pain Association has organized a number of activities. Starting in 2002, the association has conducted high-level national awareness activities, education, and training; all in cooperation with governmental and foreign organizations. It has also implemented programmes based on higher studies in medical science, such as studying the problems of scoliosis in nine-year-old school children, and the study of neuropathic pain.

Challenges and opportunities to the future development of pain services

The challenges facing the provision, organization, and delivery of pain services in Albania are similar to those in the wider region. At present there are only two highly trained pain specialists. Currently, pain medicine is a not a specialty in Albania and to become a specialist one needs to have a broad education. The optimal model for pain treament centres is to provide a multidisciplinary pain service led by a pain expert, with the provision or access to other specialty services such as psychology, neurology, physical therapy, among others. Currently there are no services that meet this criteria. In Albania, we have also seen the increasing use of anaesthetic-like medications such as morphine or lidocaine for the treatment of pain.

Innovations

There has been great progress in understanding the treatment and management of phantom pain experience, especially in the context of veterans' health. In 2010, for example, we held a seminar at the Central Military University Hospital on 'Mechanisms of Phantom Pain and its Treatment' with the support of the international research community, including local experts. This was supported by the then Albanian Minister of Health, Mr Petrit Vasili.

The next focus for the Albanian Pain Association is on the relationship between pain and nutrition in the presentation of diabetic foot pain and ulcers, which we expect to share widely in the next year.

Reference

World Health Organization (WHO) (2014). Global Health Observatory (GHO) data, Albania. Available at: http://www.who.int/gho/countries/alb/en/ [Online].

Chapter 2.2

Austria

Rudolf Likar

Background information

Austria is a democratic republic situated in central Europe. It covers a territory of about 84,000 square kilometres. Austria has nine provinces including Vienna as its capital (see Fig. 2.2.1).

Some 8.7 million people were living in Austria on 1 January 2016, according to data from Statistik Austria. The majority of the population speaks German, which is also the country's official language. A number of minority languages are also spoken in Austria, some of which have official status, such as Slovenian, Burgenland Croatian, Hungarian, Czech, Slovak, and Romanic.

At the beginning of 2016, some 1.27 million foreign citizens were living in Austria, representing a share in the population of 14.6%.

Austria's population structure has changed considerably over the last decades. The number and proportion of children and young people (persons aged below 19) has fallen in many regions, while the number and percentage of persons of retirement age (65 years and above) has increased strongly. On 1 January 2016, there were 1.7 million children and young adults (aged 0–19) living in Austria (19.65%) of the total population. Some 5.4 million inhabitants (61.90%) were of working age (between 20–64). Approximately 1.6 million inhabitants were aged 65 and above (18.65%) (Statistik Austria 2016).

Life expectancy at birth in Austria (81.2 years in 2013) has increased by 11 years since 1970 and is slightly higher than the average across Organisation for Economic Co-operation and Development (OECD) countries. Austria is, however, still lagging behind other OECD countries that have much longer life expectancy (Japan, Spain, and Switzerland all have a life expectancy of 83 years or more) (OECD, 2015).

Austrian Pain Society

2016 was an anniversary year for the Austrian Pain Society (Österreichische Schmerzgesellschaft, or ÖSG), the Austrian Chapter of the EFIC and IASP. It was founded 25 years ago, in 1991, as the first independent pain society in the country. Prior to that, Austrian pain specialists and their German and Swiss colleagues were active in a cross-border regional IASP chapter of the three German-speaking countries and took part in international activities.

Currently, the Austrian Pain Society has around 450 members, representing numerous medical specialties (anaesthesia, neurology, rheumatology, orthopaedics and

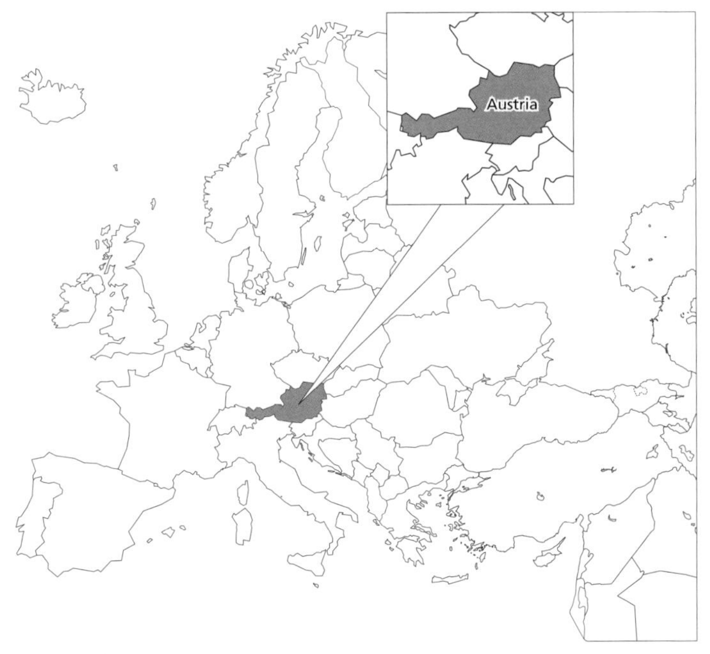

Fig. 2.2.1 Map of Austria.

traumatology, psychiatry, pharmacology, and so on), as well as other healthcare professions (e.g. nurses, physiotherapists, psychologists).

Healthcare system

The Austrian healthcare system is based on compulsory social insurance; 99% of the entire population enjoy health insurance coverage. The social insurance system includes the branches of health, accident, and pension insurance and consists of 22 social security institutions with the Main Association of Austrian Social Security (HVB) as their umbrella organization.

Access to services is regulated by law, the most important legislative basis being the General Social Insurance Act (ASVG). Because of the solidarity-based funding principle of the Austrian healthcare system, all Austrian inhabitants have equal access to healthcare services. Although statutory health insurance is linked to gainful activity, it goes far beyond that scope. Insurance cover relates not only to those directly insured, but also to family members. Roughly a quarter of health-insured individuals are co-insured family members (e.g. children, housewives, or househusbands).

The Austrian healthcare system is primarily financed through a combination of income-based social insurance contributions, public income generated through taxes, and private payments in the form of direct and indirect co-payments. Social insurance is the most important source of healthcare funding, and contributed around EUR 13.8 billion in 2011, which corresponds to around 45% of health expenditure. Whereas outpatient care is almost entirely financed by social health insurance funds, expenditure for inpatient care is shared between the public sector and social insurance. Long-term care services are mostly funded through taxes. In 2011, 10.8% of gross domestic product was spent on health. This corresponds to about EUR 32.4 billion or EUR 3 848 per capita. In 2011, about 75% of total health expenditure was generated from public sources. This includes expenditure by social health insurance funds as well as the Federal Government, provincial, and local governments. The remaining 24% is accounted for by private health expenditure: out-of-pocket payments by households, expenditure of private health insurance companies, and other private non-profit organizations, as well as expenditure by companies for services provided by occupational health physicians.

The Austrian healthcare system is quite segmented. The main actors with regard to health at federal level are the Austrian Parliament, the Federal Ministry of Health, the Federal Ministry of Social Affairs, the social security institutions, and employers' and employees' representatives, as well as associations of healthcare professionals. As far as legislation and its enforcement are concerned, the Federal Government plays a central role; however, many competencies are delegated to the provinces or to the social security institutions. Responsibility for structural policies and planning of inpatient care is a joint undertaking of the Federal Government, the provinces, and the social security institutions. Public health services and administration are jointly provided by federal, provincial, and local authorities. In addition, the provinces are in charge of ensuring hospital care for their inhabitants, as well as offering health promotion and prevention services. The Austrian Health Care Structure Plan (ÖSG) and the Regional Health Care Structure Plans (RSG) are key planning instruments in the healthcare sector. The staffing plan for physicians who are in a contractual relationship with health insurance funds is another planning instrument.

Current pain workforce

In Austria, 900 medical doctors have expanded their pain therapy skills with the 'Special Pain Therapy' diploma of the Austrian Physicians Chamber since its introduction in 2005.

Obviously, many more members of the Austrian health workforce are involved in the care of acute and chronic pain patients. These include, inter alia, a total of 2,860 generalists, 2,510 anaesthesiologists, 1.070 orthopaedists, 1.195 psychiatrists, 690 neurologists, and 305 rheumatologists (Austrian Physicians' Chamber, 2016).

'The Austrian health survey 2014' of the statistical office Statistik Austria shows that among the 'top ten' chronic diseases in Austria, several involve chronic pain: at the top are chronic back pain with 1.8 million people affected and a prevalence of 23% among women and 26% in men. Chronic neck pain is reported by 19% of respondents. Osteoarthritis affects an average of 8% of women and 15% of men (Statistik Austria 2016).

Earlier surveys of the Austrian Pain Society and extrapolations from international studies have shown a prevalence of chronic pain (i.e. pain lasting longer than three to six months), from around 20%. Accordingly, we expect more than 1.5 million patients with chronic pain in Austria.

The 2014 health survey has also analysed the prevalence of acute pain: 3.6 million people claimed to have suffered pain in the last four weeks, with women affected more often than men (54% vs. 45%) (Statistik Austria 2016).

Challenges and opportunities to the future development of pain services

The major challenge for pain medicine in Austria is the current development of pain care resources in the country. Numerous outpatient pain departments, emergency pain services, and the like have been created in hospitals over the last 20 years. But this phenomenon is not an outflow of health policy top-down planning. Instead, it is the result of a large number of dedicated people and groups working bottom-up to create institutions of this kind.

An increasing number of these institutions are jeopardized in these times of restructuring and personnel bottlenecks at Austrian hospitals, and of massive austerity pressures on the entire health system. Many outpatient pain departments have reduced their hours of service or closed altogether while acute pain services are likewise falling victim to cutbacks. In this situation, the Austrian Pain Society is needed more than ever. It must raise awareness of the current deficits in pain medicine, which it does regularly in information well-covered by the media, and it must get health policy-makers to do their duty and finally provide appropriate structures to care for people suffering from chronic pain in Austria.

In terms of collaboration among the German-speaking pain societies, a certain return to 'common roots' can now be observed after these two and a half decades of independence. The three presidents of the Austrian, German, and Swiss societies agreed to strengthen cooperation and exchange at the EFIC Congresses in 2015.

Innovations

One important goal of the Austrian Pain Society has remained unchanged since its founding in 1991, namely to unite everyone involved in pain research and pain care under a single multidisciplinary umbrella organization in order to advance pain research and the optimum care of pain patients in Austria.

The requirements and basic conditions have changed markedly in the two and a half decades since the Austrian Pain Society was founded. In the early 1990s, there was a lack of awareness of the significance of appropriate pain treatment and the possibilities for pain therapy. An 'opiod phobia' was still widespread even in medical circles back then and was among the hurdles and prejudices with which the Austrian Pain Society had to deal. It did so successfully, as we know today. In the mid-1990s, Austria was among the countries in Europe with the lowest per-capita consumption of opioids, whereas today it has top ranking for this form of therapy.

There is another important expression of this change in awareness that the Austrian Pain Society has helped to bring about. Since the turn of the millennium, the patients' right to a 'best possible pain treatment' has been anchored in the Patient Charter, an agreement with the force of law.

Since 2000, the Austrian Pain Society has teamed up with a publishing house to publish *Schmerznachrichten*, its official journal that seeks to share important medical information on pain with a broad professional readership, cutting across all medical disciplines. The broader public has been informed about the many possibilities of modern pain medicine for the past 15 years during the annual 'Österreichische Schmerzwochen', a two-week information crusade in association with the IASP and EFIC awareness campaigns. They have motivated people to seek competent help instead of simply accepting pain. This information is annually echoed in hundreds of media reports.

The Austrian Pain Society reached an important milestone in 2005 when a 'Special Pain Therapy' diploma of the Austrian Physicians' Chamber was introduced to certify solid continued training in pain therapy. In the medium term, however, the Austrian Pain Society is striving to further push postgraduate specialization in this area following the example of other European countries and is discussing details for a curriculum with all relevant medical societies, as well as other stakeholders concerned.

In 2008, the ÖSG tackled an important task when it defined quality criteria for pain institutions. The aim was to provide support to politicians and policymakers as they carried out structural planning for pain care. Unfortunately, health politicians and policymakers have failed to utilize this expertise. To date, the quality criteria are being updated and extended.

As regards international cooperation, Austrian pain medicine has received broad recognition in past years for its dedication and hard work. This is, inter alia, demonstrated by the fact that Vienna served as the venue for the IASP Congress in 1999 and the EFIC Congress in 2015 and that one of the EFIC Pain Schools is held in Klagenfurt.

References

Austrian Physicians' Chamber (2016). Verlagshaus der Ärzte, Arztadressen, Online-Übersichten. Available at: http://www.aerzteverlagshaus.at/arztadressen.html [Online].

Bevölkerungsstand und Bevölkerungsveränderung; Quartalsweise Statistik der Statistik Austria (2016). Available at: https://www.statistik.at/web_de/statistiken/menschen_und_gesellschaft/bevoelkerung/bevoelkerungsstand_und_veraenderung/index.html [Online].

Organisation for Economic Co-operation and Development (OECD) (2015). *Health at a Glance 2015: OECD Indicators*. Paris, France: OECD Publishing.

Chapter 2.3

Belgium

Patrice Forget, Susan Broekmans,
Lies de Ruddere, Conny Goethals,
Koen Lauwers, Bruno Leroy,
Marie-Claire Schommer, and Guy Hans

Background information

Belgium is a small state in Western Europe. This densely populated country covers an area of 30,528 square kilometres with a population of about 11 million people (Belgian Federal Government, 2013; The Directorate General Institutions and Population of the Federal Internal Public Service, 2016). Belgium is home to two main linguistic groups: the Dutch-speaking (mostly Flemish community, which constitutes about 59% of the population), and the French-speaking (mostly Walloon population, which comprises 41% of all Belgians). A small group of German-speakers lives in the East Cantons bordering Germany (see Fig. 2.3.1).

Healthcare system

A generalized social insurance system was introduced in 1945. Now, healthcare in Belgium is composed of three parts. Firstly, there is a primarily publicly funded healthcare and social security service run by the federal government, which organizes and regulates healthcare; independent private practitioners; and public, university and (semi)private hospitals and care institutions. Secondly, there is the insurance cover provided to patients; and finally the industry, which covers production and distribution of healthcare products and research and development, although an important part of the research effort is done in universities and hospitals. Healthcare in Belgium is mainly the responsibility of the federal minister and the '*FOD Volksgezondheid en Sociale Zekerheid/SPF Santé Publique et Securité Sociale*' ('Public Administration for Public Health and Social Security'). Anyone working in Belgium is registered to a central system, as well as the unemployed.

The government forms its tax earnings finances as part the social security system. This is a wealth redistribution mechanism and because the contributions are incremental, this means that the more someone earns, the more this person will contribute. Moreover, for health services, the compulsory health insurance and the refund system is the same for everybody (corrected for the lowest incomes). There is a complementary system of health insurance offered by the mutualities, available to all mutuality members, and there

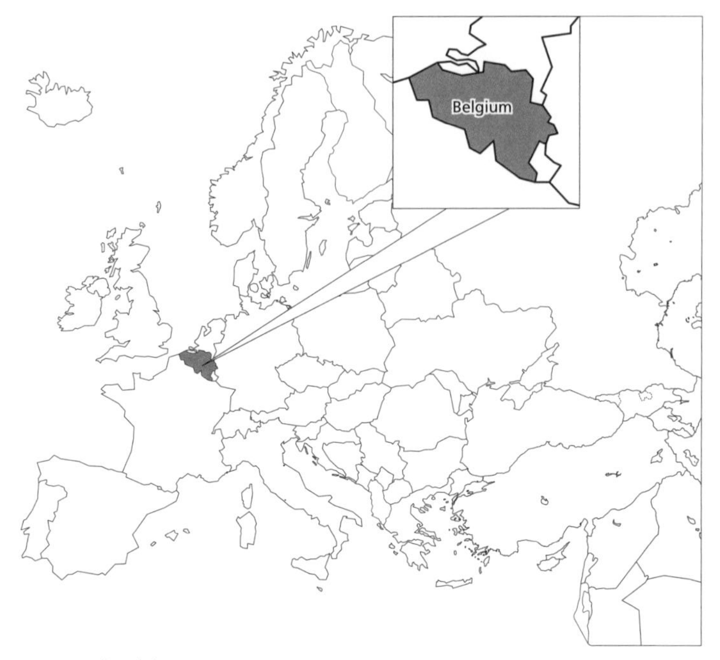

Fig. 2.3.1 Map of Belgium.
Copyright © Pyty/Shutterstock.com.

is private insurance with commercial insurance companies for extended care and for travel care. These systems are pure premium-based insurance systems.

Social security encompasses health, old-age (and other) pensions, unemployment, disability and handicap, both managing the finances (collection of contributions, subsides and payment of refunds, allowances, and so on), but also the management of different kinds of care, regulation of the market of medicines, health and safety at work, and health and safety of any public service rendered to the general public.

Current pain workforce

In 1985, the Belgian Chapter was formally established within the International Association for the Study of Pain (IASP), created in 1973. In 1993, the Belgian Pain Society (BPS) was actively involved in the creation of the European Federation of IASP Chapters (EFIC) (BPS, 1998). In 2016, the BPS had 205 members. From 1996, the following special interest groups (SIGs) and professional interest groups (PIGs) were created in Belgium and are still active: PIG Flemish Pain Nurses; PIG French-speaking Nurses; PIG Flemish Pain Psychologists; PIG French-speaking Psychologists; SIG Physiotherapists and Occupational therapists; and SIG Pediatrics. For several years we have been building a bridge between the Vlaamse Anesthesiologische Vereniging voor Pijnbestrijding (VAVP) and the Groupe Régional Interdisciplinaire Douleur (GRID) to incorporate interventional pain management as a possible treatment option, within the context of multidisciplinary pain treatment. Therefore we try always to have these organizations represented on the board of the BPS.

Currently there is no definitive specialty registration for caregivers working in the field of pain treatment (called 'algology' in Belgium). Therefore, it is impossible to provide an exact estimate of the number of physicians currently working in pain centres. It should be stated that all acute hospitals in Belgium are obliged to have a part-time medical coordinator for the multidisciplinary algological pain team within their institution (104 hospitals over the country). In addition, 35 multidisciplinary centres are recognized for the treatment of chronic pain, and they must employ a minimum number of caregivers within their centre.

Several universities have incorporated a module on the pathophysiology of pain and pain treatment within their medical training curriculum. The content and duration of these modules are, however, significantly different. In addition, all Belgian universities have joined forces to develop a postgraduate inter-university course in Algology (two years long consisting of theoretical courses, practical trainings in one of the official multidisciplinary pain centres, and workshops). Also for nurses, several specialized pain education programmes exist, and a group of psychologists are currently creating an advanced education for 'pain psychologists'.

Challenges and opportunities to the future development of pain services

In 2005, a pilot project (with nine 'multidisciplinary reference centres for chronic pain') was begun. In 2009, the Federal Public Service (FPS) Public Health launched pilot projects in cooperation with the BPS 'algological function' and 'multidisciplinary teams of chronic pain' (part-time psychologists in 36 hospitals). In 2011, a large proportion of involved centres wrote a consensus report containing several recommendations for structural funding for chronic pain teams in Belgium (Berquin *et al.*, 2011). In 2013, these projects were converted into 'multidisciplinary algology teams' in all acute hospitals and with 36 'multidisciplinary centres'. Both pain teams and pain centres have to register their activities, which are supervised by a steering committee, in which the BPS participates. This registration provides insights into how multidisciplinary an approach is adopted. The challenges will be to permit these structures to mature and to follow their missions. Opportunities are similarly linked to the awareness of the need for multidisciplinary work.

Innovations

From the 'White Book' publication in 1998, with recommendations for the management of pain in Belgium, several projects became reality (BPS, 1998). The 'White Book' was a project that involved interviews and consensus meetings, disseminated in Belgium. The creation of algology networks strengthened. In line with this, in 2005 the organization of the first inter-university course in algology started. This course is the result of discussion and debate on the development of a more structured training in algology. In all the universities, the creation of a separate branch of education of pain was adopted. In 2013, the 'multidisciplinary algology teams' and the 'multidisciplinary centres' were created, and this allowed for the regular and ongoing training of surgical and non-surgical teams in pain treatment.

In addition to the annual congress, other challenges are the ongoing support for pain research in Belgium. There is now an annual BPS award for research. Scientific Research on pain in Belgium is in need of much greater grant support. We are also working to promote discussion between our constituent members and helping to prepare, publish, and distribute various consensus documents. Moreover, the ongoing changes in the financing of healthcare, particularly in Belgium, will certainly impact the caregiver, in pain teams and centres. The way forward is, therefore, still challenging.

References

Belgian Federal Government (2013). Statistics for Belgium. Available at: http://statbel.fgov.be/fr/statistiques/chiffres/ (accessed 21 April 2017) [Online].

Belgian Pain Society (BPS) (1998). *Pain Together: Proposals for Structured Pain Treatment in Belgium*. Available at: http://www.belgianpainsociety.org/images/stories/publications/Publications_Witboek.pdf (accessed 21 April 2017) [Online].

Berquin, A. *et al.* (2011). Aanpak van chronische pijn in België: verleden, heden en toekomst. Available at: https://www.health.belgium.be/sites/default/files/uploads/fields/fpshealth_theme_file/pijnrapportstudie.pdf

The Directorate General Institutions and Population of the Federal Internal Public Service (2016). *Population Performance by Community and Community on 1 January 2016*. Available at: http://www.ibz.rrn.fgov.be/fileadmin/user_upload/fr/pop/statistiques/population-bevolking-20160101.pdf (accessed 21 April 2017) [Online].

Chapter 2.4

Bosnia and Herzegovina

Amira Karkin-Tais

Background information

Bosnia and Herzegovina sits in Southeastern Europe, located on the Balkan Peninsula. Sarajevo is the capital and largest city. It is bordered by Croatia to the north, west, and south, Serbia to the east, Montenegro to the southeast, and by the Adriatic Sea to the south, with a coastline of about 20 km (12 miles) (Fig. 2.4.1) (United Nations Environment Program, 2012). Bosnia and Herzegovina has a bicameral legislature and a three-member presidency composed of a member of each major ethnic group. However, the central government's power is highly limited, as the country is largely decentralized and comprises two autonomous entities: the Federation of Bosnia and Herzegovina and Republika Srpska, with a third region, the Brčko District, under local government. The Federation of Bosnia and Herzegovina is itself complex and consists of 10 cantons. The country is a potential candidate for membership to the European Union. The dominant languages are Bosnian, Croatian, English, and Serbian. According to data from 2013 census, the overall population is 3,531,000, with Bosniaks constituting 50.11% of the population, followed by Serbs (30.78%), Croats (15.43%), and a minority of others. As with most of the rest of Europe the general population is ageing due to declining birth rates and an increase in average life expectancy (Agency for Statistics Bosnia and Herzegovina, 2012).

The people and the country suffered greatly during the Bosnian war of 1992–1995, and health services were stretched beyond limits. However, there has been great progress since those dark days and the country now maintains high literacy, life expectancy, and education levels and is one of the most frequently visited countries in the region, projected to have the third highest tourism growth rate in the world between 1995–2020. Bosnia and Herzegovina is regionally and internationally renowned for its natural beauty and cultural heritage inherited from six historical civilizations, its cuisine, winter sports, its eclectic and unique music, architecture, and festivals, some of which are the largest and most prominent of their kind in Southeastern Europe.

Healthcare system

Before the war, the healthcare system in the former Yugoslavia was centralized. Primary healthcare was provided by general practitioners at municipal health centres and their outpatient facilities; secondary healthcare was provided at both municipal health centres and regional hospitals; and tertiary level healthcare was provided at

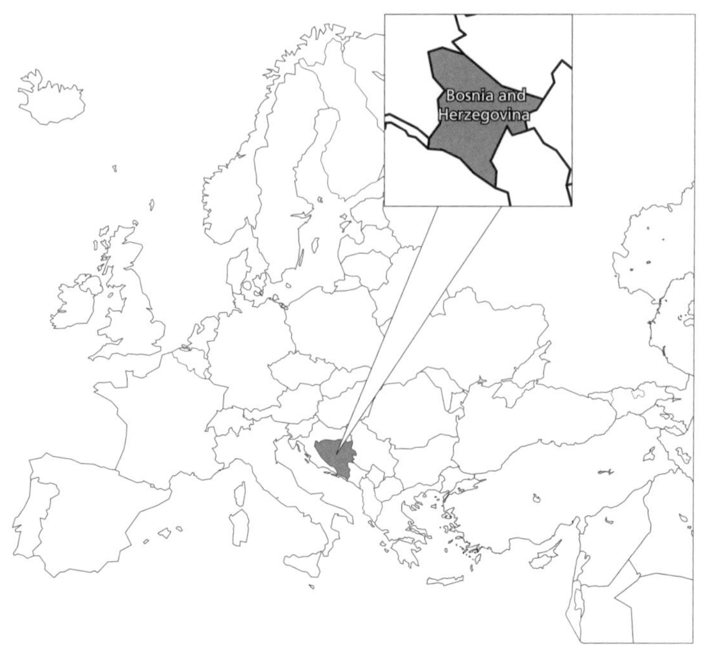

Fig. 2.4.1 Map of Bosnia and Herzegovina.

teaching hospitals linked to universities. Public health was organized through municipal, regional, and national institutes. Health insurance was state-controlled and literally everybody had complete health protection (Šimunović, 2007).

During the war, the hospitals in Sarajevo ran out of basic surgical material (dressings, bandages, sutures, cleaning solutions, and similar) within the first three months of the siege. Essential medications, oxygen, and anaesthetic gases were at a premium, and the power and water supply were cut off after several months. Some health professionals stayed and some left. The estimates are that the number of people employed in the healthcare sector dropped from around 19,300 in 1991 to 11,857 in 1996. By the end of the war in the south-west part of the country, the number of local physicians and nurses had decreased by 1,200 and 3,752, respectively. None were either prepared or trained to work under war conditions. Most injuries were caused by particles of grenades, sniper fire; mass-casualties required adequate urgent treatment, multitrauma patients had associated injuries; and the physiologic effects of trauma depended on the type and extent of injuries.

The Dayton agreement, signed in 1995, ended the worst part of the war. Subsequent health issues included shortcomings of the current healthcare system, such as the lack of communication between healthcare centres, lack of skills, and lack of uniform standards throughout the country. Smoking is a large problem, as well as increased drug and alcohol use after the war. Post-traumatic stress disorder (PTSD), as well as other psychological traumas, have appeared in high numbers after the war (Cerić *et al.*, 2001; Deletis *et al.* 1990). In 2015 it was estimated that 12.01% of the population has diabetes, costing about $523 per person per year (Diabetes UK, 2015).

Most treatment is delivered through non-governmental organizations (NGOs), who will eventually leave Bosnia and Herzegovina. The Federation Health Program of 1994 was implemented as part of the reform process (AAMC, 2007; Avdibegović *et al.* 2008; Bosnia and Herzegovina Federal Ministry of Health, 2008, 2018). This included a set of proposals by the Ministry of Health and created two new laws: the Law on Health Care and the Law on Health Insurance. The Law on Health Care focuses on the delivery of services and the family medicine model. The Law on Health Insurance ensures that each person receives a basic healthcare package regardless of income and resources available. Some of the issues that Bosnia and Herzegovina is currently facing, in terms of bettering the healthcare system in order to address the rising health concerns, includes a lack of technical infrastructure and management capacity to cause change in the short term. There is also a weak regulatory process, as well as a lack of communication between local and central levels of the healthcare system. The country is still receiving aid from international sources that are uncoordinated between international and local services and care; the two sources do not function as one but as two separate providers of care. The system of healthcare is dogged by inequality, because of the system of 'under-the-table' payments for prompt treatment, poor staff motivation due to low salary levels, little opportunity for career advancement, and an unequal system driven by specialists (Cain *et al.*, 2002).

The public healthcare system in Bosnia and Herzegovina is now organized on three levels. The first level of healthcare is provided by local first aid centres (ambulantas), which offer limited medical treatment. These facilities are located in municipalities that are unable to support a community health centre. The staff of the ambulantas is generally limited to one general practitioner and three or four nurses. The ambulantas are primarily for first aid and preventative medicine. The second level of healthcare is provided by community health centres (dom zdravlja). Usually, the 'dom zdravlja' are staffed by a team of general practitioners in addition to several specialists and dentists. The 'dom zdravlja' often provide services in the following medical fields: general medicine; paediatrics; gynaecology; tuberculosis control; occupational health; dentistry; epidemic diseases; psychiatric treatments; ears, nose, and throat; ophthalmology and radiology. 'Dom zdravlja' also offer pre-employment physical examinations, regular medical check-ups for workers, and assessments of temporary disabilities for workers. Since 2008, a family medicine system has been in place: every family has its own family doctor that should be approached initially by patients before being referred to a specialist if needed (SDC—Close-up, 2014).

The third level of healthcare is provided by general and specialized hospitals (General Hospital and Clinical University Centre in Sarajevo, Clinical Hospital Centre in Banja Luka, and other hospitals at a cantonal/regional level). General hospitals provide healthcare services for individuals suffering from diseases that cannot be treated at health centres. Specialized hospitals provide healthcare services for individuals of different age groups that focus on a particular medical specialty. Compared with European standards, the equipment of these institutions is satisfactory.

Current pain workforce

The Association for Pain Therapy-Bosnia Herzegovina (APT-B&H) is the national pain society and a Chapter of the International Association for the Study of Pain, and became a member of EFIC in June 2005. Its members come from the following fields of medical expertise: Anaesthesiology (16.4%); Physical Medicine (7.2%); Neurology and Psychiatry (3.6%); Oncology (5%); Family (2.1%); Pharmacy (2.1%). Pain medicine has been gradually developing in Bosnia and Herzegovina. The first centre for pain therapy was established in 1999, with the cooperation of the APT-B&H (Karkin-Tais, 1999). Now, with the support of the Ministry of Health there is a plan to establish seven pain units in clinics, including for children at the paediatric clinic, all with a focus on rehabilitation and education. There are three satellite units of pain therapy in Sarajevo, Mostar, and Foča, which started in 2007. The established centres/pain units are within the university centres and hospitals.

There is also effort to establish pain registration and training. At present there are about 10 students working for higher qualifications (Masters level, and PhD) in pain, and one doctor has been registered by the Medical Chamber for work and education in pain in B&H (Karkin-Tais, 1999). Otherwise, the B&H Pain Association now has 26 professionals in B&H dealing with pain and who educate others in different branches of medicine. The agreement with the faculty will enable verification of therapists for pain within their specialization. The APT-B&H, in cooperation with the medical faculty and Medical Association, will offer continuing education according to the European Pain Federation curriculum for European school. This could provide 26 new verified pain therapists.

The three specialist pain units (one in Foča, Sarajevo, and Mostar) all treat a range of pain patients including those with cancer pain, neuropathic pain, musculoskeletal pain, headache, and pelvic pain. The Centre in Foča operates part of each day, in Sarajevo three days a week, and in Mostar also daily. All of the centres work to a multidisciplinary model of care. The clinics operate a consultation model with access to specialties as needed. There are four centres for postoperative pain treatment in the university clinics at Sarajevo, Banja Luka, Tuzia, and Mostar.

Challenges and opportunities to the future development of pain services

Despite the major losses caused by war, and the difficulties of developing and managing healthcare in a post-war environment, pain services have remained robust. The next plan, spearheaded by the Association for Pain Therapy-Bosnia Herzegovina, is to expand the provision of pain services. There is currently a proposal to Ministries and Government for Action for the development of a national programme on pain control in B&H. This plan is to first establish a steering committee of experts, then plan to reactivate and incorporate existing units for pain. Currently the plan is focused on removing barriers to development, improving access to analgesics, and improving education of all those involved in pain care.

In November of 2016 we translated into Bosnian the Societal Impact of Pain (2016) policy recommendations called 'Time for Action' (SIP, 2016). Currently there are also negotiations on improving pain medicine with the Federal Ministry of Health, The Ministry of Civil Affairs, and the Medical Faculty University Sarajevo. Further, the Federal Ministry of Health has activities on a 'palliative care with pain' strategy—as a result of previous efforts. Also, we recently held a meeting with the Ministry of Civil Affairs on the 'Societal Impact of Pain, Time for Action' theme, at which it was agreed to draw up an action plan programme for pain control in Bosnia and Herzegovina. Representatives of the health authorities in Bosnia and Herzegovina have agreed to support the Association in its work on pain management.

Innovations

Bosnia and Herzegovina still shows the scars of war but there is novel research and clinical innovation here in the development of services for civil war victims based on an interdisciplinary and rehabilitative approach. In a recent study in Sarajevo over the period 2015–2017, we attempted to improve the health status of patients with complex needs including: pain, discomfort, deformities, muscle weakness, social challenges, and in some, PTSD (Williams and Baird. 2016). Pain treatment included the use of conventional and complementary and alternative medicine (CAM), opioid and non-opioid medicine, including the use of adjuvant analgesics and antidepressants. Also included was physical and psychosocial support. There was also a contract with the local medical house 'Bauerfeind AG' for physical treatment (physiatrists for home visits for those without mobility and for the making and fitting of orthopaedic devices. In addition, we provided systemic support, such as occupational therapy (e.g. hobbies, work, learning, instruction in correcting bad habits and diet, exercise self-control, information on the rights of disabled people within the system of health, pension, and social protection). The results of this largely non-invasive therapy was very positive, with a 70% success rate achieved by a combination of conventional and complementary treatment within the context of a rehabilitative approach.

There is a robust and strong workforce in Bosnia and Herzegovina working to develop pain management services, and to equip the next generation of pain practitioners with the skills and technical abilities to provide multimodal treatments for a growing population of pain patients. Although the development of pain management was disrupted by civil war, there is now a strong path for development, building on the examples of existing centres of excellence, with the support of the European Pain Federation and the Societal Impact of Pain initiative, and led by the Association for Pain Therapy-Bosnia Herzegovina.

References

Agency for Statistics Bosnia and Herzegovina (2012). Demographics of Bosnia and Herzegovina. Available at: http://www.bhas.ba/ [Online].

Association of American Medical Colleges (AAMC) (2007). Medical Informatics Advisory Panel: Report II. Contemporary Issues in Medicine: Medical Informatics and Population

Health. Available at: http://www.aamc.org/meded/msop/msop2.pdf (accessed 13 May 2007) [Online].

Avdibegović, E., Hasanović, M., Selimbasic, Z., Pajevic, I., & Sinanović, O. (2008). Mental health care of psychotraumatized persons in post-war Bosnia and Herzegovina—experiences from Tuzla Canton. *Psychiatr Danub*, **20**, 474–84.

Bosnia and Herzegovina Federal Ministry of Health (2008, 2018). Strategic Plan for Health Care Development in Federation of Bosnia and Herzegovina. National Planning Cycles. Available at: http://www.nationalplanningcycles.org/sites/default/files/country_docs/Bosnia%20and%20Herzegovina/bosnia_herzegovina_strategic_plan_for_health_care_development_2008-2018.pdf (accessed 9 May 2014) [Online].

Cain, J., Duran, A., Fortis, A., & Jakubowski, E. (2002). In: Cain, J. & Jakubowski, E. (eds). *Health Care Systems in Transition: Bosnia and Herzegovina*. Copenhagen, Denmark: European Observatory on Health Care Systems, **4**, 7.

Cerić, I., Loga, S., Sinanović, O., *et al.* (2001). Reconstruction of mental health services in Bosnia and Herzegovina. *Med Arh*, **55**(1 Suppl 1), 5–23 (in Croatian).

Deletis, V., Šimunović, V. J., & Ransohoff, J. (1990). Neurophysiologic evaluation. In: Sandel, M. E. & Ellis, D. W. (eds). *The Coma-emerging Patient—Physical Medicine and Rehabilitation: State of the Art Reviews*, pp. 421–32. Vol. **4**. Philadelphia, PA: Hanley & Belfus.

Diabetes UK (2015). Top 10: Which country has the highest rates of diabetes in Europe? The UK's position might surprise you. Diabetes UK. 27 August 2015. Available at: http://www.diabetes.co.uk/blog/2015/08/which-country-highest-diabetes-europe/ (accessed 20 December 2015) [Online].

Karkin-Tais, A. (1999). *Pain Management*. Sarajevo, Bosnia and Herzegovina: Šahinpašić.

SDC—Close-up (2014). Support for the Mental Health System in Bosnia and Herzegovina: SDC and Four Cantons Sign an Agreement. Federal Department of Foreign Affairs, 2011 (accessed 11 May 2014).

Societal Impact of Pain (SIP) (2016). 8 policy recommendations: Time for Action. Available at: https://www.sip-platform.eu/files/structure_until_2016/Symposia/SIP%202016/Materials_Programm/SIP%202016%20compiled%20recommendations%20Final.pdf [Online].

Šimunović, V. J. (2007). Health care in Bosnia and Herzegovina before, during, and after war. *Confl Health*, **1**, 7.

United Nations Environment Program (2012). Bosnia and Herzegovina: B&H Ministry of Foreign Trade and Economic Relation.

Williams, A. & Baird, E. (2016). Special considerations for the treatment of pain from torture and war. *Curr Anesthesiol Rep*, **6**, 319–26.

Chapter 2.5

Bulgaria

Atanas Temelkov

Background information

Bulgaria is located in Southeast Europe, in the northeast part of the Balkan Peninsula. It is a European, Balkan, Black Sea, and Danube country. This geographic location places it on the crossroads between Europe, Asia, and Africa (see Fig. 2.5.1). Bulgaria has been a member of the European Union (EU) since 1 January 2007.

Bulgaria has a population of 7,351,234 as of 1 February 2011, with 72.9% of its people living in either cities or villages. Approximately one-sixth of the total population is concentrated in Sofia. Bulgarians are the main ethnic group and comprise 84.8% of the population. Turkish and Roma minorities comprise 8.8 and 4.9%, respectively; some 40 smaller minorities comprise 0.7%, and 0.8% do not self-identify with an ethnic group. All ethnic groups speak Bulgarian either as a first or as a second language (RBNSI, 2015a). Bulgarian is the only language with official status and is the native language for 85.2% of the population. The oldest written Slavic language, Bulgarian, is distinguishable from the other languages in this group through certain grammatical peculiarities (RBNSI, 2015b). A great percentage of the population speaks English or Russian. The Constitution of Bulgaria defines it as a secular state with guaranteed religious freedom, but designates Orthodoxy as a 'traditional' religion (Encyclopedia Britannica, 2011). Muslims are the second largest religion (approximately 10%) (Hurriyet Daily News, 2011.)

Healthcare system

The Bulgarian healthcare system is based on a mandatory employee health insurance through the National Health Insurance Fund (NHIF), which since 2000 has paid a gradually increasing portion of primary healthcare costs. Private health insurance plays only a supplementary role. In the 1990s, private medical practices expanded somewhat, but most Bulgarians rely on public clinics and pay some additional amounts for special care. The system also has been decentralized by making municipalities responsible for their own healthcare facilities, and by 2005 most primary care came from private physicians. Pharmaceutical distribution has also been decentralized (Georgieva *et al.*, 2007).

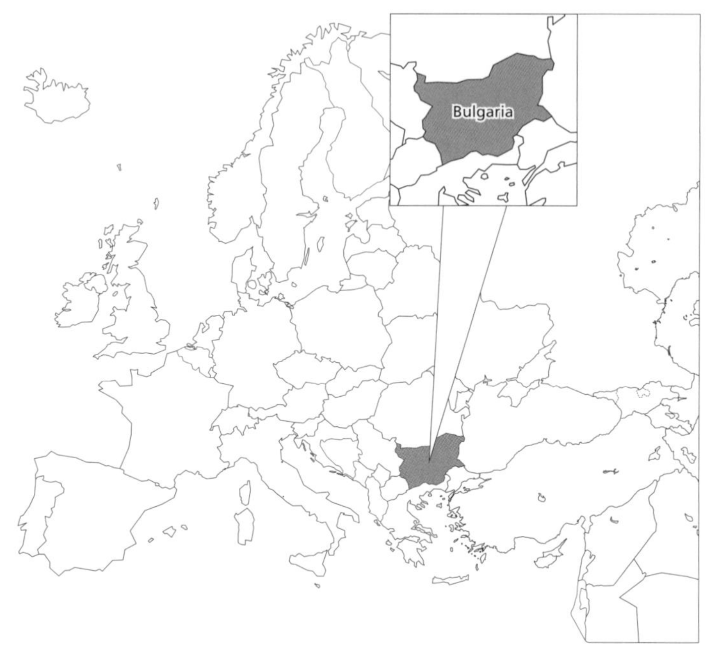

Fig. 2.5.1 Map of Bulgaria.

Current pain workforce

The Bulgarian Association for the Study and Treatment of Pain (BASTP) was found in 2002 by Professor Ivan Smilov with the support of the Israel Association and Professor David Niv, who was himself born in Bulgaria. In the same year (2002), BASTP became a member of both EFIC and IASP. Since then Professor Smilov has been the Councillor for Bulgaria in the EFIC.

Under the leadership of Professor Smilov as a chairman of BASTP for 14 years, eight National Conferences for the Study and Treatment of pain have taken place. These conferences have been very successful with more than 250 participants at each, and full multidiciplinary representation. All of the conferences were endorsed by EFIC, who approved the speakers and supported them financially. Many foreign lecturers were invited and they lectured on, and discussed problems in, the fields of rheumatology, neurology, cancer, and postoperative pain. Interested physicians from different specialties such as neurology, rheumatology, anaesthesia, and oncology attended, as well as many other healthcare professionals in fields such as physiotherapy, nursing, psychology, and ethics. The aim of these conferences was not only to share and discuss practical experiences, but also to improve strategies concerning the organization and structure of pain centres throughout Bulgaria. This was also an opportunity to alert healthcare organizations (public and private) to the problem of pain in Bulgaria, and the possibility of appropriate treatment. The efforts of BASTP over the years have been to achieve a better quality of life and greater social integration for the victims of pain.

During the 8th National Conference for the Treatment of Pain held in Hissarya in June 2016, a new chairman of BASTP was elected, Professor Atanas Temelkov, who has since been working under the supervision and guidance of Professor Ivan Smilov. The sponsorship of EFIC has made it possible for more than 20 Bulgarian trainees in the field of pain medicine to attend pain schools in Bergamo, Klagenfurt, Liverpool, and Graz. Three young trainees recieved two-month fellowships in Vienna, Berlin, and London. This education provided by EFIC has provided the opportunity to improve all the aspects of pain treatment throughout Bulgaria. At present there are several (two in Sofia and two more are being developed in Varna and Plovdiv) pain centres in Bulgaria, integrated in public or private hospitals. Specialists in anesthesiology, neurology, rheumatology, physical medicine, psychology, and cancer medicine are involved in these centres. Alternative methods for the treatment of pain, such as acupuncture and electrical stimulation, are also being developed. Local nerve blocks for the treatment of chronic and cancer pain are carried out mainly by anesthesiologists, but sometimes by neurologists and rheumatologists. Opioids have strict indications for utilization mainly for cancer pain as part of a multimodal treatment approach and combined with other drugs. Another field that has developed in recent years is the biopsychosocial rehabilitation of patients with chronic and cancer pain, which is carried out with the participation of psychologists and with full involvement of the patient's own family.

Challenges and opportunities to the future development of pain services

Unfortunately at present Bulgaria still suffers from a lack of adequate resources, such as pain centres and specialist in pain medicine. This is due to several reasons: a lack of money; lack of interest from politicians; frequent changes in the political situation and relevant ministers; and inadequate concern from healthcare providers. Bulgarian doctors with an interest in pain have been working to resolve these important issues since 2002, with the foundation of BASTP and membership in EFIC and IASP, so the future is promising. Bulgarian doctors are alert to the problem of pain management and many yearn for knowledge and experience in the field of pain medicine. Bulgarian patients deserve to have adequate pain relief and a better, more worthy quality of life and that is the main objective of BASTP. An example of this is that this year in Sofia in Alexandrovska University Hospital, and in some other hospitals, new initiatives have been started for cancer pain treatment, with epidural pumps delivering medication through catheters inserted by anesthesiologists. These are changed weekly in ambulatory practice in the patient's own home. BASTP is now seeking assistance from governmental authorities to give financial support for this initiative.

Innovation

In future, BASTP will continue to organize educational courses in the field of pain medicine for residents and doctors in different specialties, with the help of EFIC professors and speakers. It will also seek to popularize the concept of pain centres among patients and general practitioners, so that increasingly more patients with pain (acute and chronic) will be able to benefit and obtain meaningful pain relief. BASTP is also considering the concept of integrating some traditional Bulgarian medical herbs into cancer treatment and to report on their effects and outcomes.

References

Encyclopedia Britannica (2011). *Bulgarian Orthodox Church*, Encyclopedia Britannica, Inc. Available at: https://www.britannica.com/topic/Bulgarian-Orthodox-Church [Online].

Georgieva, L., Salchev, P., Dimitrova, R., Dimova, A., & **Avdeeva, O.** (2007). *Bulgaria Health System Review*. Health Systems in Transition, **9**, (1). Geneva, Switzerland: WHO. Available at: https://www.researchgate.net/publication/235975367_Bulgaria_Health_system_review [Online].

Hurriyet Daily News (2011). *Bulgarian Muslims not deeply religious: Study* December 9, 2011. Available at: http://www.hurriyetdailynews.com/bulgarias-muslims-not-deeply-religious-study.aspx?pageID=238&nid=8817 [Online].

Republic of Bulgaria National Statistical Institute (RBNSI) (2015a). Census data. Available at: http://www.nsi.bg/en [Online].

Republic of Bulgaria National Statistical Institute (RBNSI) (2015b). *Population by mother language*. Available at: http://www.nsi.bg/en [Online].

Chapter 2.6

Croatia

Mira Fingler and Ivan Radoš

Background information

The Croatian Bureau of Statistics (2011, 2012) states that the Republic of Croatia, a member of the European Union, is a sovereign state between Central Europe, Southeast Europe, and the Mediterranean. The Republic of Croatia is a parliamentary unitary state. Its capital city is Zagreb, one of the country's primary subdivisions, along with its 20 counties. Croatia covers 56,594 square kilometres (21,851 square miles) and has diverse, mostly continental, and Mediterranean climates. Croatia's Adriatic Sea coast contains more than a thousand islands (see Fig. 2.6.1).

Croatia's Bureau of Statistics reveals that the country's 2011 census showed a permanent population of 4.29 million. The population density is 75.8 inhabitants per square kilometre, and the overall life expectancy in Croatia at birth was 78 years in 2012. Since 1991, the natural growth rate of the population is negative with Croatia's death rate 4.29 million. The population density is 75.8 inhabitants per square kilometre, and the overall life expectancy in Croatia at birth was 78 years in 2012. Since 1991, the natural growth rate of the population is negative to its death rate. Croatia is in the fourth or fifth stage of demographic transition; the population is dominated by the 15- to 64-year-old segment. The median age of the population is 41.4 years, and the gender ratio of the total population is 0.93 males per 1 female (Ostroški, 2011).

While Croatian is the official language, minority languages are officially used in some local government units. Croatian is the native language for 95.60% of the population. In Croatia, there are hundreds of healthcare institutions including 79 hospitals and clinics with 23,967 beds. The hospitals and clinics care for more than 700,000 patients per year and employ 5,205 medical doctors, including 3,929 specialists. There are 6,379 private practice offices, and a total of 41,271 health workers in the country (Ostroški, 2015).

On 31 March 2000 the Croatian Pain Society was established. Prim. Dr Marijana Persoli Gudelj from Karlovac was elected president of the Association, which was founded with the intention to educate physicians, to adequately promote the treatment of pain, and to develop awareness of the need for treatment of pain. The Croatian Pain Society has become an associate member of the world (IASP) and European (EFIC) associations for pain treatment in 2002. Since 21 December 2004, it has been a permanent member of IASP and EFIC. The Croatian Pain Society has more than 200 members.

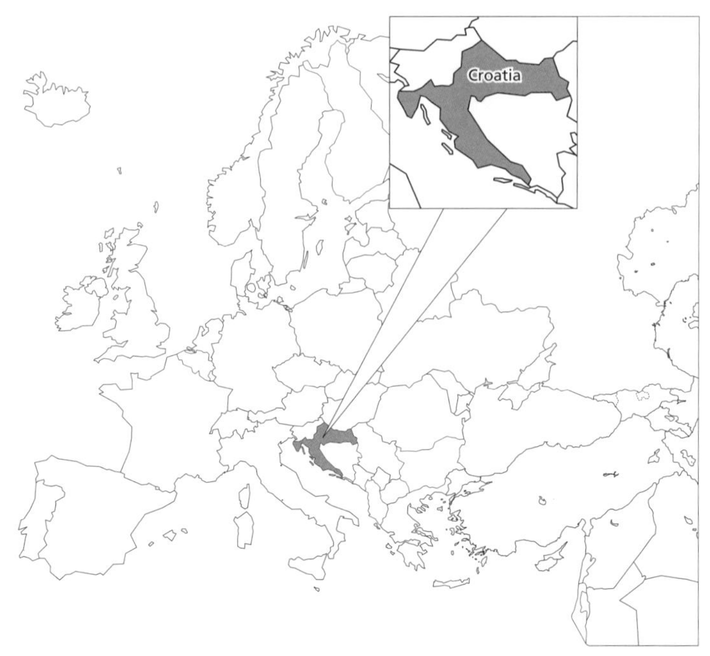

Fig. 2.6.1 Map of Croatia.

Healthcare system

Finance for the Croatian state health system comes from a variety of sources. Health insurance contributions are compulsory for all citizens in employment and for employers. Dependant family members are insured through the contributions made by working family members. Self-employed citizens must pay their own contributions in full. Vulnerable groups such as old age pensioners and low-income earners are exempted from payment. The Croatian Institute for Health Insurance (CIHI) holds the healthcare budget, made up of the working population's contributions. Some citizens supplement their state healthcare service with additional private health insurance (Croatian Bureau of Statistics, 2012).

Zrinšćak (2003) states that a minority of citizens must also pay a form of co-payment to access some health services and all patients have to pay for non-prescription drugs. Dental healthcare, as well as consultations with specialists must also be paid for. Unemployed registered expatriates may be covered by a reciprocal agreement with their home country. The population is covered by a basic health insurance plan provided by statute and optional insurance, and administered by the Croatian Health Insurance Fund. In 2012, annual compulsory healthcare-related expenditures reached 21.0 billion Kuna or 2.8 billion Euros.

Healthcare expenditures comprise 0.6% of private health insurance and public spending (Matković, 2011). In 2012, Croatia spent 6.8% of its GDP on healthcare

(World Health Organization, 2015), down from approximately 8% estimated in 2008, when 84% of healthcare spending came from public sources (Jafarov and Gunnarsson, 2008). Croatia ranks around 50th in the world for life expectancy, with 73 years for men and 79 years for women, and it has a low infant mortality rate of 6 per 1,000 live births (World Health Organization, 2015).

There are hundreds of healthcare institutions in Croatia, including 79 hospitals and clinics with 25,285 beds, caring for more than 760,000 patients per year (Ostroški, 2013). Ownership of hospitals is shared between the state and the counties within Croatia. There are 5,792 private practice offices, and a total of 46,020 health workers in the country, including 10,363 medical doctors. There are 79 emergency medical service units that performed more than one million interventions in 2012. The principal cause of death in 2011 was cardiovascular disease (at 41.7% for men and 55.4% for women), followed by tumours (at 31.7% for men and 22.8% for women). In 2012, only 20 Croatians had been infected with HIV/AIDS and six had died from the disease (Ostroški, 2013). In 2008 it was estimated by the WHO that 27.4% of Croatians over the age of 15 are smokers (Crnjak, 2008). According to 2003 WHO data, 22% of the Croatian adult population is obese (World Health Organization, 2011). The Euro health consumer index placed it as sixteenth in Europe, commenting that it did well with kidney transplants, performing more than 50 per million per year, and speculating that it might become a health tourism destination, as a state-of-the-art hip joint operation can be had for €3,000 (Health Consumer Powerhouse 2016).

Current pain workforce

Inspired by world experience and recommendations in pain medicine, the Republic of Croatia established the Croatian Pain Society. Establishment of the Society was preceded by years of work of a large number of doctors who had been encouraging a special approach to the treatment of pain. Anaesthesiologists were the first to start with organized access to pain treatment within the anaesthesiology society (Croatian Society of Anaesthesiology and Intensive Care). Anaesthesiologists were treating postoperative pain, but they also started outpatient treatment for chronic pain.

The first clinics for pain management were established in 1978 in Zagreb, 1978 in Karlovac, 1987 in Rijeka, and 1989 in Osijek. Recently the core members of the Croatian Pain Society are anaesthesiologists, rheumatologists, neurologists, oncologists, physiatrists, and specialists in general medicine. At the time of writing, the CIHI contracts 29 clinics for the treatment of pain.

The Croatian Society for pain management issues its quarterly newsletter 'Bol' ('Pain') with relevant topics on pain, and it also published two university textbooks: *The Pathophysiology, Diagnosis and Treatment of Neuropathic Pain*, and *Pain—Causes and Treatment*. As a legitimate professional society of the Croatian Medical Association, the Croatian Pain Society has published national guidelines on acute pain, cancer pain, neuropathic pain, guidance for minimally invasive treatment of back pain, as well as guidelines on the use of opioids in the treatment of non-cancer pain. Our biggest challenge for the future is to make the national curriculum for specialization in pain medicine, as well as a national strategy to manage pain.

A laboratory for the study of pain has been successfully underway at the medical school in Split for several years. The main activities of the society are education of doctors and health workers on the treatment of pain, as well as promoting and encouraging the development of clinics for the treatment of pain. The training is conducted by carrying out courses and lectures on treatment of pain to primary care physicians and other specialists. The most important courses for training are: International Course of Treatment of Pain P.A.I.N.; The Treatment of Pain in Children; Modern Approach to the Treatment of Musculoskeletal Pain; Modern Approach to the Treatment of Acute Pain; Current Treatment of Primary Headache; Acupuncture in the Treatment of Pain; Diagnosis and Treatment of Neuropathic Pain; Modern Approach to the Treatment of Chronic Pain; Modern Approach to the Treatment of Cancer Pain; EFIC European Federation-endorsed Interventional Pain Management Symposium & Cadaver Workshop. Undergraduate study in pain medicine is carried out at the department of anaesthesiology and resuscitation of medical faculties in Zagreb and Osijek.

In order to raise public awareness about the importance of diagnosis and treatment of pain, two events were held: 'Osijek and Europe Together Against Pain' and 'The Hospital Without Pain'. Their promotion was done via the media, brochures, leaflets, questionnaires, writing declarations (Osijek Declaration of 2003), and marking the week and months of pain treatment.

Challenges and opportunities for the future development of pain services

Croatia's biggest challenge for the future is to make pain care a public health priority, to raise awareness of the public about the treatment of pain as an indicator of human medicine, and encourage the government to amend the law on the availability and capabilities of pain treatment as fundamental human rights. On this track, the first and most important step is to create a national strategy, an improvement of education at all levels, and to strengthen research in pain medicine. Currently, the Croatian Pain Society offers a curriculum for subspecialization in pain medicine through the project 'Europeanization of Croatian Health 2015–2020'.

Innovations

The Croatian Pain Society currently promotes multidisciplinary pain management programmes (PMPs) as the standard of care for patients with chronic pain. The PMP is based on cognitive behavioural principles and promises significant improvement of pain impact on physical, psychological, and social function. The first such programme was established in the University Hospital Osijek under the sponsorship of the Croatian Pain Society. The first experiences showed stronger participation in daily activities and improvement in quality of life for patients with persistent pain and physical disability; reducing emotional distress, increasing mobility, improving the individual's ability to self-manage pain-associated disability, and reducing the reliance on medication or healthcare use. As an essential component, patients' return to work can be achieved, which improves the well-being of patients with chronic pain. PMP is cost-effective and significantly reduces healthcare consumption.

References

Crnjak, M. (2008). Fewer smokers in Croatia than in the EU. Zagreb, Croatia: Poslovni dnevnik (accessed 12 October 2011).

Croatian Bureau of Statistics (2011), Državni zavod za statistiku RH. Stanovništvo prema narodnosti po gradovima/općinama, popis 2011, Zagreb, Croatia. Available at: http://www.dzs.hr/Hrv/censuses/census2011/results/htm/H01_01_04/h01_01_04_RH.html [Online].

Croatian Bureau of Statistics (2012). Croatian Health Insurance. Zagreb, Croatia: Croatian Central Statistical Office.

Health Consumer Powerhouse (2016). Outcomes in EHCI 2015. Available at: http://www.healthpowerhouse.com/publications/euro-health-consumer-index-2015/ [Online].

Jafarov, E. & **Gunnarsson, V.** (2008). Government Spending on Health Care and Education in Croatia: Efficiency and Reform Options (PDF). International Monetary Fund. Available at: https://www.researchgate.net/publication/23533930_Government_Spending_on_Health_Care_and_Education_in_Croatia_Efficiency_and_Reform_Options (accessed 7 November 2011) [Online].

Matković, Ž. (2011). After the EU accession Croatia will have the maximum healthcare spending. Zagreb, Croatia: Vjesnik.

Ostroški, L. J. (2011). *Statistical Yearbook of the Republic of Croatia 2011*. Zagreb, Croatia. Available at: http://www.dzs.hr/Hrv_Eng/ljetopis/2011/SLJH2011.pdf [Online].

Ostroški, L. J. (2013). *Statistical Yearbook of the Republic of Croatia 2013*. Zagreb, Croatia. Available at: http://www.dzs.hr/Hrv_Eng/ljetopis/2013/SLJH2013.pdf [Online].

Ostroški, L. J. (2015). *Statistical Yearbook of the Republic of Croatia 2015*. Zagreb, Croatia. Available at: http://www.dzs.hr/Hrv_Eng/ljetopis/2015/SLJH2015.pdf [Online].

World Health Organization (2011). Croatia. Available at: http://www.who.int/countries/hrv/en/ (accessed 2011) [Online].

World Health Organization (2015). Croatia. Available at: http://www.who.int/countries/hrv/en/ [Online].

Zrinšćak, S. (2003). Social policy in the context of thorough social transformation of post-communist countries. *Revija za socijalnu politiku*, **10**, 135–59 (in Croatian).

Chapter 2.7

Czech Republic

Richard Rokyta and Jiří Kozák

Background information

The Czech Republic was formed as an independent state in 1918. It sits in the middle region of Europe, bordered by Germany, Austria, Slovakia, and Poland. Its population is 10,564,000. Ethnically, the majority of the population (95%) is Czech, with the remaining 5% made up from immigration, largely from neighbouring countries. Some 39.2% of the population is Roman Catholic, while 40% is atheist. The dominant language is Czech. The demographic changes in the Czech Republic are similar to those in neighbouring countries. The population is ageing due to increased life expectancy (men 75 years, women 81 years of age) and lower birth rate (average birth for one woman 1.87 children) (Ministry of Health of the Czech Republic, 2016) (see Fig. 2.7.1).

Healthcare system

The healthcare system in the Czech Republic has fundamentally changed since 1989 after the Velvet Revolution and the change of the political system. Healthcare is guaranteed by the Constitution, which in Article 31 of the Charter of Fundamental Rights and Freedoms states: *'Everyone has the right to health protection. Citizens are entitled under public insurance to free medical care and to medical aids under conditions provided by law'* (Charter of Fundamental Rights and Freedoms, 1992).

Fulfilment of constitutional rights and access to healthcare is provided by public health insurance, which functions under the Act no. 48/1997 Coll. The law is based on the principle of solidarity in healthcare (i.e. citizens contribute to the health insurance fund according to their abilities and whose healthcare according to their needs). The Act defines the participants and the payer public health insurance, and specifies their rights and obligations.

The insurance premium is set at 13.5% of gross wages. Premium payers are employers, employees, self-employed persons, persons without taxable income (e.g. housewives, students over 26 years of age) and the state. In the case of the employed insured, the employer pays 9% and the employee contributes 4.5%. Self-employed poeple pay both amounts (i.e. 13.5% of the assessment base, which is based on the average wage in the national economy), and the state pays the premium. There are also children, students under 26, pensioners, women on maternity leave, unemployed persons in social need, prisoners, and some other groups, which together represent about 55%

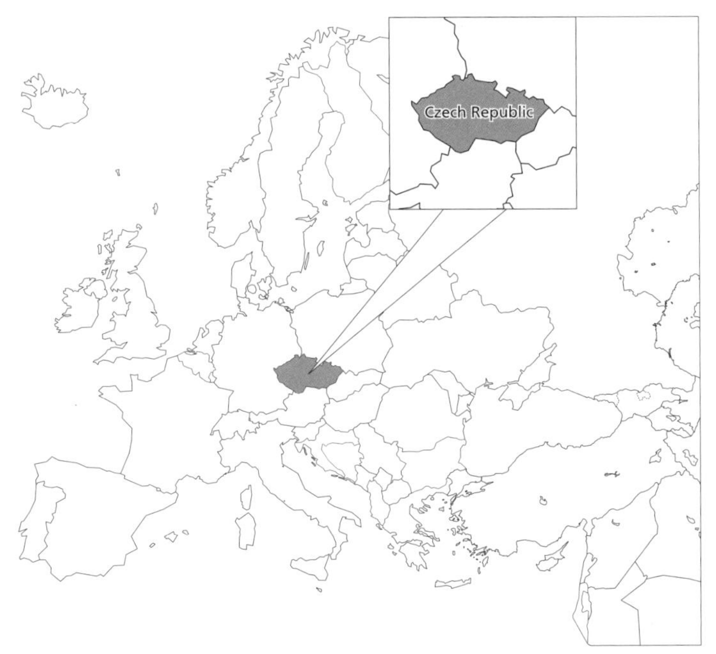

Fig. 2.7.1 Map of the Czech Republic.
Copyright © Pyty/Shutterstock.com.

of the population. The assessment base for the payment of premiums in this case, an amount equal to 50% of the minimum wage. Persons without taxable income (e.g. a housewife, a student older than 26 years) are required to pay a monthly premium of 13.5% of the assessment base equal to the applicable minimum wage. Currently it is 1,080 CZK per month.

The collection of insurance premiums, their management, and reimbursement of healthcare providers is overseen by the regions largest health insurance company VZP (Všeobecna Zdravotní Pojištovna), along with eight other employee or departmental health insurance companies. Selected premiums are collected in a special account administered by the Ministry of Finance. All of the collected premiums are redistributed among the insurers, according to the age structure of the insured. The basic duty of health insurance is to provide its insured with healthcare services in the required scope, structure, and quality. For this purpose, there are health insurance contracts with healthcare facilities (i.e. hospitals and other inpatient facilities and a wide range of specialist for outpatient facilities, including laboratories and diagnostic centres).

Public health insurance

Health insurance is mandatory in both the Czech Republic and the European Union (EU). In the Czech Republic, health insurance is paid by both the employee and employer, who together pay 13.5% of the gross income of the employee: the employee pays 4.5% and the employer 9%. If self-employed, one pays one's own health insurance: the basis of assessment is 50% of the amount of the difference between revenues and expenditures to achieve, secure, and maintain income from self-employment; the minimum assessment base is half the average wage in the national economy. For persons without taxable income, the calculation is based upon an amount corresponding to the minimum wage. This system can complement insured health supplementary insurance, which is optional.

In the Czech Republic, the compulsory health insurance scheme is for all persons who have permanent residence in the territory. They, however, must have an employer who carries out business and has its registered office in the Czech Republic. However, these employees with permanent residency only have health insurance paid for the duration of employment. Health insurance in the Czech Republic is not part of any other social insurance and is based only on a contractual agreement between a Czech citizen and their chosen health insurance. Furthermore, they must have health insurance contracts with healthcare facilities.

Public expenditure on healthcare in the Czech Republic

Public expenditure in the health sector in the Czech Republic is represented mainly by expenses such as health insurance companies. These health insurance companies are subordinate to the Ministry of Health, which annually presents an annual report, health insurance plans, and financial statements. These documents are approved by the government, VZP, and the Chamber of Deputies.

There are some private health insurance schemes which are not capped by the income of the insured, but the maximum amount is a result of a contractual relationship. Private health insurance at present rests with people with high incomes and entrepreneurs. The policyholder receives insurance benefits and premium for health services and care.

Current pain workforce

The Czech Pain Society or CPS (Společnost pro studium a léčbu bolesti ČLS JEP) was established in the Czech Republic in 1989. It was established as an independent professional company and is a member of IASP and EFIC and is a part (registration) of the Czech Medical Association JEP. Around 350 CPS members receive the Society's free journal, called *Pain*. The CPS organized the EFIC Congress in Prague, the first European pain congress in an Eastern European country. The number of participants exceeded 3,500 persons.

The separate medical specialization of Pain Management and Palliative Medicine was founded in 2002 and recognized as such by the Ministry of Health, which later became two independent specializations: Palliative Medicine and Pain Management (Algesiology). The organization of a network of pain centres in the Czech Republic follows the IASP model of four types of workplace. The workplaces are defined by CPS. In the Czech Republic, there are 10 established multidisciplinary pain centres (type I and II) (see Box 2.7.1).

Box 2.7.1 The distribution of pain centres in the Czech Republic

1. The Centre for the Study and Treatment of Pain, Second Faculty of Medicine, Charles University, University Hospital Motol, Prague. Head: Ass. Prof. Jiří Kozák, MD, PhD.
2. The Centre of Pain Management, Charles University, First Faculty of Medicine, University General Hospital Prague. Head: Jitka Fricová, MD, PhD.
3. The Pain Centre and Outpatient Clinic, University Hospital and Central Military Hospital, Department of Neurosurgery Prague, Head: Václav Masoust, MD, PhD.
4. The Pain Centre and Outpatient Clinic, Hospital Na Homolce, Department of Anaesthesiology and Resuscitation Prague. Head: Ivan Vrba, MD, PhD.
5. The Centre of Pain Treatment, Charles University, Faculty of Medicine, University Hospital in Pilsen. Head: Jan Lejčko, MD.
6. The Centre of Pain Treatment, Masaryk University, University Hospital u sv. Anny, Department of Anaesthesiology and Resuscitation. Head: Radovan Hřib, MD.
7. The Centre of Pain Treatment, Masaryk University, University Hospital FN Brno. Head: Marek Hakl, MD, PhD.
8. The Centre of Pain Treatment, Palacky University, Faculty of Medicine, Department of Neurosurgery. Head: Ivan Gabryš, MD.
9. The Centre of Pain Treatment, University of Ostrava, University Hospital Ostrava-Poruba, Department of Anaesthesiology and Resuscitation. Head: Jitka Záthurecká, MD.

The number of other types of pain treatment units (type III and IV) comes to 72. Each must have a department head qualified in Pain Management. CPS guarantees only those units that have a pain certification (qualification in Pain Management) or have a manager who acts as a guarantor—a graduate of the attestation for the Czech Republic. Teaching and preparation for the qualification is organized by the Institute for Postgraduate Medical Education (IPVZ). The emphasis is on practical training at the pain centres for type I or II. To attain the required qualification, there is mandatory theoretical training organized by IPVZ.

In 2002 the CPS introduced neuromodulation methods and created the first six neuromodulation centres. Currently the Ministry of Health supports eight neuromodulation centres. In the Czech Republic we introduced monitoring and a registry of neuromodulation practices. Those with professional competence (e.g. specialization in Pain Management) has now reached 200 medical specialists. To give a sense of scale, in the Czech Republic there are now registered a total of 5,331 (full-time equivalent) general practitioners for adults.

Challenges and opportunities to the future development of pain services

The main advances have been the improvement in pain care and the increase in accessibility to pain specialists in the Czech Republic. There are still eight operating pain centres, and there are plans to expand this to a maximum of ten, adding two additional centres in northern, eastern, or southern Bohemia. This would help with the geographic spread of specialists in the Czech Republic. Also, we are trying to improve the quality of the pain treatments offered, especially as regards extending patient access by increasing the hours the centres are open. We will continue with education of pain specialists. We have a very well-developed system of qualification (specialized training ending with an examination). The Czech Republic was, together with Slovakia, the first in Europe to officially introduce this specialty education system. This superstructure education scheme (supraspecialty) lasts for three years, with plenty of postgraduate courses that are repeated annually in different cycles. Every year a Czech-Slovak dialogue on pain is organized, with regular alternation between the Czech and Slovak Pain Societies.

In addition to the world literature, the country also has a sufficient amount of its own literature. In the years 2006 and 2012, a 730-page book of pain monographies (*Bolest*) was published, edited by Professor Richard Rokyta. Our greatest challenge is to attract young pain specialists for future work in the field of pain treatment. This issue is crucial for the development of our discipline.

Innovations

There are several innovations. Our scientific research is focused primarily on exploring the pathogenesis of pain. They are studying the underlying mechanisms and aetiologies of various types of pain. A very important part of the research is the study of neuromodulation methods, particularly non-invasive techniques (rTMS, tDCS, TES). Research in this area is closely related to the clinical realities of practice.

The CPS organizes workshops at the pain centres which cover the newly introduced invasive methods, including radiofrequency and neural blockade techniques using ultrasonography (USG) control. Neuromodulation centres (NMCs) are oriented to new procedures in NM techniques, such as peripheral nerve stimulation (PNS) and some types of non-invasive neuromodulation methods (rTMS, d TCS). NMCs promote new approaches and new indication criteria, particularly with regard to the earlier introduction of NM methods before chronification of pain after spinal surgery. For the spread of invasive methods in the treatment of pain, there were reimbursement agreements made with the insurance companies. As in the rest of Europe, new views on the value of opioid therapies for chronic, non-cancer pain have led to collaborations with addiction specialists. The CPS organizes several joint meetings with colleagues specialized in addiction and medicine use. It is, however, worth noting that in 2016 the State Institute for Drug Control (SÚKL) allowed legal prescription of cannabinoids for specific therapeutic purposes.

References

Charter of Fundamental Rights and Freedoms (1992). Resolution of the Presidium of the Czech National Council, 16 December 1992, Constitutional act No. 2/1993 Coll. as amended by constitutional act No. 162/1998 Coll.

Ministry of Health of the Czech Republic, Department of Statistic 2016.

Rokyta, R. (2006, 2012). *Bolest [Pain: Pain management monographs].* Prague, Czech Republic: TIGIS.

Chapter 2.8

Denmark

Gitte Handberg and Thorvaldur Skuli Palsson

Background information

Denmark is a Scandinavian country in Europe. The southernmost and smallest of the Nordic countries, it is southwest of Sweden and south of Norway, and bordered to the south by Germany (see Fig. 2.8.1). Denmark has a total area of 42,924 square kilometres (16,573 square miles), and a population of 5.75 million. The country is characterized by flat, arable land and sandy coasts, low elevation, and a temperate climate (Statistik D, 2016).

Healthcare system

In Denmark, the focus on pain comes naturally given the societal burden of pain-related conditions in Denmark, with the largest cause of absence from work relating to various pain conditions (The National Institute of Public Health, 2015) (Fig. 2.8.2). For individuals living with chronic pain, the common pathway through the healthcare system is that a person is referred to multidisciplinary pain management in the secondary sector when all efforts in the primary sector (e.g. GPs) have been exhausted. The clinics and centres offering multidisciplinary pain care (15 in total) are spread over the whole country and are divided into public (9 centres) and private (6 clinics) pain centres and clinics (Sundhed, 2017). The time from referral until first consultation may be up to 55 weeks at some of the centres (Sundhedsdatastyrelsen, 2017). However, if the time from referral until the consultation to the secondary sector exceeds four weeks, patients are entitled to a referral to the private sector for assessment and management of their condition.

Current pain workforce

The Scandinavian Association for the Study of Pain was formed in 1976. Ulf Lindblom from Sweden was a driving force in the process and became its first president. This organization was a common IASP Chapter for the pain societies in Scandinavia until 2009, when it separated into national chapters within Denmark, Norway, Finland, and Iceland. The Danish Chapter, the Danish Pain Society, was formed and became an IASP Chapter the same year. Therefore, even though it has matured rapidly since its establishment, the Danish Chapter in its current form is young. One of the overall goals of the Society is to support the multidisciplinary pain management approach

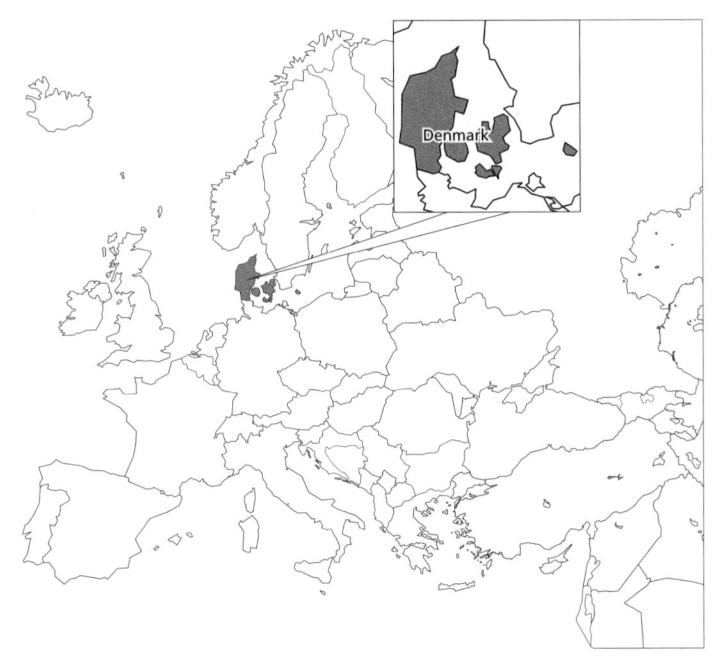

Fig. 2.8.1 Map of Denmark.

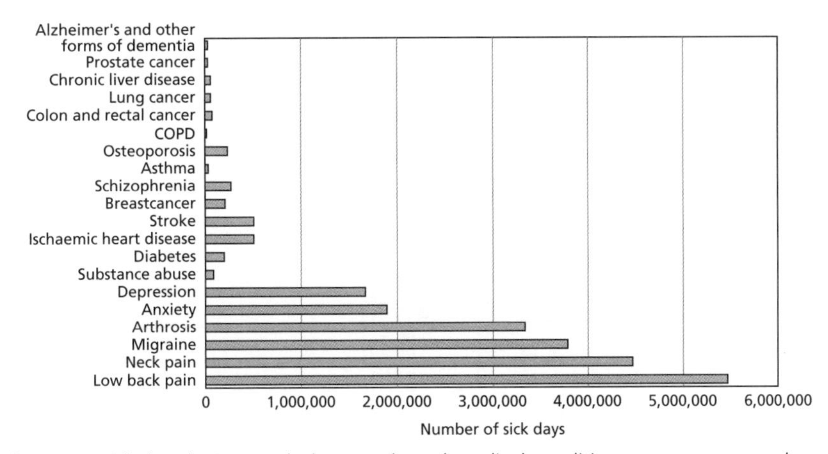

Fig. 2.8.2 Sick days in Denmark due to selected medical conditions among men and women (average values for 2010–2012).
Adapted from The National Institute of Public Health (Statens Institut for Folkesundhed S-F), *The Burden of Disease in Denmark* (Sygdomsbyrden i Danmark), Copenhagen, The Danish Health Authority, Copyright © 2015, with permission of the author.

used in the countries' pain centres, but it also aims to promote knowledge on pain science in the primary healthcare sector. To meet these goals, the Danish Pain Society facilitates a dialogue between scientists and clinicians, which is done in a formal way through the meeting programmes set up by the Society. Since its establishment, this has been done by arranging two annual meetings: a two-day meeting in the spring, and a one-day meeting in the autumn. The meetings aim at reflecting the upcoming research and clinical issues in modern pain management, both domestically and on the international scene. In the early years, the meetings were clinically focused, with clinicians and other caretakers sharing clinical experience. Over the years, the structure of the meetings has developed, with a more formal approach on evidence-based knowledge now being mediated to a greater extent. Since joining IASP as a chapter, the Danish Pain Society now invites internationally recognized scientists to the annual two-day meetings with themes typically following the Global Year Against Pain (IASP) and recently also the European Global Year Against Pain (EFIC). The programme of the annual meeting is a mixture of sessions including basic scientific presentations, in-between translational presentations, and importantly, how research knowledge can be applied in clinical practice. This gives a strong blend of topics for both scientists and clinicians. The autumn meeting is often a joint venture with other scientific or clinical associations where the focus is normally narrowed down to pain conditions that pose challenges in pain management. In 2015, the topic of the autumn meeting was music therapy for pain management, and in 2016 the focus was on: (i) pregnant women with chronic pain in collaboration with the Danish Society of Obstetrics and Gynaecology; and (ii) patients with chronic pain after gastric bypass.

Currently, the Danish Pain Society has around 280 members consisting of healthcare professionals spread over different specialties (Fig. 2.8.3). The number of formal members has grown steadily over the past five years, which is in line with the increasing numbers of participants in the annual meetings held by the Society.

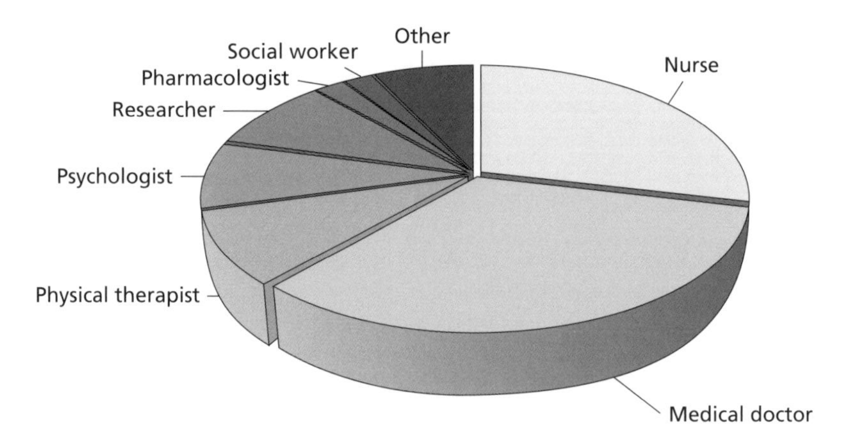

Fig. 2.8.3 Members of the Danish Pain Society divided by professions.
Source: data from Danish Pain Society registry.

Challenges and opportunities to the future development of pain services

In Denmark, there is an increased awareness of the severity of pain problems from politicians, policymakers, professionals from all over the health community, and other stakeholders. This is evident by, for example, the many initiatives of the Danish Health Authority publishing national clinical guidelines on the management of various acute and chronic pain conditions during 2015–2017 (Table 2.8.1).

Recent reports show that the existing knowledge on the mechanisms, treatment, and management of pain has not been adequately implemented into the curriculum of undergraduate medical students (Briggs *et al.*, 2015). In Denmark, the number of patients living in chronic pain has been growing steadily over time (The National Institute of Public Health, 2012). By increasing the focus on pain in the curriculum at

Table 2.8.1 Pain-related national clinical guidelines developed and published by the Danish Health Authority in the years 2015–2017

Topic	Publication year	Link to publication (only available in Danish)
Gastric bypass	2017	https://www.sst.dk/da/udgivelser/2017/nkr-fedmekirurgi
Non-surgical treatment of acute non-specific neck pain	2016	https://www.sst.dk/da/udgivelser/2016/nkr-nakkesmerter
Non-operative treatment and rehabilitation following total hip replacement	2016	https://www.sst.dk/da/udgivelser/2016/nkr-hofteartrose
Treatment of acute low back pain	2016	https://www.sst.dk/da/udgivelser/2016/nkr-laenderygsmerter
Meniscus pathology in the knee	2016	https://www.sst.dk/da/udgivelser/2016/nkr-meniskpatologi-i-knaeet
Non-operative treatment of low back pain with radiculopathy	2016	https://www.sst.dk/da/udgivelser/2016/lumbal-nerverodspaavirkning-ikke-kirurgisk-behandling
Treatment of cervical radiculopathy	2015	https://www.sst.dk/da/udgivelser/2015/nkr-cervikal-radikulopati
Diagnosis and treatment of patients with selected shoulder problems	2015	https://www.sst.dk/da/udgivelser/2013/nkr-udvalgte-skulderlidelser
Rehabilitation and management of patients with widespread pain	2015	https://www.sst.dk/da/udgivelser/2015/~/media/C2305D647E6F4E5B9229D88E96322335.ashx

Source: data from The Danish Health Authority, *National Clinical Guidelines—publications*, available from https://www.sst.dk/en/national-clinical-guidelines/publications.

undergraduate and postgraduate levels across healthcare professions, it may be possible to change this development. In this regard, the current chairman of the Danish Pain Society has invited the deans of the four Medical Schools at Danish Universities to discuss if and how more focus can be put on this topic in the undergraduate training. In the same instance, the Society's board members have encouraged and contributed to an accredited Master's programme in *Pain Science and Interdisciplinary Pain Management* run at Aalborg University, Denmark. The Danish Pain Society initiatives within promoting pain education have been welcomed by the Danish universities.

In 2015, the Danish Pain Society became a member of the Organization of Danish Medical Societies. This was another important step, as the organization engages in postgraduate medical education and the development of good clinical quality in Danish healthcare. It is the purpose of the Society to become acknowledged as a professional partner of consultation in all aspects of pain and pain management. With the unique position as member of the international scientific organizations, as well as being a member of the Danish Medical Societies, the Danish Pain Society will be able to support future development within the pain field.

Innovations

From what has been discussed here, it is clear that credit should be given to the hard work of all regular members, board members, Chairs and Founders past and present. As a result of their contribution, the Danish Pain Society has developed a solid base with a sound clinical, scientific, and educational profile. Furthermore, the Society has established itself as an organization that is heard by clinical and political policymakers. This joint effort on improving educational standards and sharpening the focus on pain will likely promote many future improvements in pain management in Denmark.

References

Briggs, E. V., Battelli, D., Gordon, D., *et al.* (2015). Current pain education within undergraduate medical studies across Europe: Advancing the Provision of Pain Education and Learning (APPEAL) study. *BMJ Open*, **5**, e006984.

Statistik D (2016). Denmark in numbers 2016 (Danmark i tal 2016). Agerskov, U., Bisgaard, M. P. (eds), Copenhagen, Denmark: Danmarks Statistik.

Sundhedsdatastyrelsen (2017). Available at: http://sundhedsdatastyrelsen.dk/da (accessed 20 March 2017) [Online].

Sundhed (2017). Official portal for the public Danish Healthcare Services. Available at: https://www.sundhed.dk/ (accessed 20 March 2017) [Online].

The National Institute of Public Health (2012). Health and disease in Denmark in 2010 and its development since 1987 (Sundhed og sygelighed i Danmark 2010—og udviklingen siden 1987). Copenhagen, Denmark: The National Institute of Public Health (Statens Institut for Folkesundhed).

The National Institute of Public Health (2015). Statens Institut for Folkesundhed S-F: The Burden of Disease in Denmark (Sygdomsbyrden i Danmark), Copenhagen, Denmark: The National Institute of Public Health (Statens Institut for Folkesundhed).

Chapter 2.9

Estonia

Maksim Kunevich and Aleksandra Shilova

Background information

The Estonian Republic is in the Northern Europe, situated on the northeastern coast of the Baltic Sea, and bordering the Gulf of Finland and the Gulf of Riga (see Fig. 2.9.1). Geographically the country is divided into 15 counties. Estonia has been a member of the European Union since 1st May 2004. The population of Estonia is more than 1,300,000 people. The gender distribution is 54% female and 46% male. The economically active population comprises 67% (16–65 years). Children make up 18% of the population (up to 15 years). Senior citizens constitute 18% of the population. The average life expectancy for women is 81.5 years, and for men, 72.3 years. Residents of Estonia by ethnicity are: 69% Estonians, 25% Russians, 2% Ukrainians, and other nationalities (Finns, Belorussians, Latvians, Jews, Lithuanians, Poles, and others) (Tammur, 2017). The official language is Estonian, although the Russian language is widespread, especially in the northeast of Estonia and in Tallinn.

Healthcare system

The foundation of the current healthcare system in Estonia was laid down in 1992, after the restoration of independence. The Swedish healthcare system was used as a prototype. The Estonian healthcare system is based on the principle of compulsory solidarity and general access to medical services. The Ministry of Social Affairs is responsible for the management and general oversight of the system. The total expenditure on health amounts to 5.8% of GDP. Hospitals and private property related to the public sector, legal medical institutions of the first level, as well as some non-governmental organizations and professional associations are part of the complex organizational structure of the health system. Basic regulations and initiatives to prevent losses related to health are based on the law of the organization of medical services and on the Law of Obligations Act.

The main source of health financing in Estonia is an independent public-law institution of the Health Insurance Fund, the funding of which is included in the state budget. To a lesser extent, some items of expenditure are financed through the state treasury. Medical licensing of the hospitals is governed by the Department of Health. The licence is based on the type of hospitals and takes into account the

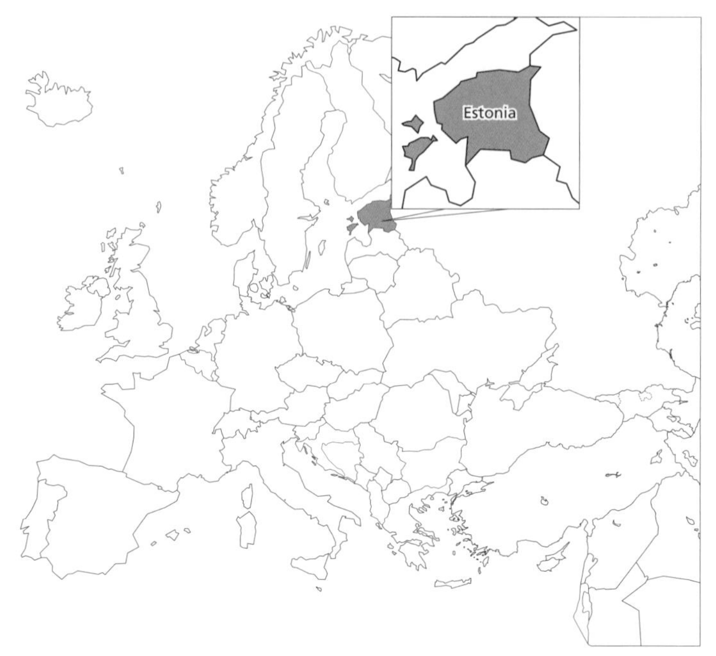

Fig. 2.9.1 Map of Estonia.

availability of staff, the number of hospital beds, and available equipment, which in turn are stipulated by the law. Funding is provided through a contract with the Health Insurance Fund, which takes into account the type of hospital and permission to work.

After the restoration of independence in 1991, the structure of the hospitals were changed—smaller hospitals were closed and/or integrated into bigger ones. Some parts of the hospitals were redesigned into nursing care hospitals. Private medicine has been permitted in Estonia since 1992. At present, there are several types of hospitals in Estonia: regional, central, general hospitals, local clinics, private hospitals, rehabilitation centres, and nursing care hospitals. Private clinics do not take more than 5% of the market of all medical services. The boundary between public and private medicine is blurred, because: (i) there are no government medical institutions in the country; (ii) the large public hospitals are joint-stock companies or public organizations that belong to the municipalities, being legally private entities; and (3) many private clinics have a contract with the Estonian Health Insurance Fund for the provision of medical services.

In private hospitals, all medical services are paid for. In public hospitals, the payment for medical services is covered by the Health Insurance Fund and indirectly by patients through the social tax, which is payable by the working population.

Current pain workforce

The Estonian Pain Society was established in 1990 as a non-profit and non-governmental body. At the same time, it established contact with the EFIC by joining the organization. At the moment, there are more than 75 active members in the Estonian Pain Society. It mainly consists of anesthesiologists and neurologists, and also of medical nurses working in the field of pain management and nursing care. It also includes palliative medicine specialists (physicians and nurses).

The administrative structure of the Estonian Pain Society is the following: the President and the Board, who are elected by all members; nurses and physicians can enter the society freely; meanwhile, the Society Board consists of representatives of Estonia's main hospitals. The Estonian Pain Society's membership consists of doctors and nurses from different specialties such as anesthesiology, neurology, rehabilitation, surgery, oncology, and others.

The main objective of the Society is to create optimal conditions for professional education and practice in the pain treatment. The activities of the society also aim at familiarizing healthcare professionals and the general public with the problems of people suffering from pain.

The Estonian Pain Society was founded in 1990 by Professor of Neurology Rein Zupping, who also organized the first pain clinic in Estonia. Professor Rein Zupping made an enormous contribution to the development of cooperation with the international organizations in the areas of neurology and pain management. He was also the first president of the Estonian Pain Society. The next president was Ursula Koorits, an anesthesiologist, who continued the active development of the society and participated in the creation of the first pain management standards and guidelines.

At the moment, the president of the Estonian Pain Society is Dr Boris Gabovich, who developed the first education course for the training of specialists in the field. Contributions to the society were also made by Dr Yuri Alex Kolesnikov, who defended the first dissertation devoted to pain treatment in the territory of the former USSR.

The Board of the Estonian Pain Society consists of six members who are practitioners in the pain management fields. The Board members are elected and they represent the main hospitals in Estonia, where there are offices or pain management services. At the moment, the number of the public members is about 76. The number of members is dynamically changing due to the fact that some doctors have stopped practising, but while some migrate to other countries, new specialists are joining too.

Unfortunately, the specialty or subspecialty for Pain Management in Estonia does not exist. But there is a list of doctors with additional competence in pain treatment, who are able to treat pain and prescribe strong opioids. The list is made and updated by the Estonian Pain Society and submitted to the Ministry of Social Affairs. Because of the lack of a Pain Managment specialty in Estonia, the main specialties of the doctors involved in the pain treatment are anesthesiologists and neurologists, but there are also surgeons, oncologists, and physiotherapists.

At the moment, there are about 25–30 doctors working in outpatient pain departments and pain offices in Estonia. These offices and clinics are uniformly distributed in the large hospitals of the county with a calculation that from any point in Estonia and from each patient there is no more than 50 km to the pain management doctor. This helps to comply with the principle that analgesia should be accessible for all patients. The admission and treatment of patients is conducted in eight public and one private pain treatment offices. Both outpatient and inpatient medical treatments are provided in clinics and hospital departments. The emphasis is on an integrated approach that includes pharmacological and, non-pharmacological therapies, invasive, and rehabilitation techniques. Separately, there is the Estonian Headache Society, which cooperates and closely communicates with the Pain Society.

Currently, there is almost no research work in the area of pain management in Estonia. At the moment, two major studies are underway: one in the areas of pain genetics and pharmacology under the direction of Dr Yuri Alex Kolesnikov, and the other on the topic of opioid use.

Challenges and opportunities to the future development of pain services

Despite the lack of pain specialty in the country, the Estonian Pain Society has developed a system of additional training for all physicians interested in pain treatment. The system includes theoretical lectures at the university and a practical one-month course at one of the central hospitals, mainly for anesthesiologists, but also available for other doctors. Due to a small number of experts, the focus is on individual training with an internship in different countries of the EU. Additionally, there are lectures on various topics of pain treatment for doctors and nurses. The lectures deal with the following topics: chronic pain, cancer pain, neuropathic pain, acute pain, perioperative analgesia, opioids, and so on.

Further objectives of the Pain Society are to seek (i) recognition of a subspecialty in pain for physicians and for nurses; (ii) separate funding from the Estonian Health Insurance Fund (currently there is no separate funding, it is carried out on the residual principle and the patient's basic disease, such as back pain—neurology, pain in the joints—orthopaedics); (iii) the introduction of a separate training system at the university followed by residency; (iv) legislative improvement concerning opiate trafficking. And (v) the development of the national guidelines for the treatment of various pain syndromes. At the moment, there is only one national guideline in perioperative analgesia.

Innovations

Existing achievements in the last five years include several changes in legislation, optimizing prescribing rules. They include a 100% discount on strong opioids for patients with non-oncological and chronic pain; and permission for GPs to prescribe strong opioids for patients with oncologic pain syndromes. These changes are the result of lengthy negotiations with the Ministry of Social Affairs.

Unfortunately due to the lack of adjustment at the state level, the financing of the residual principle and undeveloped private practice in pain management, innovation has been delayed. However, the society is constantly considering options for further development and patient care. At the moment, the focus is on educational programmes for doctors and patients, which may further contribute to a more active development of the Estonian Pain Society.

Reference

Tammur, A. (2017). *The population of Estonia increased last year—Statistics Estonia*, News Release No. 8, January 2017. Available at: http://www.stat.ee/news-release-2017-008 [Online].

Chapter 2.10

Finland

Juha Nevantaus

Background information

Finland has about 5.4 million inhabitants and an average population density of 17 people per square kilometre (see Fig. 2.10.1). This makes it the third most sparsely populated country in Europe, after Iceland and Norway. The distribution of the population is very uneven: the population is concentrated on the small southwestern coastal plain. About 85% of Finns live in towns and cities, with one million living in the Helsinki Metropolitan Area alone. In Arctic Lapland, on the other hand, there are only two inhabitants to every square kilometre (OSF, 2012).

Until recently the country has been ethnically homogeneous, the dominant ethnicity being Finnish. The official languages are Finnish and Swedish, the latter being the native language of about 5% of the Finnish population.

The Finnish Association for the Study of Pain (FASP) was founded in 1996 as a multiprofessional organization to promote multidisciplinary research and treatment of pain in Finland. Other objectives of the organization are to increase awareness of pain within the general public, healthcare professionals, and policymakers; to legitimize diseases associated with pain; and to improve the education and working conditions of professionals working with pain patients. FASP became a national chapter of IASP in August 2010 and thereafter joined EFIC. Collaboration with SASP (Scandinavian Association for the Study of Pain) is also frequent. There were 1,062 regular members of FASP at the end of the year 2015. These were physicians of various disciplines, dentists, psychologists, nurses, physical therapists, social workers, and other professionals.

Healthcare system

Healthcare in Finland consists of a highly decentralized, three-level publicly funded healthcare system and a much smaller private sector. Although the Ministry of Social Affairs and Health has the highest decision-making authority, the municipalities (local governments) are responsible for providing healthcare to their residents.

Finland offers its residents universal healthcare. Health promotion, including prevention of diseases has been the main focus of Finnish healthcare policy for decades. This has resulted in the eradication of certain communicable diseases and improvement in the health of the population. Finland's infant mortality is nowadays one of the lowest in the whole world.

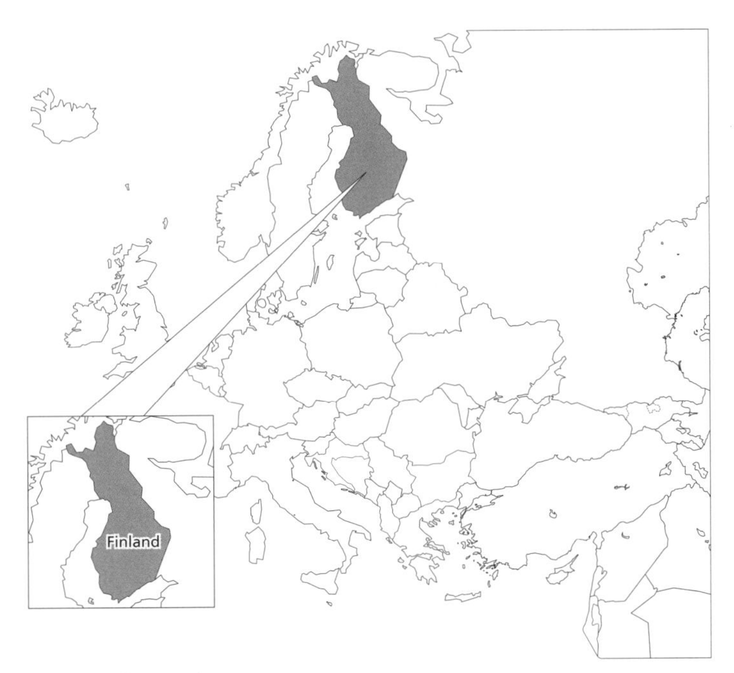

Fig. 2.10.1 Map of Finland.

The quality of service in Finnish healthcare is considered to be good; according to the survey 'Health and long-term care in the European Union' published by the European Commission in 2000, Finland belongs to the top five countries where the citizens are most satisfied with their healthcare. An average of 88% Finnish respondents were satisfied compared with the EU average of 41.3%.

At the moment, the Finnish healthcare system is in the middle of a major reform. The goal of the social welfare and healthcare reform is to secure services of sufficient quality and to make them available on an equal basis under conditions of limited resources. The goal is to reinforce first-line services—that is, new types of basic level services. This means that it will hopefully be easier to get an appointment to see a physician in the future.

This basic goal also implies that in the first phase all central services would be available close to where the people are. In addition to the current services of primary healthcare, higher level specialist services, both medical and social, should be easily available to the customers.

Current pain workforce

In Finland there are five universities with a medical faculty. All university hospitals have multidisciplinary pain clinics. Only the University of Helsinki has a professor in Pain Medicine. Most regional hospitals have outpatient pain clinics, and also some of the largest local health centres have specialist physicians working in the field of pain management.

At the moment there are about 100 physicians in Finland who have gained special competence in pain medicine (the total number of actively working physicians in Finland is about 21,000). Almost half of them are anesthesiologists. However, among them there are physiatrists, neurologists, general practitioners, psychiatrists, neurosurgeons, and dentists. At the moment, ageing of these pain specialists is a challenge to be solved. There are plans to make specialization in pain medicine more attractive among younger physicians. It has also been under discussion if the responsibility of training pain specialists should be transferred from the Finnish Medical Association and the Finnish Association for the Study of Pain to medical faculties. In the basic medical education of doctors, the EFIC core curriculum for medical schools is to be followed. New methods of teaching have also been introduced into practice; for example, Internet-based learning and the so-called 'flipped classroom' methods are in use at the Helsinki University.

There are about 100–150 nurses working mainly in the field of pain at present. A problem is that currently there is no possibility for the nurses to get special education in pain medicine.

FASP is a co-organizer in a course programme providing special education in pain psychology for psychologists. At the moment, about 70 psychologists have accomplished this course of 30 academic credits (one credit equals 27 hours of work).

There are about 100 physiotherapists who have completed a diploma course in pain physiotherapy. FASP is a co-organizer also for these courses of 15 academic credits.

Challenges and opportunities for the future development of pain services

The Finnish Ministry of Social and Health Services recently commissioned a task force, in collaboration with FASP, to survey the availability of treatment in chronic pain and cancer pain, and to recommend actions for the improvement of pain treatment in Finland in the future. This report shows that in both cancer pain and chronic pain, the resources do not meet the treatment needs. There are also great differences in the availability of treatments in different parts of the country.

The task force made a national blueprint, which recommends procedures to create equal, patient-centred, and good-quality services for the multidisciplinary and multiprofessional management of chronic and cancer pain. The blueprint recommends that pain management be organized at three different levels of expertise, and suggests the minimum resources for the services. An audit and guidance group should be established to ensure the implementation of this plan.

It is a necessity to improve the possibilities for primary healthcare professionals treating pain following the national guidelines. One important focus is in the prevention of pain chronification by promoting a healthy lifestyle, ensuring rapid access to pain management, and maintaining the patient's function and ability to work.

Efficient pain treatment is economically profitable. Disability due to chronic pain creates huge costs to society. The price Finnish society paid just from low back pain was calculated to be €469 million in 2013. The productivity losses multiply this sum.

Remarkable savings can be reached by investing in prevention of pain, early rehabilitation, and renewal of both basic and special healthcare systems.

Pain treatment for patients with incurable cancer is part of holistic palliative care. The European Association for Palliative Care has set several guidelines for the treatment of cancer patients. Treatment of cancer pain through a three-level model is a goal reached through education and also sufficient resources.

Innovations

The Finnish Medical Society Duodecim is providing Current Care Guidelines in many medical fields. Current Care Guidelines are independent, evidence-based clinical practice guidelines. These cover important issues related to Finnish health and medical treatment, as well as the prevention of diseases. The guidelines are intended as a basis for treatment decisions, and can be used by physicians, healthcare professionals, and citizens (www.kaypahoito.fi) (The Finnish Medical Society, 2017). The guidelines are developed in association with various medical specialist societies and are produced by the Current Care editorial teams, which are publicly funded.

Members of FASP have actively participated in the writing of the guidelines for pain management. The guidelines cover the main aspects of the management of patients suffering from chronic pain and they were released in late 2015. The following aspects are covered in these guidelines:

- definition of chronic pain;
- prevalence of pain;
- pain in healthcare services, costs of pain;
- meeting of a pain patient;
- evaluation of pain, adults/children;
- evaluation of pain patients' performance and ability to work;
- principles of treatment:
    - non-pharmacological—exercise, therapeutic training, cognitive-behavioural therapy, physiotherapeutic treatments;
    - pharmacological—pain medication in common chronic diseases (in elderly patients and in severely ill patients, and children) during pregnancy and breast-feeding, principles of opioid use;
    - guidance of a patient;
    - treatment arrangements;
    - follow-up of a patient;
    - treatment of most common chronic pain states (e.g. fibromyalgia, neuropathic pain, complex regional pain syndrome, and so on);
    - rehabilitation of a pain patient;
    - prevention of chronic pain.

Helsinki University Hospital is the first institution in the world which has started an outpatient clinic for patients who are at risk of chronification of acute postoperative pain (APS-OPC). The APS-OPC is an outpatient clinic for subacute postoperative pain management. Pain medication, including strong opioids, is tapered off. It also enables an easy transfer to chronic pain services, if pain persists. The results of the first year of this clinic are also published (Tiippana *et al.*, 2016).

Research in the field of pain in Finland is presently active, taking place mainly at pain clinics at the university hospitals. In addition to clinical research and epidemiological studies, also basic research in pain is conducted. FASP supports research with various grants. It is also about to start a Pain School for researchers, and tries to improve communication between investigators by providing an Internet forum for communication.

References

European Commission (2000). Health and long-term care in the European Union. (accessed 3 August 2015).

Official Statistics of Finland (OSF) (2012). *Population structure* [e-publication]. ISSN=1797-5395. Annual review 2012. Helsinki, Finland: Statistics Finland

The Finnish Medical Society (2017). Current Care Guidelines 2017. Available at: www.kaypahoito.fi [Online].

Tiippana E., Hamunen, K., Heiskanen, R., Nieminen, T., Kalso, E., & Kontinen V. (2016). New approach for treatment of prolonged postoperative pain: APS Out-Patient Clinic. *Scand J Pain*, **12**, 19–24.

Chapter 2.11

France

Didier Bouhassira and Nadine Attal

Background information

France is a large European country covering 643,801 square kilometres (metropolitan France) with 13 metropolitan regions and 5 overseas regions. Its population comprises 66,990,826 inhabitants and has grown every year for the last century (NISES 2017). The median age of the French population is 40.4 years (33.8 for males, 41.8 for females) and has increased since 2004 (NISES, 2017). French is the official language (Fig. 2.11.1).

According to a French epidemiological survey, approximately 20% of the French general population suffers from chronic pain of at least moderate intensity (Bouhassira *et al.*, 2008). Such prevalence has been estimated to affect up to 60% of elderly subjects, one-third of whom suffer from severe chronic pain (French National Authority, 2000). According to another French survey, 44% of the patients with chronic pain feel isolated and two-thirds suffer from anxiety or depression symptoms because of their pain (Pain Story Survey, 2009). The impact of chronic pain encompasses all aspects of quality of life and is worse for neuropathic pain as compared to other types of pain (Attal *et al.*, 2011). Furthermore, 45% of chronic pain subjects have taken sick leave because of their pain, for which the cumulative mean duration outlasts four months per year (Lanteri-Minet, 2006). This typically illustrates the major burden of illness associated with chronic pain in France and the necessity of multidisciplinary management (Becker *et al.*, 2000).

Healthcare system

In France, multidisciplinary and pluriprofessional structures involved in pain management have been developed specifically to better assess and manage the most hard-to-treat chronic pain patients, since general practitioners and most specialists have difficulty managing these patients by themselves. A large number of recommendations related to the assessment and management of pain have been proposed over the last 15 years under the auspices of ANAES, which recently became the French National Authory for Health (Haute Autorité de Santé, HAS) (French National Authority for Health, 2008; Recommendations from ANAES, 1999, 2000, 2002, 2005). Similarly, the French scientific societies have promoted several therapeutic recommendations (French Society of Pain, 2013, 2014; Perrot *et al.*, 1999; Moisset *et al.*, 2016). The large dissemination of these recommendations has helped to significantly improve the

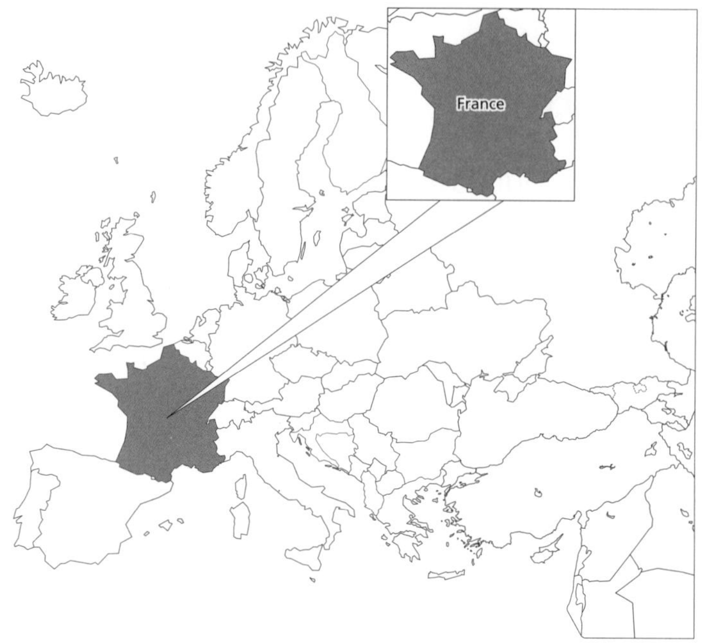

Fig. 2.11.1 Map of France.

quality of healthcare management of chronic pain patients in France and reduce medical expenses.

In the present chapter, we will first describe the care resources regarding chronic pain, then will present the various laws and regulations relative to the pain management system in France. This has been the subject of two books edited by the French Society of Pain in France in 2005 and 2015 (Serrie and Queneau, 2005; Creach, 2014).

Current pain workforce

The initial organization: 1998–2012

In 1998, French health authorities proposed the first official criteria for the identification of multidisciplinairy pain clinics (circular DGS/DH n° 98/47 from 4 February 1998 relative to the identification of pain clinics devoted to refractory chronic pain). Such criteria have allowed us to identify three distinct types of pain clinics:

- Multidisciplinary consultation, encompassing the majority of cases.
- Multidisciplinary unit, including access to technology platforms and/or hospital beds.
- Multidisciplinary centre in a university hospital including teaching and research activities on pain.

Furthermore, public health law dating from 2 March 2002, relative to patients' rights has recognized pain relief as a fundamental right for patients (Ministry of Employment and Social Affairs, 2002–2005).

In keeping with these advances, three successive national pain plans proposed between 1998–2010 (High Public Health Committee, 2011) have facilitated the development of specialized pain clinics, whose number has climbed from 96 in 2001 to around 250 in 2010–2011. The third national pain strategy has emphasized several areas of improvement, including reducing the time for consultation in a pain clinic and increasing visiblity of pain clinics for the lay public and for healthcare professionals.

In 2012, new requirement specifications for the identification of pain centres have appeared (Circular DGOS/PF2/2011/188 from 19 May 2011): the label 'pain unit' has been abandoned and only the labels 'pain consultation' and 'pain centre' have remained.

The updated organization: 2016

Since 23 May 2016, new requirement specifications for pain centres and consultations in France have been proposed by Directorate-General of Care supply (DG care supply) (Direction Générale de l'Offre de Soins (DGOS) (SFETD, 2016). Some of the criteria previously proposed in 2012 are unchanged, while others have been added to make a further distinction between pain centres and pain consultations.

Common criteria for multidisciplinary pain consultations or centres include the following:

- Be part of a health institution.
- Propose at least 500 medical consultations per year.
- The premises must be grouped together.
- There should be a dedicated telephone reception.
- There should be at least two consultation boxes.
- The responsible officer should have a specific official training in pain.
- Medical activity should be at least 50% full-time equivalent for doctors and 1.5 full-time equivalent for paramedics.
- The team should be able to consult a social worker.
- There should be regular medical team staff meetings.
- Medical activity should be diversified except for child care.
- Medical consultations should be traceable.

Prior criteria to become a pain centre still include the following:

- Several medical specialties, access to technical facilities and hospital beds, and at least part of the staff affected fully or partially to pain management.

The new 2016 requirements for pain centres have become more stringent and now also include the following:

- At least one medical pluridisciplinary medical staff meeting per month including at least three doctors from distinct specialties;
- Coordination of university teaching in pain; and/or

- Research activity with at least three PubMed publications by members of the medical staff within the last five years.

Regarding paediatric pain centres, criteria should also include the necessity for the responsible officer to have a specialty in pain and in paediatrics, and at least one medical pluridisciplinary medical paediatric staff meeting per month.

Challenges and opportunities to the future development of pain services

Geographic distribution of pain centres and consultations in France

According to DG care supply, each region should have at least one centre and one paediatric pain centre or consultation. Furthermore, pain consultations with less than 1,000 consultations per year should be funded only if there is no multidisciplinary pain centre within less than one hour of transportation.

To date, according to the data from the Ministry of Health (21 May 2015) there are 245 pain consultations or centres in France, including 39% centres and 61% consultations. These organizations are well distributed in general, although there is a trend towards fewer pain centres or consultations in three distinct French regions (Corsica, Limousin, and Champagne Ardennes).

Funding of pain centres and consultations in France

The funding of health institutions in France is generally based on clinical activity. Such funding concerns activites related to diagnosis, treatment, and care, but is generally unfavourable to pain because pain consultations are usually very long and necessitate multidisciplinary management. Therefore, a specific source of funding has been proposed and is integrated in the financing of general interest missions and contractual elements, called *MIGAC* (Mission d'Intérêt Général et d'Aide à la Contractualisation). The objectives of *MIGAC* are to fund a certain number of missions that cannot be adequately covered by financing on the basis of clinical activity.

General interest missions called *MIG* (Missions d'Intérêt Général) aim to fund the costs related to specialized and long multidisciplinary and pluriprofessional specialized consultations (https://www.sante.gouv.fr). These have been based for years on the annual number of external medical consultations and in 2014 represented a total amount of €62.7 million. However, the allocation of MIG varies heavily from one health institution to another. If there are fewer than 500 consultations per year, then no funding is proposed and the pain organization cannot be identified by health regional agencies (DGOS/FP2/2011/188, 19 May 2011). Starting from January 2017, and based on new criteria proposed by DGOS on 23 May 2016, this funding will still require a minimun number of consultations but will also be based on the number of patients per year (total active file), rather than on the number of consultations.

Pain consultations or centres involved in medical research can also receive specific funding relative to missions of teaching, research, and innovation called

MERRI (Missions d'Enseignement, de Recherche, de Recours et d'Innovation) which are based on scientific publications, teaching activity (students), and clinical trials.

Innovations

The management of pain has been subject to several national plans and legal texts in the public health code in France and is part of patients' rights. The importance attributed to pain has been developed in the law n°2002.303 dating from 4 March 2002, relative to the patient's rights and the quality of the healthcare system. According to this law (L11105): 'Every person has the right to receive care aiming to relieve pain. Such pain must be in any circumstanes prevented, evaluated, managed and treated', and 'Every health professional must implement all means to insure for everyone a decent life until death'. Box 2.11.1 presents a number of major circulars or laws regarding the organization of pain management in France since 1988.

Box 2.11.1 Main circulars and laws regarding the organization of pain management in France since 1988

- Circular DGS/3D (26 August 1988) relative to the healthcare organization and to support patients in terminal illness.
- Report of the task force of the Directorate-General for Health (Direction Générale de la Santé) 'chronic pain: specialized structures for treating pain', Bulletin Officiel, n° 3 bis 1991.
- Relief of pain, special leaflet N° 86–32 bis of the Official Bulletin (Ministry of Health and Social Affairs).
- General report 'Health in France' from the High Public Health Committee (HPHC, France).
- Law n° 91–748 from 31 July 1991 relative to patients' rights.
- Circular DGS/DH n° 3 from 7 January 1994 relative to healthcare organization and management of chronic pain.
- National survey from the Directorate-General for Health conducted in 1994 and published in 1995: 'Pain organizations in France'.
- Report 'Manage pain' from the senate group of pain studies directed by Mr Lucien Neuwirth (October 1994, n° 138).
- Law n° 95–116 from 4 February 1995 proposing various social disposiions (Official Journal of 5 February 1995), articles 31 and 32, p. 1998.
- Circular DGS/DH n° 95–22 from 6 May 1995 relative to the hospital patients' charter.

- Circular DGES/DGS n°15 from 9 May 1995 relative to teaching for undergraduate and postgraduate medical students, p. 7.
- Decree n° 95–100 from 6 September 1995 relative to the code of medical practice (Official Journal, 8 September 1995), articles 37 and 38, p. 13306.
- Recommandations from the National Agency for the development of medical evaluation (ANDEM): 'Pain assessment and treatment organizations', November 1995.
- Bylaw dated 4 March 1997 relative to postgraduate medical students (Official Journal, 26 March 1997), Article 7, p. 4685.
- Bylaw dated 4 March 1997 relative to postgraduate medical students, proposing the core curriculum including pain (Official Journal, 26 March 1997), article 1, p. 4686.
- Circular dated 29 May 1997 on 'Organization of pain control in health institutions'.
- Circular DGS/PS n° 97/412 dated 30 May 1997 in accordance with the decree n° 93–345 dated 15 March 1997 regarding the professional acts and the nurse practice, paragraph V.
- Circular DGS/DH n° 98/47 dated 4 February 1998 relative to the identification of structures for treating persistent chronic pain.
- Circular DGS/DH/AFS n° 98–213 dated 24 March 1998 relative to organization of care in oncology: includes a chapter on pain control and palliative care.
- Circular DGS/DH n° 98/586 dated 22 September 1998 regarding the implementation of the triennal action plan relative to pain control in public or private health institutions.
- Circular DGS/DH/DAS n° 99/84 dated 11 February 1999 relative to the implementation of acute pain management protocols by multidisciplinary medical or nurse teams in health institutions.
- Decree n° 99–49 dated 31 March 1999 relative to poisonous substances and organization of the evaluation of pharmacodependancy.
- Circular DGS/DH dated 8 April 1999 relative to the implementation of protected orders in health institutions.
- Law n° 99–477 dated 9 June 1999 aiming to guarantee the right to access to palliative care.
- French National Authority for Health (HAS) professional recommendations regarding the diagnosis of peripheral neuropathies including a section on pain, May 2007.
- HAS professional recommandation on chronic pain: 'Chronic pain: diagnose chronic pain, assess, and orient the patient' (Professional consensus, December 2008).

- Circular n° DGOS/PF2/2010/463 dated 27 January 2010 relative to the funding for modernization of public and private health institutions (FMESPP) of the national programme of improvement of the management of pain 2006–2010.
- First triennal government plan of pain control 1998–2001.
- Second triennal government plan of pain control 2001–2006.
- Third quadrennial governmental plan of pain control 2006–2010.
- Circular n° DGOS/PF2/2011/188 dated 19 May 2011 relative to the identification of the requirement specifications for the structures treating persistent chronic pain.
- Circular n° DGOS/PF2/2016/160 dated 23 May 2016 relative to the identification of the requirement specifications for the structures involved treating chronic pain and their clinical activity in 2016.

The management of chronic pain in France is based on a large number of multidisciplinary pain centres or consultations disseminated throughout the French territory. Requirements relative to the identification of pain clinics have been edicted and pain consultations or centres receive specific funding. Furthermore, the management of pain has been subject to several national plans and legal texts in the public health code in France and is part of patients' rights. Nevertheless, although pain is now largely taught to undergraduate and postgraduate students in France, it is not yet considered as a full medical specialty, but as a subspecialty.

References

Attal, N., Lanteri-Minet, M., Laurent, B., Fermanian, J., & Bouhassira, D. (2011). The specific disease burden of neuropathic pain: results of a French nationwide survey. *Pain*, **152**, 2836–43.

Becker, N., Sjøgren, P., Bech, P., Olsen, A. K., & Eriksen, J. (2000). Treatment outcome of chronic non-malignant pain patients managed in a danish multidisciplinary pain centre compared to general practice: a randomised controlled trial. *Pain*, **84**, 203–11.

Bouhassira, D., Lanteri-Minet, M., Attal, N., Laurent, B., & Touboul, C. (2008). Prevalence of chronic pain with neuropathic characteristics in the French general population. *Pain*, **138**, 380–7.

Creach, C. (2014). Livre blanc structures douleur. Management of chronic pain in France. French Society of Pain, 2014–2015.

High Public Health Committee (2011). Assessment of the improvement of pain management 2006–2010. Collection Evaluation. Available at: http://www.sfetd-douleur.org/plans-douleur [Online].

Lanteri-Minet, M. (2006). ECONEP: Assessment of cost related to management of neuropathic pain patients: 6th Congress of the French Society of Pain. Nanters 17 November 2006.

Ministry of Employment and Social Affairs (2002–2005). Delegate Ministry of Health Pain Management Programme 2002–2005.

Ministry of Health (n.d.). Available at: http://www.sante.gouv.fr (accessed 21 May 2015) [Online].

Moisset, X., Trouvin, A. P., Tran, V. T., *et al.* (2016). Use of strong opioids in chronic non-cancer pain in adults. Evidence-based recommendations from the French Society for the Study and Treatment of Pain. *Presse Med*, **45**, 447–62.

Pain Story Survey (2009). Pain Study Tracking Ongoing Responses for a Year—September 2009. Available at: https://painstory.org.fr [Online].

Perrot, S., Bannwarth, B., Bertin, P., *et al.* (1999). Use of morphine in nonmalignant joint pain: the Limoges recommendations. The French Society for Rheumatology. *Rev Rhum Engl Ed*, **66**, 571–6.

Recommandations from French National Authority for Health (HAS) (2000). Assessment and therapeutic management of pain in elderly subjects with communication disorders. Available at: https://www.has-sante.fr [Online].

Recommendations from French National Authority for Health (HAS) (2008). Chronic pain: recognize chronic pain, assess and orient the patient. Formal consensus, December 2008 Available at: https://www.has-sante.fr [Online].

Recommendations from ANAES (1999). Assessment of chronic pain in adult in ambulatory care. Available at: https://www.has-sante.fr [Online].

Recommandations from ANAES (2000). Diagnosis and management of patients with chronic low back pain. Available at: https://www.has-sante.fr) [Online].

Recommendations from ANAES (2002). Diagnostic and therapeutic management of migraine in adult and child: clinical and economic aspects. Available at: https://www.has-sante.fr [Online].

Recommendations from ANAES (2005). Chronic daily headache: diagnosis, role of drug abuse and management. Available at: https://www.has-sante.fr [Online].

Recommendations from French Society of Pain (SFETD) and Pain Committee of the French Society of Anesthesiology (2013). Loco-regional analgesic techniques and chronic pain. Nice, France: French Society of Pain, notebook n°2.

Recommendations from French Society of Pain (SFETD) (2014). French Society of migraine and headache (SFEMC) and Association of French Liberal Neurologists (ANLLF): Diagnosis of chronic daily headache—management in migraine patients; medication overuse headache and chronic migraine. Nice, France: French Society of Pain, notebook n°3.

Serrie, A. & Queneau, P. (eds) (2005). Livre blanc de la douleur. Comité d'organisation des états généraux de la douleur (COEGD).

The French Society for the Study and Treatment of Pain (SFETD) (2016). Chronic pain structures. Available at: http://www.sfetd-douleur.org/les-structures-douleur-chronique [Online].

The National Institute of Statistics and Economic Studies (NISES) (2017). Statistics. Available at: https://www.insee.fr/fr/statistiques [Online].

Chapter 2.12

Germany

Thomas Tölle, Michael Schäfer,
and Thomas Isenberg

Background information

Germany, officially called the Federal Republic of Germany, is one of the largest European countries with a geography of 357,021 square kilometres, and a population of 82 million people. Germany is governed as a federal parliamentary republic, divided into 16 states. It is a well-developed and stable economy. Life expectancy is currently 77 years for men and 82 years for women, and infant mortality is low at 4 per 1,000 births. German is the dominant and national language and the protected minority languages are Sorbian, Romany, Frisian, and Danish. However, the majority of people speak two languages (Busse and Blümel, 2014) (Fig. 2.12.1).

Healthcare system

Healthcare in Germany is a universal system, and its origins can be traced to the late nineteenth century. Individuals have a health insurance plan with the option to pay privately for some care. As with other European nations, cardiovascular disease, complicated by lifestyle, with obesity as the observable marker, is the major cause of death. There are approximately 500,000 hospital beds, of which half are in the public hospitals. Hospital beds and length of stay in hospitals have both been declining.

Current pain workforce

On a voluntary basis, general or specialized physicians may undertake further training in 'pain therapy'. If they achieve this qualification, they may take part in a remuneration scheme accepted by the statutory health insurance (SHI) schemes. At present, roughly 1,100 doctors qualify for this. However, reviews show that this is not enough to deal with all the patients in pain. Often it takes several years for patients to present for appropriate chronic pain treatment. In the field of acute pain treatment, national reviews also show a lack of appropriate treatment in hospitals. Currently, there are 3,400 members in the German Pain Society, and Germany was an early member of EFIC, joining in 1993.

In 2013 the German Pain Society started a process to substantially change the bylaws of the Society. The president and the executive board campaigned to clear away the German Interdisciplinary Pain Association (DIVS), which had been established

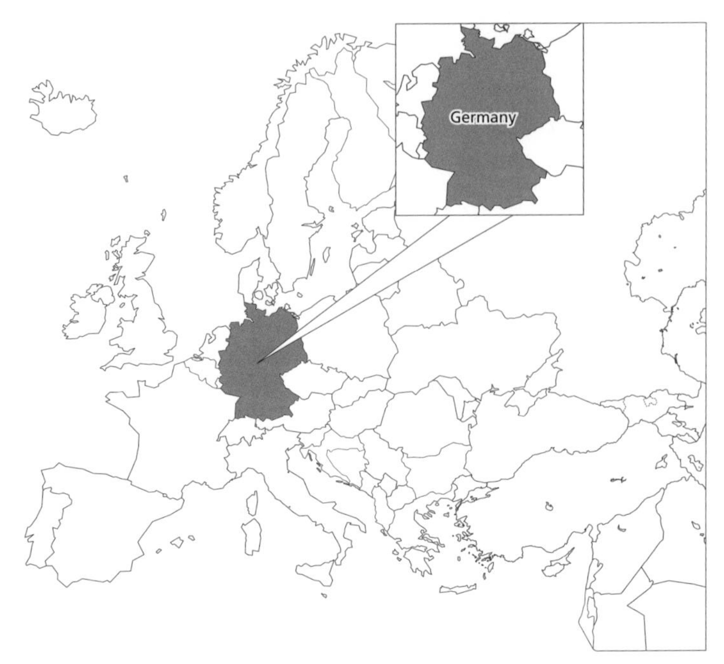

Fig. 2.12.1 Map of Germany.

years before in order to install a system that allowed German doctors to specialize for pain medicine. The DIVS collected many forces from all disciplines of medicine in Germany in order to stand up in the highest general assembly of all German doctors ('Deutscher Ärztetag') for the right of a specialization in pain medicine in addition to any other medical specialization (e.g. anesthesiology, neurology, and so on). This was achieved in 1996 and no other task had been established for the DIVS since then.

The goal of the process of change for the German Pain Society was to bring those scientific organizations directly into the German IASP Chapter and with this also into EFIC. The motto was: 'Greater voice from a broader base.' The idea behind this was to allow the German Pain Society not only to speak for its 3,400 ordinary members, but also for all forces in the medical societies in Germany that were interested in pain medicine. The scientific societies selected to participate in the 'Board of Societies' had to be accredited in the AWMF (Arbeitsgemeinschaft der Wissenschaftlichen Medizinischen Fachgesellschaften) and had to be responsible for the curricula of medical specialization in their particular fields. In 2015 the general assembly of the organization affirmed a most fundamental change in the bylaws of the society (see Fig. 2.12.2). The new structure now allows the society—after internal discussions and negotiations between the societies (in the Board of Societies) and in the Executive Board of the German Pain Society—to present a consistent view on the developments of pain medicine in Germany to politicians and all other stakeholders, also in discussion with the EU. This also allows the society to speak for its members, and to speak on

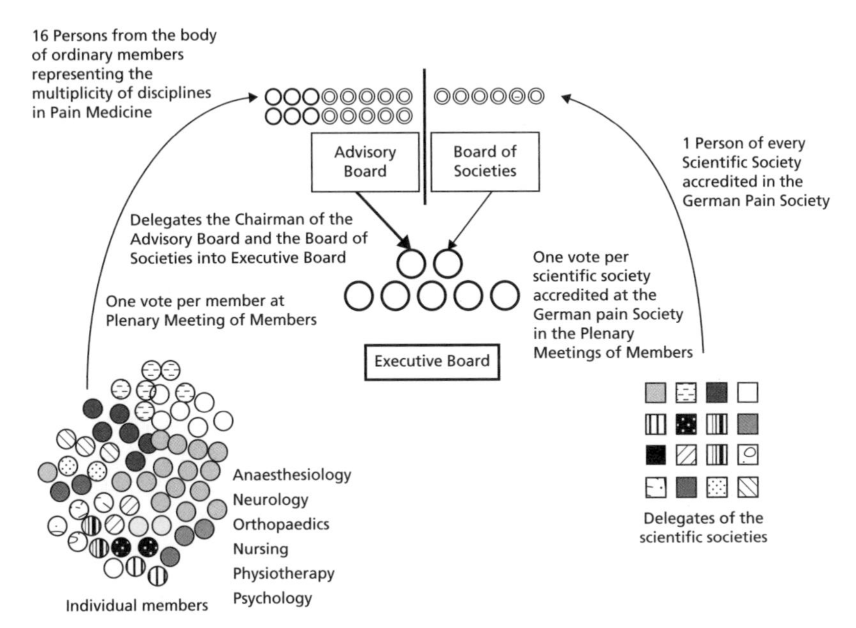

Fig. 2.12.2 Structure of the Executive Board of the German Pain Society.
Reproduced courtesy of Thomas Tölle.

behalf of the 50–100,000 specialized medical doctors from other disciplines and their special interests in pain medicine.

The schematic drawing demonstrates the new structure of the society. All individual members vote in the Plenary Meeting of members the Executive Board and the delegates for the Advisory Board (currently 16 board members from all disciplines represent the society and great care is taken that all medical disciplines and healthcare professionals are represented). The Advisory Board appoints a chairman who is sent into the Executive Board. The accredited scientific societies delegate a spokesman of their society into the general assembly. He also has one vote per society in the general assembly. The spokesmen of the societies are assembled in the Board of Societies and send a chairman into the Executive Board. This organization of the Executive Board with permanent inclusion of a chairman from all different parties within the society (Advisory Board) and the input via the chairman for the scientific societies (Board of Societies) guarantees an exchange of knowledge and vision, both top-down and bottom-up, as the basis for decision-making by the Executive Board.

Challenges and opportunities for the future development of pain services

The German Pain Society has most recently been involved in raising interest in the use of 'pain' as a quality indicator. At the Society's first National Pain Forum in September 2014, a broad array of stakeholders of the country's healthcare system met in Berlin.

This is now an annual meeting with the 2017 meeting focused on the quality agenda. Already this is proving effective. As a result of all these efforts and high-profile gatherings, the Permanent Conference of Health Ministries of the Germany Federal States passed a resolution requiring the introduction of a 'pain indicator' in hospitals.

Hospitals should have departments with an acute pain service for complex patients. Specialist pain doctors and nurses would be employed. A mandatory pain structure and process would be required, put in place by the federal states, as they are responsible for the infrastructure of hospitals. Alternatively, or in addition, the Federal Joint Committee (GBA) could make it mandatory for each hospital to adhere to pain quality indicators before being able to apply for reimbursement. The Federal Joint Committee, a kind of self-governing administrative structure under the supervision of the ministry, is made up of doctors' associations, hospital organizations, statutory sickness funds, and patients. This institution decides on the details of healthcare delivery in Germany and has been mandated by law to set up indicators in several areas. We urge the committee to work on criteria for good pain care in hospitals; in fact, such a proposal is just being prepared and will be put forward by the patient representatives officially. This process has started and now the task is to get pain, eventually both chronic and acute pain, included in this regulatory framework.

In regard to acute pain, ongoing studies assessing pain during different surgical procedures have revealed that with certain procedures patients still feel pain after three months. This is often a consequence of not receiving adequate pain treatment during or after surgery. If the pain persists, it inevitably develops into chronic pain. In Germany, we have different benchmarking systems for acute pain called, for example, QUIPS/PainOut or Certcom. These projects feed back in an anonymous way patient-reported outcomes on postoperative pain management to hospitals. Pain levels are assessed depending on different surgical procedures. There is a large variability between good hospitals and those that need to be improved, and the feedback gives the necessary incentive for change. However, only 10% of German hospitals participate in this. Nowadays, due to increasing economic pressure and the way hospitals are paid for their services, more and more of these institutions are considering reducing pain services, as a short-term way of saving money.

Innovations

It is pleasing to see that the issue of pain is being raised at a Pan-European level (e.g. the Societal Impact of Pain Campaign). The EU could take on an advisory role or it could use its instruments of the official 'Open Method of Coordination' (OMC). For example, they could set up workshops at a European level to address these issues and to collect information from member states and look at where there are already existing indicators. Also, it might be worthwhile implementing such issues in several departments and programmes of both the health and research directorate. In the long run, one might even put forwards a separate 'pain' programme, given budgets for specific tasks. The Parliament could ask the Commission to develop an appropriate strategy. To raise the issue might be an important public health concern as such, not the same, but similar to hygiene, for example. There, nearly all member states have hygiene indicators and often it is possible to see how good or bad a hospital is. Transparency will be key. Patient information forums and (voluntary) benchmarking systems could be set up or co-funded on a European level. Finally, one could consider inviting the European Observatory on Health Systems to implement pain monitoring into its working programme.

We think it important that pain organizations all over Europe work to achieve resolutions on pain care passed within their own medical boards and scientific committees. This is not only an issue for the legislative framework; it is also an issue for those within our healthcare systems. Medical experts in hospitals, in outpatient care, in health insurance schemes, in research, and so on, need to be saying, 'Yes, we need such processes for pain and pain indicators'. This would also be a message to the European platform Societal Impact on Pain (SIP). It is far too easy just to tell politicians what they have to do. We forget sometimes that the majority of politicians tend to follow what large parts of the medical fraternity think would be worthwhile doing. So hospital and medical organizations have to convince their members and other relevant stakeholders in the healthcare system to make this issue their issue, otherwise society will not change fast enough.

Reference

Busse, R. & Blümel, M. (2014). Germany Health System Review. *Health Systems in Transition*, **16**, 2, 1–331. Available at: http://www.euro.who.int/__data/assets/pdf_file/0008/255932/HiT-Germany.pdf [Online].

Chapter 2.13

Greece

Emmanouil P. Anastassiou

Background information

Greece has a population of approximately 11 million people (see Fig. 2.13.1). The Greek National Health System (GNHS) was established in 1985. Nowadays the public sector is only 50% of the total health sector. Some 138 general hospitals all over Greece covers this NHS.

Today the dire economic situation in Greece has dramatically reduced the funding of the National Health and Social Welfare services, which are diminishing on a daily basis. In this challenging environment, the healthcare professionals involved in the treatment of pain patients have difficulties in offering meaningful help.

Healthcare system

The Greek National Health System was founded in 1985. Until then, all the doctors working in the state hospitals were allowed to work in the private sector as well. Prior to 1985, there were not any pain clinics running in either the public or the private health sector but, since then, such clinics have been established in the state hospitals under the initiative of the corresponding anaesthesia departments. Today, there are 62 established pain clinics in the GNHS, run by doctors who are specialized in dealing with patients with chronic pain. The private sector has a much smaller number of pain clinics.

Referral and access to, as well as provision of therapy in, the state pain clinics are all free of charge at the point of delivery for all people, and their running costs are covered by the respective state insurance funds. However, in the private sector the respective process and fees are met by the individual patient either in full or partly, provided that sufficient cover is in place by an insurance fund.

The relationship between pain experts and the Ministry of Health is best characterized as poor and ineffective. There is no support or understanding of the importance of pain within national government, and despite ongoing work at influencing health planning, there is little engagement.

Despite this planning it is clear that the need for effective pain management services continues to grow. The National Statistical Service (data for 2006 and 2011) estimates that there are >30,000 new cancer patients every year. Cancer is the second cause of

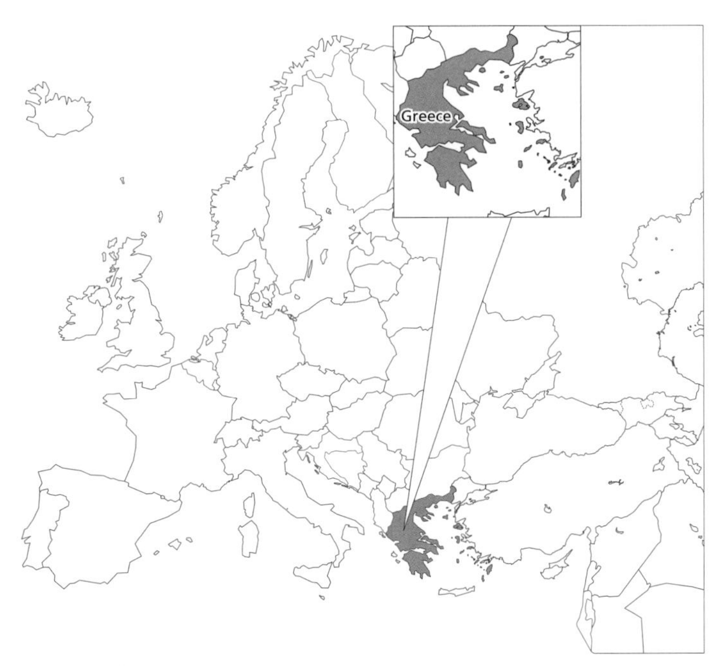

Fig. 2.13.1 Map of Greece.

death in Greece (24.4%) after cardiovascular diseases (29.4%). Pain control of cancer patients depends on the stage of their malignant tumour. It is easy for cancer patients suffering from pain to approach pain clinics, but in some areas of Greece, especially in continental distant areas or in small islands of the Aegean Sea, it is very difficult because there is an unequal distribution of pain clinics. The pain clinics in Greece have developed only in public hospitals and there is no possibility of following up the pain clinic patients on an outpatient basis (e.g. at home) because the organization and the support of home care does not exist.

The provision of palliative care in Greece is currently at very low levels. There are neither public hospices, nor care. There is a legislative framework, but this has not yet been applied. Only three or four hospitals with pain clinics have the ability to follow up the patients at home and to offer basic home care. The opioids available in Greece are: morphine, fentanyl, alfentanyl, nalbuphine, pethidine, dextropropoxyphene, tramadol, tapentadol, oxycodone, and codeine.

There is some difficulty in the prescription of opioids in regard to the use of morphine (a prescription can only be made for five days—all forms of morphine). There is a great bureaucracy involved in opioid access, which is very frustrating for patients and their relatives. In Greece, there is a general belief in the need to use opioids sparingly, especially for non-cancer pain.

Current pain workforce

The Hellenic Pain Society (HPS) is a relatively new scientific society which was founded in 1994 by 27 Greek anaesthesiologists. Its main objective is the promotion of the scientific treatment of patients suffering from acute and chronic pain, as well as preventing and dealing with the consequences of these diseases.

At the end of 1994, the Hellenic Society of Pain became an official member (Chapter) of IASP and some months later, a member of the European Pain Federation (EFIC) (1995). The General Assembly of 6 June 2005 decided to modify the bylaws of HPS and it was thus renamed the Hellenic Society of Algology (HSA). The HSA is the unique scientific society in Greece with the responsibility to defend the human right of all people to have access to pain management without discrimination.

Today, the HSA has 1,120 members, the majority of whom are anaesthesiologists (approximately 75%). The remaining 25% are physicians of other specialties (orthopaedic, general surgery, neurosurgery, internal medicine, psychiatry, neurology, physical medicine and rehabilitation, and so on). Other health professionals such as dentists, psychologists, social workers, physiotherapists, pharmacists, are also members, as well as a large number of nurses working in anaesthesia departments and pain clinics or pain centres. Dr Vassiliki Chimonitsy-Cypriou was the first president and served for two terms (1994–1999), and was followed by Dr Karathanos Achilleas for three terms (1999–2003), Dr Emmanouil Anastasiou for three terms (2003–2011), Dr Helen Plesia for one term (2011–2013), and then again by Dr Emmanouil Anastasiou for a further two terms (2013–2019).

The principal purpose of the Hellenic Society of Algology is to encourage the study and investigation of the mechanisms of pain and pain syndromes, and to promote theoretical and practical training in the field of coping with and treatment of chronic pain. It is a scientific society, and aims to widely disseminate scientific knowledge about pain. The HSA meets these goals by establishing regular scientific exchange and training, postgraduate education, the production of a scientific journal, and the provision of advice and consultation, both nationally and locally.

The Panhellenic Congresses that have been held since the establishment of the Hellenic Society of Pain have now run 11 meetings, with the first held in 1996. In 2010 (27–30 May) the HSA hosted the Third International Congress for Neuropathic Pain in Athens. This congress under the presidency of Professor Chris Wells enjoyed great success and more than 1,800 doctors from all over the world participated.

In previous years, the Hellenic Society of Algology has organized the annual programme of Continuing Education in Algology (CEA) in the field of pain management (4 courses—50 hours total of theoretical and practical training and 20 daily attendances in selected pain centres or pain clinics). The programme was held under the auspices and endorsement of the EFIC and has been credited by the Panhellenic Medical Association in accordance with UEMS EACCME criteria, with 33 credits of continuing medical education (CME-CPD). Thirty-five members of the HSA completed the seminar in 2011, 45 in 2012, 52 in 2013, 61 in 2014, 72 in 2015, and 60 in 2016. The estimate for 2017 is 55 members.

Challenges and opportunities to the future development of pain services

When the Hellenic Pain Society was established in 1994, only eight pain clinics were active all over Greece. Today 62 pain clinics operate throughout Greece, 26 of these are in Attica, 3 in Thessaloniki, and 33 in the rest of the country. The Hellenic Society of Algology encourages the establishment and operation of pain units or pain clinics or pain centres in hospitals of the National Health System, as well as in university and military hospitals. The pain clinics belong to anaesthesia departments, which operate them staffed mainly by anaesthesiologists on a voluntary basis. In these clinics, we treat thousands of patients suffering from acute and chronic pain syndromes, including cancer pain, musculoskeletal pain, headache and migraine, rheumatological, neuropathic, and idiopathic pain syndromes.

Pain clinics in Greece have to overcome numerous obstacles to their day-to-day running. In national hospitals, there is usually a subgroup of anaesthesiologists interested in pain therapy and they are the ones that try to cover the pain clinic as well. Given their expertise, the priority of hospitals is often to use their anaesthetic skills for patients in surgery, and given that presently anaesthesia departments in most hospitals are understaffed, the anaesthesiologists are primarily needed in the operating theatres. Other specialties are involved in pain therapy such as neurologists, neurosurgeons, orthopaedic surgeons, and specialists in physical medicine and rehabilitation, but they are equally pulled into other service provision.

Training for the next generation of pain practitioners is inadequate. Pain management has a wide range of treatments and techniques and is related to a variety of health problems. We believe that there is a great need to create a subspecialty in Greece as in some other countries. Doctors who are interested in pain management try to educate themselves by attending pain educational programmes, pain seminars, pain fellowships in other countries, and so on.

Innovations

Our society organizes seminars and conferences in Greece and, with the approval of EFIC, a one-year programme of Continuous Education in Algology to give the opportunity to doctors interested in pain management to broaden their knowledge. This programme started in 2010 and is now in its seventh year. Every year more than 50 physicians and others health professionals participate in this programmeme. However, we believe it is time for pain education to be more organized and specific qualifications to be required in order to work in a pain clinic.

There seem to be many opportunities for private physicians, since there are still only few private pain clinics and therefore a lot of space for new doctors. The problem is that pain therapy is still not widespread in Greece. Its therapeutic range is not familiar to patients, but even some doctors of other specialties are not fully aware. Since most pain clinics work by referrals from other specialties, this is an obstacle to overcome. We must educate both doctors and patients as well, so that the latter can receive the best treatment possible.

Despite the difficulties and obstacles that exist under these conditions, and the current severe socioeconomic crisis, the Greek doctors involved in the treatment of chronic pain are passionate about their work and committed to providing the highest quality of pain care, for now and in the future.

Reference

The National Statistical Service (data for 2006 and 2011). Hellenic Society of Algology archives. Available at: http://www.algologia.gr [Online].

Chapter 2.14

Hungary

János Tajti, Délia Szok, and János Szolcsányi

Background information

Hungary is located in Central Europe within the Carpathian tube, with an area of 93,000 km^2. The country has lowlands and mountains in an approximately equal ratio. Hungary has two main rivers, the Danube and the Tisza, representing the main sources of water within the country. The biggest lake of Hungary, Balaton, is at the same time the largest fresh water lake in whole of Central Europe. Hungary is surrounded by Slovakia in the north, by Ukraine and Romania in the east, by Serbia and Croatia in the south, and by Slovenia and Austria in the west (Fig. 2.14.1).

The population of Hungary was 9,937,628 according to the 2011 census, with a population density of 107/km^2. More than 25% of the population lives within or in the close vicinity of the capital, Budapest, and some 69.5% of people live in towns throughout the country. In terms of ethnic distribution, 83.7% (8,314,029) declared their ethnicity to be Hungarian, 3.1% (308,957) to be Roma, 1.3% (131,951) to be German, 0.3% (29,647) to be Slovak, 0.3% (26,345) to be Romanian, and 0.2% (23,561) to be Croatian, whereas 14.7% of the population (1,455,883) did not provide information. The population of Hungary has continuously decreased since the beginning of the 1980s, and the number of people above 65 years is increasing. The expected lifespan was 72 and 80 years for men and women, respectively, in 2015. The official language is Hungarian.

Healthcare system

The first infirmaries, which were established and run by monasteries, have been documented from as early as the eleventh century. Selmec, located in the northern region of the former Hungarian Kingdom, was the first town to build a hospital in Hungary in 1224, with its main objective being to take care of injured employees of a nearby mine. The first documented mutual fund was established in 1496. At that time, municipal physicians provided healthcare services for the poor. From 1752, each county of the Kingdom was ordered to provide such a service. In the nineteenth century, mutual assistance funds for industrial workers were set up on a voluntarily basis, and subsequently, the General Fund of Sick and Disabled Workers was established as a healthcare provider and an institute responsible for the management of the personal contributions, with the financial commitments guaranteed by the Emperor. In 1891, health insurance was made compulsory for all industrial employees, which provided cash benefits as well as benefits in kind, via an act, it being only the third in Europe of its type.

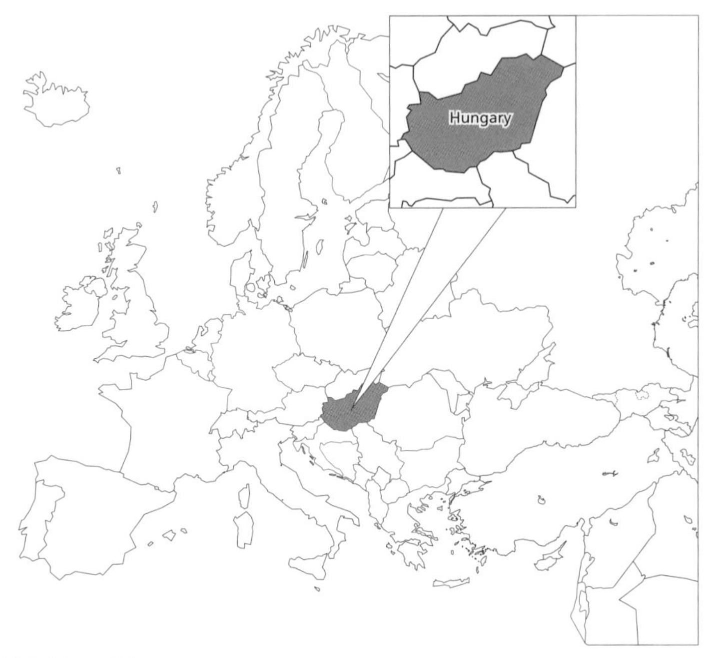

Fig. 2.14.1 Map of Hungary.

Following the establishment of the National Social Insurance Institute covering healthcare of approximately 30% of the total population, general healthcare services were provided predominantly by private and certain state-run hospitals. This system worked until the late 1940s during the communist era, when its leadership nationalized the related institutions, either in terms of funding or healthcare provision. Since then, the latter task was considered to be the responsibility of the state, whereas the remaining issues were assigned to the National Council of the Trade Unions. All private healthcare providers were shut down, with services fully provided by centralized institutes run by the state. After the fall of the communist regime in 1990, the Health Insurance Municipality was established, and the healthcare system including primary care underwent serious modifications and rearrangements. General practitioners were promoted to establish private practices in offices financed by the local municipalities, a generally applied solution in Hungary of the time often referred to as 'functional privatization'. In 1992, the Social Insurance Fund was divided into separate institutes of the Pension Insurance Fund and the Health Insurance Fund (Országos Egészségbiztosítási Pénztár, OEP). In the period of 2004–2008, a series of major attempts aimed to reorganize and reform the system of healthcare in Hungary, including also the increase of the budget financing the Health Insurance Fund.

In 2010, an agenda was published by the government highlighting the main plans as regards the reform of healthcare system in Hungary (Gaál *et al.*, 2011). These included the enhancement of the role of outpatient care, the preservation of a single-payer insurance system, the increase of budget expended on health, the reduction of the waiting lists by half, as well as the introduction of a novel system for the regulation of financial capacities based on objectivized health necessities. This corresponds with what is known as the Semmelweis Plan, a discussion paper published by the Secretary of State for Healthcare of the Hungarian Ministry of National Resources under the title '*Resuscitated Health Care—Recovering Hungary—Semmelweis Plan for Saving Health Care*' (Ministry of National Resources, 2011). The plan proposes the application of the following levels:

- Level 0—Microregional outpatient care office: provides outpatient care in small hospitals and outpatient clinics close to populated areas by specialists transferred there, and it provides patient pathway management at the subregional level.
- Level 1—Inpatient and outpatient care institution at the town level: provides inpatient and associated outpatient care in the fields of 'basic professions' in town hospitals and outpatient centres close to the target population.
- Level 2—Inpatient and outpatient care centre at the county level: provides county-level specialized care in county hospitals and their outpatient centres.
- Level 3—Inpatient and outpatient care centre at the supraregional level: provides almost full care in the determined area, apart from services provided only by level 4 institutes.
- Level 4—National professional centre and subcentre: provides costly, highly specialized, equipment-demanding, and/or infrequent services centralized at the national level.
- The overall level of revenue of the Hungarian National Health Insurance Fund in 2011 was 1,370,937 (million HUF) (NISHR, 2011).

Current pain workforce

The Hungarian Pain Society was established in January 1996 and has been a member of EFIC since its establishment. Its objectives are to promote the comprehensive and full care of patients suffering from acute or chronic pain syndromes (including surgical and/or conservative care, as well as rehabilitation) by means of professional scientific approaches. It brings together researchers, physicians, and other healthcare personnel in the field. The Society also supports basic research related to pain. The Hungarian Pain Society currently has about 150 members, including specialists from theoretical (anatomy, neurophysiology, and pharmacology) and practical (anesthesiology, neurology, oncology, rheumatology, orthopaedics, rehabilitation, oral surgery, paediatrics, family medicine, psychology, and psychiatry) specialties dealing with pain management.

The Hungarian Pain Society and the Federation of Hungarian Medical Societies (Magyar Orvostársaságok és Egyesületek Szövetsége, MOTESZ) are full members of the IASP. Hungary is represented by the current president of the Society or its delegatee within the IASP Committee of Presidents of Chapters. For issues related to the EFIC, the councillor is the legal representative. The leadership of the Hungarian Pain Society comprises nine people (past president, president, president elect, secretary, treasurer, and four board members). The supervisory committee includes three members. The past presidents are granted with the title of Honorary President. The Hungarian Pain Society organizes congresses on a yearly basis, in the autumn period. The location of the congress varies from year to year targeting different regions of the country, so as to promote the education of fellow physicians of the particular region. Each congress follows the topic of the campaign announced by the IASP in the current year (Global Year Against Pain). The congresses are organized either independently or within the framework of an interdisciplinary forum (e.g. in 2014, it was organized in association with the neurostimulation symposium). The official journal of the Society, entitled *Fájdalom/Pain*, is published annually and contains the abstracts of the yearly congress talks.

Membership of the Hungarian Pain Society requires a high-level education (i.e. college or university diploma). The diagnosis and the treatment of pain disorders are definitely multidisciplinary tasks, necessitating team work. Medical experts from several different fields are involved in the diagnostic work-up and the care of pain patients. Given that pain syndromes are chronic diseases, rehabilitation approaches play a role in the therapy of such disorders and in the enhancement of patients' quality of life.

Outpatient pain clinics are working in Hungary, with the first opening on 1 January 1988 in the National Institute of Oncology, Budapest. The establishment of a state-run outpatient pain clinic now requires official authorization (by the National Public Health and Medical Officer Service) and approval by the Health Insurance Fund (i.e. a unique nine-digit identifier provided by the Health Insurance Fund).

The initiation of a private pain office likewise requires official authorization. Physicians working in such outpatient pain clinics may come from various fields of medicine (neurology, anesthesiology, psychology, neurosurgery, and orthopaedics). The number of specialists working in the field of pain is about 100, whereas that of the generalists are up to 30,000 persons in Hungary.

The *Analgesic Guidelines* (*Analgetikai útmutató*), is a periodical national publication with reviews on pain management as part of the *Handbook of Clinical Guidelines* (Klinikai Irányelvek Kézikönyve) series, with the latest issue published in 2011 (Budai and Hatfaludy, 2011). The book covers the diagnostic work-up of patients suffering from chronic pain, the potential therapies aiming at the alleviation of pain caused by malignant tumours, and the current perspectives of opiate therapy. Besides, the chapters of the guidelines also provide information about the proper way of prescribing analgesics based on the legislations in force, the pathomechanism and therapy of neuropathic pain, the national experience as regards the treatment of diabetic neuropathy, and the therapy of post-herpetic neuralgia. The book discusses the potential therapeutic options of postamputation chronic neuropathic pain, the therapy of complex regional pain, the tunnel syndromes, the chronic low back pain and its therapeutic possibilities, trigeminal neuralgia, and migraine as well. Furthermore, it reviews the options of postoperative analgesia, as well as that of the pharmacological alleviation of pain in rheumatological disorders.

Challenges and opportunities for the future development of pain services

Hungary is proud of her excellent medical education and specialist training system. However, there is a paucity of appropriate subdisciplinary education, including the training of pain specialists. It would be desirable to create a post-specialty training system through which the basic professions (of neurology, anesthesiology, neurosurgery, orthopaedics, or rheumatology) could be supplemented with an expertise in pain, by means of an algologist specialty exam or licence exam. Such a training should include both the theoretical and the practical fields of education, and should be based on unified criteria in accordance with the European accreditations. It might be sufficient to create the necessary institutional background for the training of pain specialists in only one of the four medical faculties in Hungary. The invited lecturers should be gathered from the experienced and skilled colleagues currently working in outpatient pain clinics.

Chronic pain, as a disease entity, has significant social and economic impacts. It represents a remarkable disease burden for both the affected individuals and their environment, an important aspect also necessitating specially trained physicians and healthcare personnel (including pain nurses, physiotherapists, and psychotherapists). At the administrative level, the approval of chronic pain as an independent disease entity and the provision of an ICD (International Classification of Diseases) identifier for the disease are necessary. Furthermore, it would be imperative for the decision-makers in health politics to understand the importance of care for patients with chronic pain and the training and continuous education of specialists with expertise in the field. To achieve this, health policy should be proactive and supportive, and the economic policy should provide the proper financial background, which should include the provision of high-standard inpatient and outpatient care, and an appropriate salary for the healthcare personnel. The leadership of the Hungarian Society of Pain has a duty to represent these interests in front of the decision-makers, and to make steps towards improving the quality of care as regards pain care in Hungary in both the short and the long term (Hungarian Pain Society, 2016).

Innovations

Hungary has a long tradition of preclinical pain research (e.g. that related to capsaicin). With the introduction of capsaicin patches onto the market, training sites could be established where academic experts can prepare the clinicians with a specific programme and can put their theoretical knowledge into medical practice. Subsequently, colleagues participating in the specialist pain training would be educated about the clinical and practical aspects by expert clinicians in the field. These educational sites would be present in each of the four medical faculties, with the tutors working in rotations.

In order to keep the current practice state-of-the art, lectures by pain specialists from abroad could be presented in form of video conferences. The experts would be invited based on the recommendation of the leadership of the IASP and the EFIC. This could enable the improvement of the relationship between the pain specialty training in Hungary and the IASP and EFIC.

Taking an overview of the past and current state of the Hungarian Pain Society, we believe that there is a need for a high standard of post-specialty algology training organized within institutional frameworks.

References

Budai & **Hatfaludy** (2011). *Analgetikai Útmutató. Klinikai irányelvek kézikönyve.* Budapest, Hungary: Medition Kiadó.

Gaál, P., Szigeti, S., Csere, M., Gaskins, M., & **Panteli, D.** (2011). Hungary Health System Review. *Health Systems in Transition*, **13**, 1–299.

Hungarian Pain Society (2016). Available at: https://www.fajdalom-tarsasag.hu (accessed 26 August 2016) [Online].

Ministry of National Resources (2011). State Secretariat for Health. Resuscitated Health Care Recovering Hungary. Semmelweis Plan for the Rescue of Health Care. A professional concept. Budapest, Hungary: Ministry of National Resources.

National Institute for Strategic Health Research (NISHR) (2011). Borbás, I., Mihalicza, P., Ajtonyi, Z., Lux, L., Szirmai, L. (eds), *Hungarian Health System Scan*, **4**, 1.

Chapter 2.15

Ireland

David P. Finn, Brona M. Fullen, Brian E. McGuire, Joanne O'Brien, Laserina O'Connor, Raymond Victory, and Shelagh Wright

Background information

Ireland is located in the continent of Europe on the eastern part of the North Atlantic covering 68,883 square kilometres of land and 1,390 square kilometres of water, making it the 121st largest nation in the world with a total area of 70,273 square kilometres. Ireland has a population of 4.76 million, with Dublin, Meath, and Laois the fastest growing counties, and there are slightly more women than men (97.8 males for every 100 females). The ethnic mix is White Irish: 85.1%, other White: 9.5%, Asian: 2.1%, Black: 1.4%, other: 2.2%, not stated: 2.6% (Census, 2016). The age profile is 0–24 years (34%), 25–44 years (32%), 45–64 years (22%), and those over 65 years (12%) (Census, 2011). The most dominant language is English but Irish is the first official language of the state. The population is growing by an average of 0.8% annually. Ireland has been a member of the European Union (EU) since 1973 (see Fig. 2.15.1).

The Irish Pain Society is the largest professional and multidisciplinary pain society in Ireland and has 167 members made up of: anaesthetists (49), nurses (31), physiotherapists (33), psychiatrists/psychologists (7), dentists (2), general practitioners (3), pharmacologists (5), radiologist (1), and others, for example, PhD students, healthcare students, and researchers. The Irish Pain Society was formed in the mid to late 1990s, under the auspices of its first president, Dr Hugh Raftery, and joined EFIC in 2002.

Healthcare system

In Ireland, the Department of Health was established in 1947. Subsequently, a government proposal to implement a national social insurance and health service similar to that being implemented in post-war Great Britain failed due to high-level opposition in Irish government, church, and the medical profession. A state-sponsored health insurance scheme, Voluntary Health Insurance, was introduced in 1957. Funded by the hospital sweepstake lotteries, public health services were delivered through the local government system until 1970. About one-third of the Irish population was eligible for free medical care through a medical card system introduced in 1970. For the remainder, access to healthcare involved a combination of subsidized services, state, and private health insurance (Harvey, 2007). Currently, the Health Service Executive

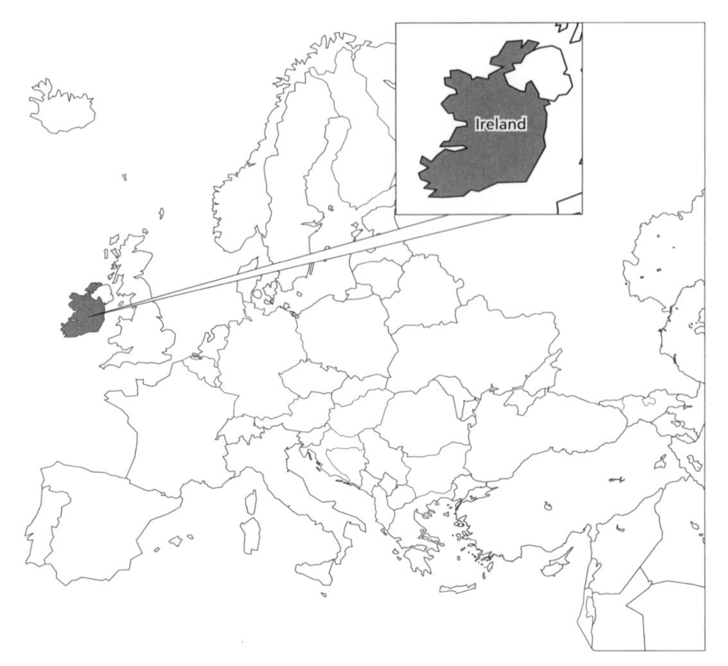

Fig. 2.15.1 Map of Ireland.

has responsibility for the provision of population health, social care, community, and hospital services across Ireland.

For the most part, the Irish healthcare system is tax-funded. In 2013, 77% of total healthcare expenditure was funded by general taxation revenues, 9% by private insurance, and 12% by household out-of-pocket expenditure. In the hospital context, publicly and privately funded care is usually delivered by the same staff in the same facilities. Ireland delivers hospital care through public and private hospitals. In public hospitals, consultants can also treat private patients (Connolly and Wren, 2016).

Prior to the economic recession of 2008, Ireland enjoyed one of the highest economic growth rates in Europe, with public expenditure rising rapidly between 2005–2008. In the last decade, public spending on health in Ireland has been in line with spending in other countries. However, the cost of delivering health services has become higher in Ireland than in comparable countries (Thomson *et al.*, 2014). A recent analysis of the Irish healthcare system by the World Health Organization concluded that Ireland is the only EU health system that does not offer universal coverage for primary care and is an extreme outlier among EU countries with regard to user charges (Thomson *et al.*, 2014).

Ireland was one of the most severely impacted countries in the Organisation for Economic Co-operation and Development (OECD) following the 2008 recession and, due to austerity measures, long-term aims to introduce universal health insurance are currently not feasible. In recent years, the health budget has been slightly increased and free general practice (GP) care for children under 6 years old and people over

70 years old has been introduced. However, penalties have been introduced for people who first take out private health insurance after the age of 35 years (Burke *et al.*, 2016).

In Ireland, large amounts of health data are collected through several information systems, which include the Hospital Inpatient Enquiry System (HIPE), the National Cancer Registry of Ireland (NCRI), the National Screening Service, Immunization Uptake Statistics, and the Computerized Infectious Disease Reporting (CIDR) system. Patient experience measures and appropriate data collection methodologies are currently being developed by the National Patient Experience Steering Group and the National Patient Experience Advisory Group. Patients are also represented on the steering group (National Health Quality Report System, 2016).

Current pain workforce

The specialty of pain medicine in Ireland has its roots in the 1980s with the formation of pain clinics which were run by consultant anaesthetists in co-operation with Nursing, Physiotherapy, Psychology, and Occupational Therapy Departments. Initially, practitioners in the area of pain management were associated with the British Pain Society, but subsequently the Irish Pain Society was founded. The College of Anaesthetists formed a Committee to oversee pain medicine in 2000, and the first Diploma in Pain Medicine was launched in 2002. The Fellowship in Pain Medicine was established in 2007. Residents in Anaesthesia must complete six months in pain medicine before sitting the Diploma (part 1) and subsequently spend two years training before sitting the Fellowship (part 2).

There are now 28 consultants [16 whole time equivalent (WTE) posts] involved in overseeing pain medicine in pain centres around Ireland and 30 residents in Pain Medicine in Ireland.

With regards to Nursing, University College Dublin (UCD) offer a Professional Certificate and Diploma in Pain Management and an MSc in Advanced Pain Management (+/− Prescriptive Authority) for nurses and the University of Limerick offer a multidisciplinary post graduate course in pain medicine within their Health Sciences Department. There are 33 nurses involved almost exclusively in chronic and acute pain services (29 WTE).

There is a very low number of psychologists directly involved in pain medicine. There are 5.2 WTE state-funded posts and a number of psychologists in private practice provide pain management services.

Similarly, very few dedicated state-funded posts have been established for physiotherapists to support pain clinics. Currently there are five WTE posts. Table 2.15.1 summarizes the current pain workforce across the seven hospital groups in the Republic of Ireland involved in both acute and chronic pain management.

Challenges and opportunities to the future development of pain services

Prevalence rates for Irish people suffering with chronic pain range 13–35.5% of the population (Breivik *et al.*, 2006; Raftery *et al.*, 2011). Services for managing chronic

Table 2.15.1 Pain management service provision according to professional discipline

Hospital group	No. of hospitals	Academic partner	Pain consultants	NCHD	RANP/ ANPc	CNS/CNM	Physiotherapy	Psychology	PMP
Dublin North East	7	RCSI	1 WTE	1 WTE	1 WTE	1 WTE	1 WTE	None	1 × MDT pain workshop
Dublin/Midlands	6	TCI	3.5 WTE	1 WTE	None	5.5 WTE	1 WTE	1 WTE	1× MDT PMP
Dublin East	11	UCD	3 WTE	4 WTE	0.5 WTE	3 WTE	1.5 WTE	2 WTE	1 × MDT PMP
South/South West	9	UCC	4.5 WTE	1 WTE	None	4.23 WTE	1.0 WTE	1 WTE	
West/North West	6	NUIG	2.5 WTE	1 WTE	1 WTE	4.5 WTE	0.5 WTE	0.2 WTE	
Midwest	6	UL	1 WTE	1 WTE	None	2.35 WTE	None	0.5 WTE	
Children's	2	All	0.5 WTE	1 WTE	1x WTE ANPc	1.8 WTE	None	0.5 WTE	
Totals	47		28 (16 WTE)	10 WTE	4 (3.5 WTE)	29 (21.38 WTE)	6 (5 WTE)	7 (5.2 WTE)	

(WTE = whole time equivalent; NCHD = non-consultant hospital doctor; RANP = registered advanced nurse practitioner; ANPc = advanced nurse practitioner candidate; CNS/CNM II = clinical nurse specialist/manager; PMP = pain management programme; No.= number.)

Source: data from Irish Pain Society, 2016

pain have traditionally been under-resourced, with prolonged waiting times for patients to attend specialized pain clinics (Fullen *et al.*, 2006). Healthcare costs are also significant, with estimates of up to €5.34 billion (or 2.86% of GDP) per year (Raftery *et al.*, 2012). The significant burden of chronic pain both to the individual and to the economy highlights the need for integrated, cost-effective, multidisciplinary primary and secondary care services.

The Irish healthcare system is currently undergoing profound changes, with healthcare reform offering new opportunities to prevent and treat pain more effectively. In 2014, The Irish Pain Society appeared before the Oireachtas Joint Committee on Health and Children Debate (Irish Parliament) to propose the development of a National Strategy for Chronic Pain Management in Ireland. Core to the discussion was prioritizing chronic pain management in healthcare reform, offering new opportunities to prevent and manage chronic pain more effectively in both primary and secondary care (Oireachtas Report, 2014). A follow-up meeting was held with the Chief Nursing Officer in the Department of Health to discuss the need for advanced nurse practitioners in pain management.

In 2014, pain medicine was officially recognized as a medical specialty within the Irish Medical Council's Register of Medical Practitioners, thereby enabling doctors to pursue specialist training and registration in the specialty of pain medicine. The well-established Fellowship in Pain Medicine (established in 2007 by the College of Anaesthetists of Ireland) underpins this training initiative.

By continuing to fight for improved healthcare services for patients, the Irish Pain Society hopes that the Irish Government's white paper on the 'Path to Universal Healthcare' (Department of Health, 2014), recognizing health as 'a state of complete physical, mental and social well-being and not merely the absence of disease or infirmity', will be realized and implemented.

Innovation

Research

With regards to research in the field of pain science, a number of initiatives have been developed:

1. *Academic research centres*

Two multidisciplinary pain research centres have been developed in academic institutions: the Centre for Pain Research (CPR) at the National University of Ireland, Galway, and the UCD Centre for Translational Pain Research (CTPR), University College Dublin. Both have close links with clinical sites, facilitating high quality research and innovations in service delivery (e.g. Internet-delivered interventions).

2. *The Irish Pain Research Network*

The Irish Pain Research Network (IPRN) is a special interest group of the Irish Pain Society. Founded in 2015 by National University of Ireland (NUI) Galway researchers Professor David Finn and Professor Brian McGuire, and University College Dublin (UCD) researchers, Dr Brona Fullen, Dr Catherine Doody, and Dr Catherine

Blake, it was launched by Professor Rolf-Detlef Treede, president of the International Association of Pain, at the 15th Annual Scientific Meeting of the Irish Pain Society in Dublin in September 2015.

The IPRN brings together all active pain researchers on the island of Ireland (north and south) for the purposes of sharing research results and ideas, and facilitating closer cross-institutional collaboration in the area of pain research in academic institutions, hospitals, other healthcare practices, or industry. Pain researchers at any level of seniority are welcome to join, and students and early-career researchers are particularly encouraged.

Specialist training in pain management

Diploma in Pain Medicine

The Diploma in Pain Medicine, established in 2002 by the College of Anaesthetists of Ireland, was the first of its kind in the European Union. It was followed by the successful establishment of a Fellowship in Pain Medicine (Part 2) by the Faculty of Pain Medicine within the College of Anaesthetists.

Clinical practice

National Clinical Care Programme

In 2010, the National Clinical Care Programme was established by the Health Service Executive to improve and standardize patient care by bringing together clinical disciplines to develop more efficient and appropriate clinical care pathways. This included programmes in Orthopaedics, Rheumatology, and Primary Care. In an important innovation, advanced physiotherapy roles were established to work alongside consultant medical specialists to autonomously triage and manage patients with benign musculoskeletal dysfunction. These roles have helped to reduce orthopaedic waiting lists and ensure appropriate treatment for patients that can be managed without specialist orthopaedic intervention. The long-term plan is to establish similar roles in the primary care setting, minimizing the need for referral to secondary care.

References

Breivik H., Collett B., Ventafridda V., Cohen R., & Gallacher, D. (2006). Survey of chronic pain in Europe: prevalence, impact on daily life, and treatment. *Eur J Pain*, **10**, 287–333.

Burke, S. A., Normand, C., Barry, S., & Thomas, S. (2016). From universal health insurance to universal healthcare? The shifting health policy landscape in Ireland since the economic crisis. *Health Policy*, **120**, 235–40.

Census (2011). Results. Central Statistics Office (CSO). Available at: www.cso.ie (accessed April 2017) [Online].

Census (2016). Summary Results—Part 1. Central Statistics Office (CSO). Available at: www.cso.ie (accessed April 2017) [Online].

Connolly, S. & Wren M. A. (2016). The 2011 proposal for Universal Health Insurance in Ireland: Potential implications for healthcare expenditure. *Health Policy*, **120**, 790–6.

Department of Health (2014). The Path to Universal Healthcare: White Paper on Universal Health Insurance. Dublin, Ireland: Department of Health, Government Publications.

Fullen B., Hurley D. A., Power C., Canavan D., & O'Keeffe D. (2006). The need for a national strategy for chronic pain management in Ireland. *Irish J Med Sci*, **175**, 68–73.

Harvey, B. (2007). Evolution of Health Services and Health Policy in Ireland. Combat Poverty Agency. Available at: http://www.combatpoverty.ie/publications/EvolutionOfHealthServicesAndHealthPolicyInIreland_2007.pdf [Online].

National Health Quality Report System (2016). Department of Health. Available at: http://health.gov.ie/wp-content/uploads/2016/07/NHQRS_AR16-Final-July-2016.pdf [Online].

Oireachtas Report (2014). Available at: https://www.oireachtas.ie/parliament/media/committees/healthandchildren/Irish-Pain-Society-opening-statement.pdf [Online].

Raftery M. N., Ryan P., Normand C., Murphy A. W., de la Harpe D., & McGuire B. E. (2012). The economic cost of chronic noncancer pain in Ireland: results from the PRIME study, part 2. *J Pain*, **13**, 139–45.

Raftery M. N., Sarma K., Murphy A. W., de la Harpe D., Normand C., & McGuire B. E. (2011). Chronic pain in the Republic of Ireland-community prevalence, psychosocial profile and predictors of pain-related disability: results from the Prevalence, Impact and Cost of Chronic Pian (PRIME) study, part 1. *Pain*, **152**, 1096–1103.

Thomson, S., Jowett, M., & Mladovsky, P (2014). Health system responses to financial pressures in Ireland: Policy options in an international context. Geneva, Switzerland: WHO.

Chapter 2.16

Israel

Elon Eisenberg and Silviu Brill

Background information

Israel sits in the Middle East bordered by Lebanon, Syria, Jordan, Saudi Arabia, and Egypt. It has a parliamentary democracy governing system, established in 1948. It has a population of 8.63 million people, with a median age of 29.7, and a life expectancy of 81.7 years (Israel Central Bureau of Statistics, 2017). The population is getting older, and is expanding. Israel's population is predominantly Jewish with minorities of Muslims, Christians, and Druze. The dominant language is Hebrew, but languages also spoken are Arabic, Russian, and English (Fig. 2.16.1).

Healthcare system

The healthcare system in Israel is based on a national health insurance law. It is universal and participation in a medical insurance plan is compulsory. All Israeli citizens must join one of four official health insurance organizations, and are entitled to basic healthcare. Israelis can increase their medical coverage and improve their options by purchasing private health insurance. The major public health issues are related to the fact that Israeli national healthcare spending per capita is relatively low and therefore Israelis cover about a quarter of their healthcare expenses out-of-pocket.

Current pain workforce

The first pain clinic in Israel was established by Prof. Mark Chayen, director of the Department Anesthesiology at Ichilov Hospital (Tel Aviv University Medical School) in 1967. At about the same time, at least two additional clinics began operating under Prof. Florella Magora at the Department of Anesthesia of the Hadassah-Hebrew University Hospital in Jerusalem, and by Prof. Jesmond Birkhan, director of the Department of Anesthesiology at Rambam Hospital (Technion Medical School) in Haifa. All three groups began to train anesthesiology residents in pain management. Consultations and treatments mainly took place in the hospital emergency rooms or operating theatres. These clinics were mainly 'block clinics'. For a number of years, pain clinics were run by these pioneer anesthesiologists. Although more professionals from additional disciplines became involved in pain management in those clinics, no substantial changes in the awareness of pain and its treatment took place so, in essence, pain remained an overlooked field in medicine in Israel for those years.

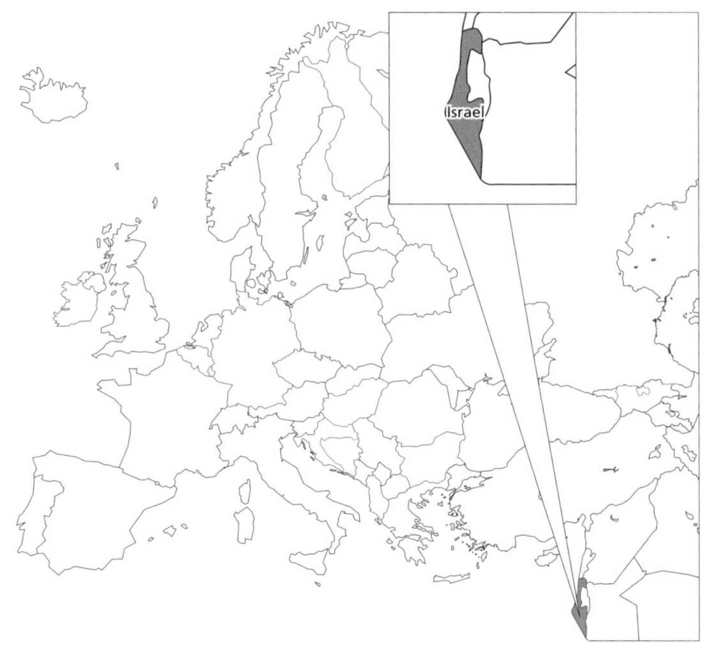

Fig. 2.16.1 Map of Israel.

Two decades later, the Israeli Pain Association (IPA) was established in 1984. The mission of the IPA is to serve all Israeli professionals interested in pain, including both physicians and non-physicians such as psychologists, nurses, physiotherapists, and investigators in the basic sciences. One of the key founders of the IPA was Prof. David Niv, who was its second president and also the third president of EFIC. Tragically Prof. Niv was murdered in 2007. Gradually, pain clinics grew in number and in the types of provided services and became more multidisciplinary in their profile. More and more caregivers and researchers from different disciplines became interested in pain, annual pain meetings of the IPA were held, and the 'voice of pain' could be heard.

However, it wasn't until 2010 that the Israeli Medical Association (IMA) officially announced that pain medicine had become a recognized medical profession in Israel.

The Israel Pain Association

The Israel Pain Association is a multidisciplinary professional organization and is the only official professional organization in the field of pain research and treatment in Israel. The IPA has been an official IASP Chapter since 1984. This was announced at the 4th IASP World Congress on Pain, held in Seattle, Washington. Nonetheless, an Israeli representative was elected in 1975 as member of the first IASP Council. The IPA has been an active EFIC member Chapter since EFIC's establishment.

The IPA has 352 members. The vast majority are physicians from different disciplines including anesthesiology, neurology, family medicine, orthopaedic surgery, neurosurgery, and more. A considerable number of nurses are IPA members, but unfortunately only a small number of other professionals are members, such as physical therapists, psychologists, basic science researchers, and so on. Fortunately, the number of researchers and research students grows steadily. The IPA executive board consists of seven members (honorary president, secretary and treasurer plus four other board members) who are elected every three years. The IPA organizes a three-day annual meeting with both local and international speakers. A semi-annual one-day meeting has been held since 2010. Several regional meetings, usually devoted to one or two selected topics, also take place every year. In collaboration with other medical societies, IPA has released several position papers on important topics such as radicular back pain, pain and kidney failure, pain in osteoarthritis, and neuropathic cancer pain. These position papers are well-read by physicians from other disciplines and most of them have been adopted by the IMA and appear on its website. Last but not least, the IPA is responsible for the pain residency programme. It is also the official consultation body for the Israeli Ministry of Health in relation to the introduction of new medicines, treatments, and technologies and including them in the Israeli 'health services basket'.

Pain residency in Israel

As mentioned earlier, the IMA announced in 2010 that pain medicine was an official medical profession in Israel. This happened only after 10 years of struggle between IPA and IMA. Briefly, IMA believed that there were too many medical professions in Israel and that additional medical specialties will further augment what they called 'fragmentation of medicine'. We in the IPA believed that pain medicine is exactly the opposite, a wide profession, just like infectious disease medicine, which leads to defragmentation of the medical profession. This argument, along with the growing need for pain specialists in the country, led eventually to the desired change.

Our pain medicine residency is open to physicians who are specialists in any clinical medical profession. The residency programme itself consists of 21 months of full-time work in an acknowledged (by the IMA and by Ministry of Health) pain clinic plus six months of obligatory rotations in anaesthesiology and neurology (three months each). All residents have to take a board examination which has a multiple choice question written part and an oral part, and is being held annually.

Thus far, we have 84 pain specialists in Israel, 28 of whom have completed the above formal training program. There are 13 residents who are at different stages of their training.

EFIC and Israel

Even though Israel is not geographically located in Europe it has had a tight relationship with EFIC. As mentioned earlier, Israel has been a member in EFIC since its foundation in 1993. Prof. David Niv was EFIC's third president between the years 1999–2002. Prof. Elon Eisenberg is currently EFIC's Honorary Treasurer. Israeli physicians and researchers (Dr Siviu Brill and Prof. Dorit Pud and Prof. Elon Eisenberg) teach in EFIC's Pain Schools. EFIC's congresses are always heavily attended by Israeli professionals. Notably, the Pain Institute at Tel Aviv Medical Center was recognized as an EFIC centre of excellence in 2014.

Challenges and opportunities to the future development of pain services

Perhaps the most challenging aspect of pain medicine in Israel is the shortage of pain clinics and long waiting times which can be as long as 3–12 months. The awareness of pain medicine and the 'right to be pain-free' has increased significantly among the population and by other caregivers, who refer many of their patients to pain specialists. The availability of pain therapy is therefore low and is not expected to change in the near future, even with the current pain residency programme. This unfortunately affects the quality of pain medicine and increases frustration and other negative feelings among both patients and caregivers.

One possible solution is in changing the structure of pain medicine in the country so that it will have three levels of care: the first level will be in the hands of primary care physicians; the second level will consist of community pain clinics; and the third, are full capacity pain clinics. The idea behind this model is that better care at the community level will dramatically reduce the demand on tertiary pain clinics and allow them to treat only patients who truly need their services (i.e. multidisciplinary therapy, complex pharmacotherapy, invasive procedures). It also takes into account the need for accessible consultations for patients with pain problems which require a somewhat deeper level of expertise than primary care physicians would normally have. This model seems to be accepted by various levels of decision-makers. Consequently, huge efforts to improve education on pain in medical schools, residencies, and among practising physicians is being made. In order to establish community pain clinics, a number of 'pain schools' have been opened to provide advanced knowledge and practice in pain medicine to interested physicians. Notably, this is not a formal residency programme for GPs. Some health maintenance organizations in Israel have already opened such clinics.

A second growing challenge in Israel is the issue of medical cannabis. The Israeli Ministry of Health approved the use of medical cannabis several years ago, primarily for pain control. Initially, only patients with cancer-related pain or chemotherapy-induced nausea were allowed to use cannabis. However, fairly quickly patients with other forms of (chronic) pain applied for its use. Thus far, about 25,000 licences to use medical cannabis have been issued by the Israeli Ministry of Health, and the vast majority are for the control of chronic pain (Israeli Medical Cannabis, 2017). Since marijuana is illegal in Israel and no national or international clinical guidelines for its medical use are available, there is a lot of confusion around this issue in the country. While some doctors see a clear advantage in adding cannabis to their analgesic armamentarium, others emphasize the potential harms associated with its use (diversion, addiction, encouraging smoking, medical side effects, and so on) and are reluctant to recommend it for their patients. This is clearly an ongoing medical, legal, and societal challenge to the country.

Innovations

- Most general hospitals in Israel have pain clinics and acute pain services. At least two hospitals are involved in the PAINOUT European project.
- Most large pain clinics in Israel are truly multidisciplinary clinics and are located in referral hospitals throughout the country.
- Pain research in Israel is fairly substantial. A Medline search using the words: 'Pain', 'Israel', and '2015' revealed 2,086 hits.
- The International Narcotic Control Board (INCB) releases data every year on opioid consumption in many countries worldwide. According to its last report, the equivalent morphine consumption in Israel in 2013 was a little over 100 mg/capita (International Narcotics Control Board, 2017). This is about one-fifth of the consumption in the United States, a quarter of what Germany is consuming, half of the Netherlands' consumption, and a little less than France. Israel therefore does not face a major opioid crisis like some Western European countries and North America.
- Nurses play a growing role in pain management in Israel. About 1,000 nurses are members in the Israeli Pain Nursing Forum, which was established in the year 2000. One of the main topics on their agenda is receiving an approval of the new role of 'Pain Specialist Nurse' in Israel.
- Teaching of pain pathophysiology and treatment is already included in the syllabus of all medical schools in Israel. Yet, more needs to be done in the area of education on pain in medical schools and in post-graduate courses.

References

International Narcotics Control Board (2017). Report of the International Narcotics Control Board for 2016, United Nations Publications, 2017. Available at: https://www.incb.org/documents/Publications/AnnualReports/AR2016/English/AR2016_E_ebook.pdf [Online].

Israel Central Bureau of Statistics (2017). Israel in figures. Available at: http://www.cbs.gov.il/reader/cw_usr_view_Folder?ID=141 [Online].

Israeli Medical Cannabis (2017). Good Clinical Practice. Jerusalem: Israeli Medical Cannabis Agency.

Chapter 2.17

Italy

Stefano Coaccioli and Antonella Paladini

Background information

Italy, or officially the Republic of Italy, sits in the Mediterranean sea and is bordered by its neighbours in Austria, France, Slovenia, and Switzerland. It has approximately 60 million people, the majority of whom speak Italian, although there are many dialects, and there are a number of other official minority languages spoken. The Italian Chapter of IASP is named Associazione Italiana per lo Studio del Dolore (AISD—Italian Association for the Study of Pain). It was established in February 1976, just a few months after the first IASP Congress, held in Firenze (September 1975). Hence it is one of the oldest IASP Chapters in the world (Fig. 2.17.1).

AISD is one of the seven IASP European Chapters that, invited by Ulf Lindblom as President of the IASP, agreed to establish the European Federation of IASP Chapters on 27 August 1993, in Paris, during the IASP Congress. The other countries were Germany, Romania, Scandinavian countries (at that time they just had one single IASP Chapter), Slovakia, Switzerland, and the United Kingdom.

AISD represents all scientists interested in the study of pain, in Italy. Its official language is Italian. It has around 1,200 members, mainly represented by the specialty of Anesthesiology (around 65%). The second most represented specialty is Neurology (20%). There are also 5–6% from Rheumatology. The rest is equally divided between Physiology, Gerontology, General Practice, and others.

Healthcare system

The Italian healthcare system experienced a profound modification at the beginning of the 1970s. The previous organization, based on mutuality providing healthcare assistance for the different professions and classes of population, was replaced by a general public assistance, managed at the regional level. This means that any of the 20 Italian regions has the possibility to provide a different quality/quantity of care, always following the general recommendations established by the national government. At the moment, all healthcare is public, with just small private hospitals providing care funded privately or by private insurance.

The Italian Agency for the Quality in Health Care (AGENAS) monitors the quality for both private (very few) and public hospitals.

The Italian Agency for Drugs (AIFA) monitors the entire pharmaceutical system, also deciding on the reimbursement for any drugs. They also have a very strict monitoring system for the use (and abuse) of drugs, via a personal microchipped card,

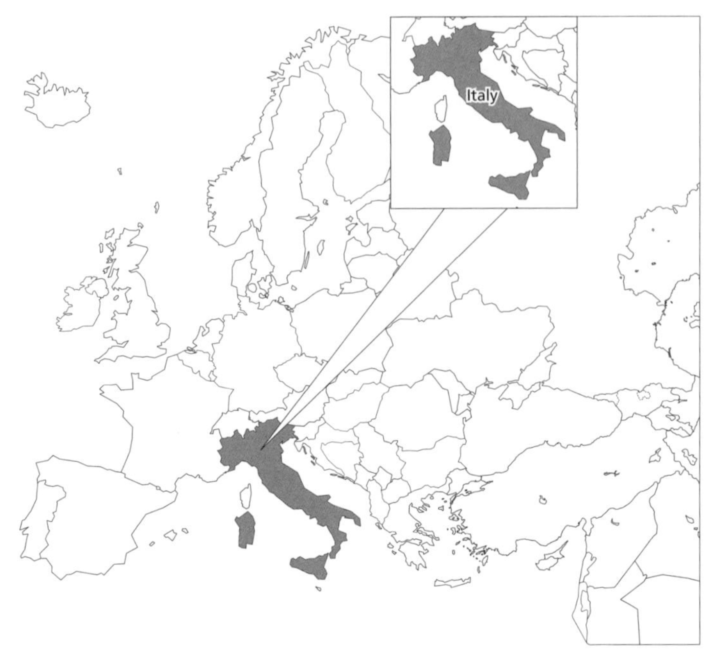

Fig. 2.17.1 Map of Italy.
Copyright © Pyty/Shutterstock.com.

which can be owned by any Italian citizen. It is impossible to obtain any drug without the registration via the microchip, even privately.

Current pain workforce

Pain medicine has a long history in Italy. It was not by chance that the first IASP Congress was organized in Firenze. In the university of that city, pain was largely studied already in the 1960s, at many levels. The most famous studies coming from that institution were on visceral pain and on headache.

Immediately after the Firenze IASP congress, the diffusion of pain management spread very rapidly, while also education on pain medicine spread quickly. As an example, in 1983 the University of Verona established a residency programme in Pain Therapy. This was in the Department of Anesthesiology, chaired by Professor Stefano Ischia. In the same year, two different Italian universities (Milano and Trieste) opened a full course on Pain Therapy, taught by two full-time professors, Mario Tiengo and Giuseppe Mocavero, respectively. The first one became president of the AISD immediately afterward. In the academic year 1985–1986, there were at least 10 Italian medical schools with a course in Pain Therapy, by choice, and not mandated. In 1989, after the reform of the Medical Schools, the course on Pain Therapy officially became mandatory for the students in their sixth year at the medical school. It means that all the students graduating in Medicine after 1995 have received some education in pain management in their undergraduate courses.

Unfortunately, with the European unification of the postgraduate education for physicians, the residency programme in Pain Therapy taught in the University of Verona was officially closed in 1999. Since then, we are still debating with the European Union of Medical Specialists (UEMS) if the medical specialty in pain medicine should exist or not.

At a clinical level, pain medicine is largely diffuse at the moment in Italy. In the 1970s and 1980s there were individual physicians interested in pain management at a number of hospitals. At the end of the 1980s there was a huge project underway to open the network of hospices for terminally ill patients. This was followed in 1999 by a first official initiative by the Ministry of Health, with a project called 'Pain-Free Hospitals'. The main aim was to spread more widely the idea of the necessity to treat pain in the hospitalized patient. Meanwhile, the network of hospices was increasing, and especially in the northern part of the country there were numerous hospices, both private and public. Since March 2010, following a law aimed to protect the rights of the pain patients; the national healthcare system has three different national networks: one for the pain patients (organized as a hub-spoke system); one for palliative care; and one for the paediatric palliative cares.

The first one, the most important for our purposes, has been largely implemented, and is almost complete in the majority of regions in the country.

Challenges and opportunities to the future development of pain services

From a public health perspective, chronic pain has a major impact on a person's physical and mental capacity to function in everyday life, their quality of daily life, and on the economic balance sheet of the population. Therefore, in Italy we must consider why chronic pain is not sufficiently recognized as an important public health problem. From a population perspective, pain—especially chronic pain—is a major public health problem and a clear priority for planning and problem-solving. Once again it seems more helpful to consider chronic pain as a disease in its own right.

Defining chronic pain as a public health problems represents, in Italy, the organized response by society and the public health system to protect and promote health, to prevent illness and disability, and to pass from the concept of 'cure' of pain towards a real 'taking care' of patients suffering from acute as well as chronic pain.

Innovations

All effort must be raised in order to increase as well as ameliorate a huge number of issues, including for example:

- increasing knowledge of pain (and about chronic pain, in particular);
- teaching of pain medicine in the academic courses;
- increasing the prevention strategies of chronic pain in the population, supported by epidemiological studies;
- standardizing and spreading a national hub-spoke system;

- establishing and maintaining update and refresher courses in pain medicine for general practitioners;
- ensuring constant contact and cooperation with the authorities involved in the field;
- and, finally, the complete implementation of the two Italian laws about the '*Hospital and Territory Without Pain*' (promulgated in 1999) and the '*Access to Pain Therapy and Palliative Cure*' (promulgated in 2010).

Chapter 2.18

Kosovo

Adem Bytyqi, Agron Bytyqi, and Bashkim Sylaj

Background information

Kosovo has an area of 10,887 square kilometres. It is bordered by the Republic of Albania to the south, Montenegro to the west, and the uncontested territory of Serbia to the north and east (Fig. 2.18.1). Its capital and largest city is Pristina. Based on data from the Kosovo Agency of Statistics (2016), the total population of Kosovo is 1,804,944. According to this agency, the ethnic mix of Kosovo is largely Albanian at 92%, Serbs 4%, Bosnians and Gorans 2%, Turks 1%, and Roma 1%. The average age of the population in Kosovo is 29.5 years. The official languages are Albanian and Serbian, and recognized regional languages are Bosnian, Turkish, Gorani, and Romani (Kosovo Agency of Statistics, 2016).

The Professional Health Association (PHA) is one of the largest professional associations for the multidisciplinary treatment of pain in Kosovo. This association in itself includes various health professionals who are actively involved in the diagnosis and treatment of pain. The PHA was registered in the Ministry of Public Service of the Republic of Kosovo on 20 January 2009. The president of the PHA is Adem Bytyqi MD, the vice-president is Fadil Kryeziu, MD, PhD, the secretary is Agron Bytyqi, MSc, and the treasurer is Bashkim Sylaj, MSc. The executive committee has 17 members. Its central office is located in Prizren, the second largest city in Kosovo, but operates all over the country.

During the EFIC Council meeting on 29 May 2012 at the Bella Sky Hotel and Conference Centre, Copenhagen, the Kosovo Chapter (PHA) was accepted as a new EFIC Chapter. There are 85 members in the Chapter from different specialties like anaesthesiology, neurology, orthopaedics, surgery, cardiology, public health, family medicine, and nursing.

Healthcare system

The healthcare system in Kosovo is organized in three sectors including primary, secondary, and tertiary healthcare. Primary healthcare is organized in family medicine centres and ambulatory care units. Secondary healthcare is decentralized in seven general hospitals, although Prishtina itself does not have any hospitals and instead uses the University Clinical Centre of Kosovo for healthcare services. The University Clinical Centre of Kosovo provides its healthcare services in 12 clinics, where 642 doctors are employed. At all three levels in public institutions (as of 2014) there are 19,100 employees, while at the primary level there are 5,420 employees, of which 1,068 are

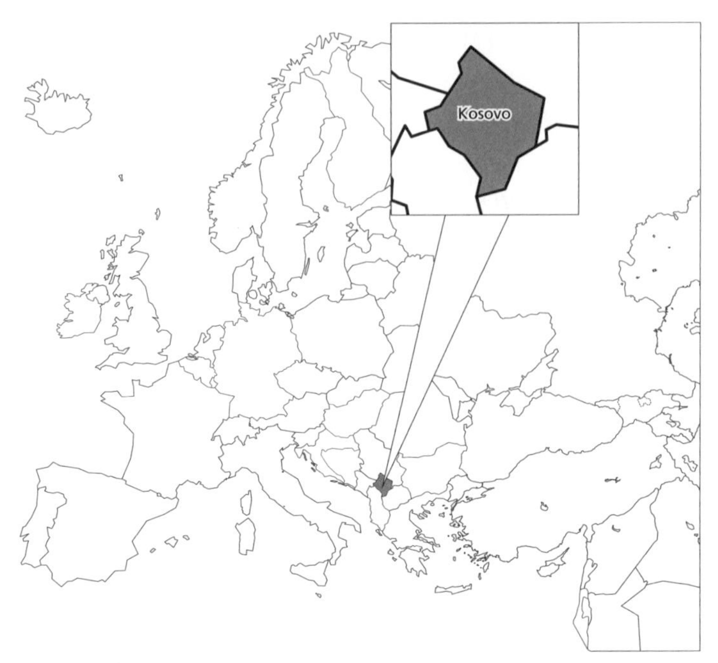

Fig. 2.18.1 Map of Kosovo.

doctors, 285 dentists, 3,151 nurses, and 916 are other workers. The second and tertiary level is organized in the Hospital and University Clinical Service of Kosovo (HUCSK) where in total there are 13,680 workers, of which 5,560 have a higher education, 7,392 have an upper secondary education, and 728 are non-professional associates (Kosovo Agency of Statistics, 2015).

At a lower level, home services are provided for several vulnerable groups which are not able to access healthcare premises. Kosovo healthcare services are now focused on patient safety, quality control, and assisted health. At present, healthcare institutions are going through some profound reforms that focus on providing decentralized services and covering all community residents by health insurance packages. The total healthcare budget (last noted in 2014) was €85,917,619,92 and donations added a further €4 million. The number of licensed private health institutions is now 1,069, and 305, or 28.5% of the licensed institutions are local dental practices. The Ministry of Health in Kosovo is responsible for planning and monitoring the delivery of services. Agencies that are involved in planning and delivery of healthcare services are WHO, UNICEF, UNFPA, USAID, and so on.

Current pain workforce

In our country there are no specialists for pain management, but other specialists, mostly anesthesiologists, deliver pain management. In Kosovo there is no centre or institutions that deal with pain management.

The PHA is keen to increase awareness of pain and pain management, and to deliver training where possible. It has organized and held five international conferences and five workshops about pain management. It has also delivered specific courses on cancer pain management and on neuropathic pain. As part of the countrywide 'train the trainer' initiative, we have also delivered pain education for primary healthcare professionals. During 2014–2015, the team at the Prizren hospital undertook a research project aimed at improving the practice of postoperative pain management in surgery and gynaecology. In collaboration with a non-professional high school, the department of nursing has introduced a module on 'Pain and Its Management'.

Challenges and opportunities to the future development of pain services

For the future development of pain services, there are some challenges and opportunities. The first challenge is for the allocation of a pain subspecialization or specialization for pain specialists by the specializations committee in the Ministry of Health. Another challenge for our country is the establishment of psychological services for patients with pain, and a public centre for the diagnosis and treatment of chronic pain.

There are also opportunities to improve general knowledge and skills about pain by teaching 'Pain and its Management' in schools of medicine and in the University of Prishtina, Faculty of Medicine (general medicine, dentistry, pharmacy, and nursing). There is also a good opportunity to have better information about pain management in the establishment of an informative and scientific journal for health professionals, a journal which can address topics on the management of acute and chronic pain.

Although the treatment of pain is a basic human right, to us with a Balkan mentality, there is a tradition that one should endure pain and that this is normal. If you are young, 'you must endure pain', and if you are older, 'you must expect pain', If you are operated on 'it is normal to have pain', if you are injured 'it doesn't matter it will pass'. While pregnant 'you know maybe what do you expect'. While there are people who complain of pain throughout the body, 'it happens at this time of life'. Challenging this dominant view of pain as acceptably untreated is a major challenge, not only for the PHA, but for Kosovo as a nation.

Innovations

There is much to be proud of in Kosovo. There have been many activities such as national and international conferences, courses, workshops, and various meetings with local and international experts, all of which have positively influenced the approach to pain management in Kosovo. A major change has been in the shift from viewing pain as always a symptom explained by a disorder, to understanding the unique causes of pain. In assessment, we have shifted from using pain as a symptom, to documenting the whole pain experience itself. Through organized courses, the assessment of pain was improved by making use of both objective and subjective data, using documentation in several places such as on the ward, and using that assessment to guide treatment. Through briefings from other conferences and meetings, we have been successful in sharing the idea of the need to assess postoperative acute pain as the fifth vital sign.

Methods of pain treatment are constantly being discussed, and there is now growing interest in expanding the treatment choices available to clinicians and patients, including conservative and interventional methods, increasing the number of drugs available for pain in Kosovo, and exploring non-drug-based and non-surgical interventions.

References

Kosovo Agency of Statistics (2015). General Statistics, Kosovo in Figures, pp. 33–43. Available at: http://ask.rks-gov.net/media/2362/kosova_shifra-2015-ang.pdf [Online].

Kosovo Agency of Statistics (2016). Women and Men in Kosovo 2014–2015. Published in Prishtina, December 2016. Available at: http://ask.rks-gov.net/media/2582/women-and-men-ang-2014-2015.pdf, Professional Health Association, 2017; and http://www.pha-ks.com/en/about_us/about_us [Online].

Chapter 2.19

Latvia

Iveta Golubovska, Mihails Arons,
Aleksejs Miscuks, and Inara Logina

Background information

The Republic of Latvia (short form Latvia) is one of the Baltic countries and a European Union Member State from 2004. Latvia is situated by the Baltic Sea between Estonia and Lithuania. The total land area is 64,589 square kilometres. The population was 1.989 million as of 2014 (Central Statistical Bureau of Latvia, 2014). Approximately 60% of the population are Latvians. The official language is Latvian. The political system of the state is a parliamentary democracy. The capital of Latvia is Riga, with the population of 1.15 million in the metropolitan area. The state currency is the Euro (see Fig. 2.19.1).

The Latvian Association for the Study of Pain (LASP) was founded in 1995 under the name of the Latvian Association for the Study and Treatment of Pain. The founder was a neurologist, Professor Juris Berzins. There were 44 members in the association at its founding moment. From 2004, LASP has been associated with EFIC and IASP. In 2005, the association was reorganized and given a new name. The current membership is 116 people, 58 of whom are certified pain specialists, named algologists.

The members of LASP include professionals from various disciplines. The majority or 49 are neurologists. There are also 21 anaesthesiologists, 13 internists, 10 physical and rehabilitation medicine doctors, 6 oncologists, 3 neurosurgeons, 2 psychotherapists, 2 psychiatrists, 2 surgeons, 1 orthopaedic surgeon, and 1 public health expert.

The following guidelines have been prepared with the participation and on the initiative of the association: *Neuropathic Pain, Headache, Back Pain, Rational Pharmacotherapy of Reimbursable Medicine System for Cancer Patients, Rational Pharmacotherapy of Neuropathic Pain and Low Back Pain in Primary Care*, and so on. Books on pain mechanisms and certain types of pain and diseases have also been issued. The Medical Publishing House also issued Professor Inara Logina's book titled *Pain* in 2013.

Healthcare system

The healthcare system is run by the Ministry of Health of the Republic of Latvia. The Ministry of Health in its current form was established in 2003, and it is responsible for the health sector and public healthcare and its funding. The Ministry develops the

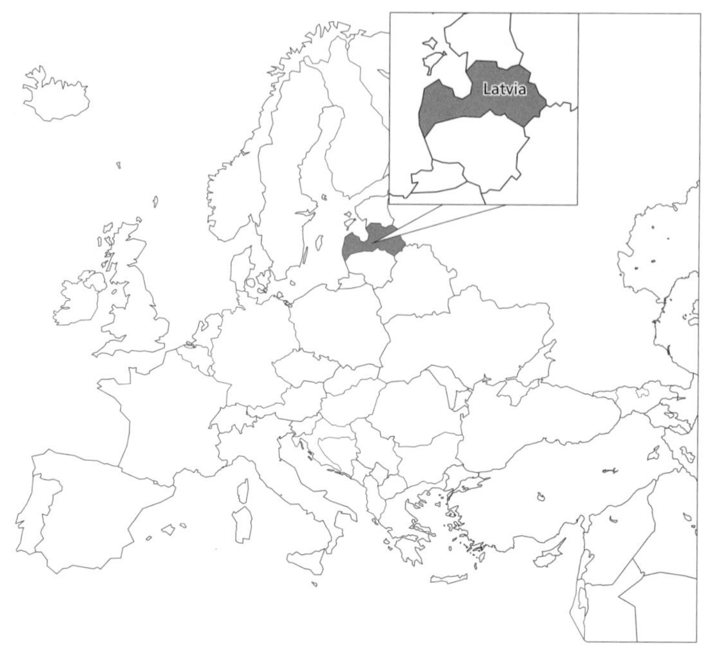

Fig. 2.19.1 Map of Latvia.

national health policy as well as organizes, coordinates, and monitors its implementation; drafts regulations and planning documents; evaluates projects developed by other institutions; represents state interests in international institutions; informs the society about health policies and about the work of other healthcare institutions; and develops and defends national positions in the area of healthcare in the European Union.

The healthcare system in Latvia is based on the residence principle. Its funding consists of governmental subsidies, patient fees, and co-payments, and voluntary insurance. The public funding is a negative list of benefits: the state pays for all services, except those that are excluded from the scope (the latter is a majority). The healthcare benefits are available at the state, municipal, and some private inpatient and outpatient healthcare institutions. Patients should pay a co-payment to receive medical services. The following services are provided as part of the state budget and patients' own co-payment system: healthcare provided by general practitioners and their staff; healthcare provided by specialist doctors in chronological order based on a waiting list; laboratory tests and medical investigations with a family physician's or specialist doctor's referral; outpatient healthcare; some types of home care; emergency medicine; care at a hospital after an acute treatment phase at an emergency care unit, as well as in cases of exacerbation of chronic diseases; rehabilitation after the hospital treatment; and selected types of reimbursed drugs and medical devices. The primary healthcare is provided by a primary healthcare doctor, assisted by a nurse and/or doctor's assistant.

The Ministry of Health has several subordinate institutions, including the National Health Service (NHS), the Centre of Disease Prevention and Control, the Health Inspectorate, the State Emergency Service, the State Agency of Medicines, the National Medical Service, the State Centre for Forensic Medical Examination, the Latvian Sports Medicine State Agency, Pauls Stradins Museum of the History of Medicine, and Riga Stradins University.

The NHS is the acting direct administrative institution subordinate to the Ministry of Health. It was established in 2011. The main tasks of the NHS are to implement the state policy for the availability of healthcare services; to manage the state budgetary funds earmarked for healthcare; to implement the state policy in the planning of healthcare services; to ensure the most rational and effective use of state budget for healthcare; and to implement the e-health programme.

The scope of activities and functions of NHS are to supervise the expenditures of NHS-managed budgetary funds in medical institutions and pharmacies; to analyse the financial and quantity indices of healthcare services; to inform the society about healthcare services and the procedures to receive them, as well as to consult the country's residents on their rights while receiving healthcare services; and to organize and carry out public procurements of medicinal products and medical equipment. The NHS also calculates service tariffs, develops, maintains, and updates the list of reimbursed drugs; determines the types of healthcare services funded from the state budget; approves and registers medical technologies, develops and evaluates clinical guidelines; develops guidelines for rational pharmacotherapy; manages the Medical Treatment Risk Fund; and implements the e-health programme in accordance with the state policy.

Current pain workforce

For qualified care and treatment of patients with pain, it is not enough just to have internists and other specialists with good knowledge. It is extremely important to prepare highly qualified pain specialists. The Cabinet Order No. 251 of 2003 approved the regulations for the specialty of algology, which was included as an additional specialty with code PP16 on the list of medical treatment professions in the Classification of Professions. In order to acquire an additional specialty, a two-year long postgraduate specialization is required. An algologist or pain specialist should be familiar with pain anatomy and physiology, chronification mechanisms, and treatment methods. In 2015, a one-year residency programme for pain specialist education was founded at the Riga Stradins University. The specialties qualified for this postgraduate programme are: neurologist, family physician, orthopaedic surgeon, physiotherapist, anaesthesiologist, neurosurgeon, oncologist, surgeon, and others.

Challenges and opportunities for the future development of pain services

Considering pain epidemiology in the Latvian population in recent years, pain in different body areas is the main complaint among the Latvian adult population.

According to research, 46.5% of females reported headache occurring during last month. The percentage was even higher among females in the age group of 25–34 years (i.e. 52.3%). Backache is widespread in all populations: in 31% of males and 33.5% of females; 20.8% of female and 16.1% of male patients noted joint pain; and 22.1% of females and 14.4% of males experienced pain in the cervical and thoracic spine. Overall, 25.7% of respondents had been using medications for different kinds of pain (27.5% of females and 23.9% of males) (Pudule *et al.*, 2013).

We know that, compared with other European Union Member States, a high proportion of the Latvian working population report having regular backache or muscular pain (Giaccone, 2007). Up to 64% of the general population report that their health is affected by musculoskeletal conditions. Spondylosis and radiculopathy were the top occupational diagnosis at a rate of 92.1 per 100,000 employees in 2009, compared to 60.8 in 2008. The Fourth European Survey on Working Conditions (Parent-Thirion *et al.*, 2007) shows that over 44% of the Latvian working population report work-related back pain. Country-specific studies also suggest an increase in the number of individuals with backache symptoms: the FINBALT Health Monitor reported 42.4% of employees having back pain complaints in 2008 compared to 35% in 2004 (Pudule *et al.*, 2010). This increase can be partially explained with employers' increased awareness of the need to monitor the health of their employees. According to the Fourth European Survey on Working Conditions (Parent-Thirion *et al.*, 2007), up to 36% of the Latvian working population report that they have experienced muscular pain in their neck, shoulders, and upper limbs.

Tracking the changes in complaints in the child and adolescent populations from 1994 to 2010, one can see significant changes in the chronic pain statistics. The number of teenagers who complain about having backache in the last sixth months had increased from 8.3% in 1994 to 20.3% in 2010. Overall, females in these populations have higher pain prevalence compared to males, whereas chronic back pain tripled among males and doubled among females in the period of 1994–2010 (Pudule *et al.*, 2012).

The list of benefits partially includes only primary consultations by pain specialists, but not any invasive manipulations. Most of the clinical guidelines and medical technologies are approved and included in the register of NHS: from the methods of investigation and examination, to treatment and follow-up. Foraminal and translaminar epidural blockades, radiofrequency procedures, intrathecal drug delivery for the treatment of pain and spasticity, spinal cord stimulation—all of these are included in the register. Yet, in the circumstances of insufficient funding, they are not covered by the state and are only partially covered by private insurance companies. In the situation of insufficient funding, interventional pain management manipulations are not funded by the state, while private insurance companies cover, or partly cover only cheapest technologies and do not cover the costs associated with such manipulations as spinal cord stimulation or first-time implantation of an intrathecal drug pump.

The major challenge for pain management service in Latvia is to reduce morbidity associated with acute pain and chronic pain conditions in the Latvian population. This could be facilitated by establishing a multidisciplinary unit under one roof, partially funded by the state and investments and partially covered by patient co-payments. The functions of such a multidisciplinary centre could be to publish information leaflets, to arrange public lectures and activities in public media, to organize primary consultations of different medical specialists—such as neurologists, orthopaedic surgeons, and pain specialists, who could provide conservative and invasive treatment (i.e. prescribe medications and perform invasive manipulations if necessary). A primary consultant could refer patients to a physiotherapist or a rehabilitation specialist, or, optionally and if necessary, to a psychotherapist. The consultant could also organize individual and group physiotherapy exercise workouts.

Presently, the main establishments of pain patient care consist of separate pain units in hospitals, medical centres, and clinics. To establish a multidisciplinary pain centre or clinic in Latvia is not an easy task. At the same time, several pain management units are already working with success. Stradins University Hospital Pain Service, headed by Dr M. Malina from the very beginning, has been successfully operating since 2006. Multidisciplinary pain management consilia are organized in difficult cases. One of the main goals of the Association for the Study of Pain is to attract state funding for neuromodulation and radiofrequency procedures.

Innovations

One of the most recent developments related to the provision of care and training is a 44-week postgraduate education programme to prepare pain specialists. The programme is available for the graduates of certain medical specialties, so that they could acquire an additional specialty by state funds. The first two residents graduated in 2016. The Undegraduate Core Curriculum were developed and two compulsary and two optional programmes of pain medicine have been implemented in Riga Stradin's university.

The acquisition of innovative state-of-the-art technology will facilitate pain research as the University of Latvia has procured equipment for remote monitoring of pain sensation by humans. The technology is based on a real-time analysis of thermal images and photoplethysmography data obtained from human skin and visualization of these data directly on the skin surface using a real-time projection mapping technique. This technology can be used for the assessment of dysfunction of body surface innervation in patients with localized or diffuse pain (Marcinkevics *et al.*, 2016).

References

Central Statistical Bureau of Latvia, Statistics Database (2014). Available at: http://www.csb.gov.lv/en/dati/statistics-database-30501.html [Online].

Giaccone, M. (2007). *Managing Musculoskeletal Disorders.* European Foundation for the Improvement of Living and Working Conditions, pp. 39–44. Available at: http://www.eurofound.europa.eu [Online].

Marcinkevics, Z., Rubins, U., Zaharans, J., Miscuks, A., Urtane, E., & Ozolina, L. (2016). Imaging photoplethysmography for clinical assessment of cutaneous microcirculation at two different depths. *J Biomed Optics*, **21**, 1–12.

Parent-Thirion, A., Fernández Macías, E., Hurley, J., & Vermeylen, G. (2007). *Fourth European Survey on Working Conditions*, pp. 61–6. Dublin, Ireland: European Foundation for the Improvement of Living Standards.

Pudele, I., Velika, B., Grinberga, D., Gobina, I., & Villerusa, A.. (2012). *Latvian Student Health Habit Research, Year 2009/2010. Survey Results and Trends*, p. 11. Riga, Latvia: Centre of Disease Prevention and Control.

Pudule, I., Villerusa, A., & Griberga, D. (2010). *Health Behaviour among Latvian Adult Population*, p. 9. Riga, Latvia: Health Economics Centre.

Pudule, I., Grinberga, D., Velika, B., Gavare, I, & Villerusa, A. (2013). *Health Behaviour among Latvian Adult Population*, p. 12. Riga, Latvia: Centre of Disease Prevention and Control.

Chapter 2.20

Lithuania

Arunas Sciupokas

Background information

The Republic of Lithuania is a country in Northern Europe, situated along the south-eastern shore of the Baltic Sea, bordered by Latvia to the north, Belarus to the east and south, Poland to the south, and Kaliningrad Oblast (a Russian exclave) to the southwest (Fig. 2.20.1).

Lithuania has an estimated population of 2,849,317 people (2015), 84% of whom are ethnic Lithuanians. Several sizeable minorities exist, such as Poles (6.6%), Russians (5.8%), Belarusians (1.2%), and Ukrainians (0.5%). The official language is Lithuanian, which along with Latvian, are the only two living languages in the Baltic branch of the Indo-European language family. Lithuania has been a member of both the European Union and NATO since 2004. The capital of Lithuania, and largest city, is Vilnius (542,990 in 2015) (Statistics Lithuania, 2017).

Lithuania has been a Chapter of the International Association for the Study of Pain (IASP) since 1995, and became a member of EFIC since 1996. The Lithuanian Pain Society was founded at its first congress in 1998, and is successor became the Lithuanian chapter of IASP and EFIC.

The membership of society is 64 people (2016) including physicians, nurses, physiotherapists, psychologists, pharmacologists, with core specialties of anesthesiology (13) and neurology (14).

Healthcare system

The Lithuanian health system is a mixed system, predominantly funded from the National Health Insurance Fund through a compulsory health insurance scheme supplemented by state budget contributions. Public financing of the health sector has gradually increased to 6.6% of GDP in 2011. The state healthcare system is intended to serve the entire population, and the Health Insurance Law requires all permanent residents and legally employed non-permanent residents to participate in the compulsory health insurance scheme (typically paying 6–9% of taxable income), without an option to opt-out. Compulsory health insurance provides a standard benefits package for all beneficiaries. Emergency care is provided free of charge to all permanent residents irrespective of their insurance status. For pharmaceuticals, drugs prescribed by a physician are reimbursed for certain groups of the population (e.g. children, pensioners,

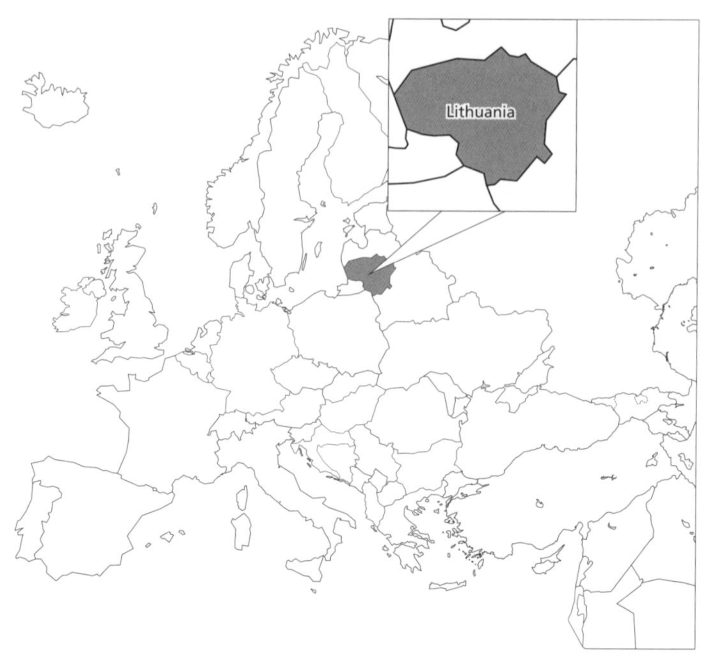

Fig. 2.20.1 Map of Lithuania.
Copyright © Pyty/Shutterstock.com.

the disabled) as well as for patients suffering from certain diseases but not for pain. All other insured adults must pay the full cost of both prescribed and over-the-counter drugs out of pocket. Primary care is financed predominantly through capitation, outpatient care is financed mainly through case payment, and through fee-for-service for diagnostic tests. Inpatient care is financed mainly through case payment. More than 70% of out-of-pocket (OOP) payments are for pharmaceuticals.

Primary care is delivered by a general practitioner (GP) or a primary care team having the GP gatekeeping function. Emergency care is commonly provided by GPs during working hours. Alternatively, or during out-of-hours for GP service, it is provided by the emergency departments of hospitals. Specialist outpatient care in Lithuania is delivered through the outpatient departments of hospitals or polyclinics as separate legal entities, as well as through private providers. Day care, day surgery, and outpatient rehabilitation services have been significantly developed.

The health system management authorities are governance institutions (the government, ministries, and municipalities, as well as other specialist governance and control bodies), providers of healthcare services, and health system resources and services. The Ministry of Health has been a major player in health system regulation through setting standards and requirements, licensing, and approving capital investments. Municipalities became responsible for organizing the provision of primary and social care, and for public health activities at the local level. Privatization of the health sector has been limited, particularly in inpatient care.

The vast majority of healthcare providers are not budgetary institutions but public non-profit-making enterprises. Healthcare institutions and professionals are mainly concerned with meeting the minimum requirements (e.g. the minimum number of hours of professional training for retaining their licence). Obligatory licensing of healthcare professionals has four major categories: physicians, nurses, dentists, and pharmacists. The State Health Care Accreditation Agency licences and registers healthcare professionals. At present, citizens have a formal choice of primary and secondary care providers, while their actual opportunities to choose depend on the availability of providers. There are seven day care units located in big towns: county centres providing pain management services. Those services are mainly patient consultations and invasive treatment procedures. Such an order is specified by the Decree of the Ministry of Health (2003).

Current pain workforce

There are no physicians currently licensed for pain management in Lithuania, and pain management services are provided mainly by anesthesiologists working together with intensive care nurses. Thus, there is no Pain Management specialty on the list issued by the State Health Care Accreditation Agency. A team approach for pain services does not exist. The total number of anesthesiologists currently working in pain management services is 9–10.

Meanwhile, the national survey for chronic pain (Sciupokas, 2009) performed by the similar methodology as the EFIC survey (see Chapter 1.2 'Epidemiology of pain: Its importance for clinical management and research') found that the prevalence of chronic pain in Lithuania is 20.98% among adults. The most common chronic pains are musculoskeletal, joint pain (34%), and low back pain (34%).

Challenges and opportunities to the future development of pain services

The Lithuanian Pain Society regularly organizes annual meetings with the participation of invited speakers from abroad. The last annual meeting (the 14th) was held in 2015. The society also organizes one or two conferences a year, and one of them is always related to the topic of the Global Year Against Pain. During the period 2001–2010, the society was organizing regularly in October the 'Week Against Pain' campaign for the general public, which was devoted to the movement 'Europe Against Pain', as established by the European Pain Federation (EFIC).

Since 1996, the Society always has representatives at the European and World Pain congresses to present its achievements in the field of pain medicine. The Lithuanian Pain Society has received international grants: (i) from IASP, for the project 'The development of palliative care and pain medicine in the Baltic countries' (2001); (ii) from EFIC, for the project 'The fifth vital sign is discovering Lithuania' (2006). The Society has organized a Baltic course on neuropathic pain (2014), and was the main organizer of the 6th International Symposium 'Pain in the Baltics 2017' has been held in Kaunas, April 2017. The Lithuanian Pain Society publishes its magazine 'Skausmo medicina' (Pain medicine), which since 2002 has regular issues twice a year. The bulletin '*Skausmo naujienos*' (*Pain updates*) was issued quarterly and published during 1999–2009.

Innovations

In the last 18 years of the Lithuanian Pain Society, there have been many attempts to achieve recognition of pain medicine as subspecialty and thus to develop pain services. At the beginning, our efforts met with support from health politicians and produced results. During 2002–2005, the Ministry of Health (MOH) issued some important decrees related to pain services: (i) endorsement of the EFIC declaration of chronic pain as a disease in its own right; (ii) day care units as pain service institutions to perform invasive procedures; (iii) a decree on emergency care with clinical cases including severe pain as an emergency case to be treated immediately; (iv) a decree on opioid analgesics and psychotropic medications use with rules for prescriptions. Seven pain clinics as day care units have started their activities following MOH decrees.

However, there has been no further development since that time. Therefore, the major challenges facing the development of pain medicine in Lithuania remain and are as follows:

1. Establishment of a postgraduate medicine introductory course on pain medicine for all specialty doctors, to be completed at the medical schools of universities;
2. Inclusion of pain medicine into the list of special healthcare services and approval by State Health Care Accreditation Agency of licensing regulations for doctors;
3. Issuance of a decree on pain medicine services, including a multidisciplinary team approach to pain management.

References

Decree of the Ministry of Health (2003). Decree Order 1032250ISAK000V-430, 11 July 2003, enacted by Ministry of Health Republic of Lithuania. Available at: https://www.e-tar.lt/portal/en/legalAct/TAR.FC1A3CCB6E15 (accessed 8 May 2017) [Online].

Sciupokas, A. (2009). National survey of chronic pain patients. *Skausmo Medicina*, **1**, 40–1 (in Lithuanian).

Statistics Lithuania (2017). Official Statistics Portal Population and Social Statistics, Resident population at the beginning of the month. Available at: https://osp.stat.gov.lt/ [Online].

Chapter 2.21

Moldova

Adrian Belîi

Background information

The Republic of Moldova is a parliamentary republic, situated in the southeastern part of Europe. It borders with Romania to the west and the Ukraine to the north, east, and south (Fig. 2.21.1). The Republic of Moldova has an area of 33,843 square kilometres and a population of 2,998,235. Administratively, it is divided into 32 regions, five municipalities, and two regions with special status. The Transnistria region (4,163 sq. km, 500,000 population) is currently under Russian army occupation. Out of the total population, 10.9% are older than 65 years old, and 23.3% are younger than 20. The ethnic structure of the country is the following: Moldovans (Romanians) (82.0%), Ukrainians (6.6%), Russians (4.1%), Gagauz (4.6%), Bulgarians (1.9%), other (0.8%) (National Bureau of Statistics of the Republic of Moldova, 2014, n.d.). Spoken languages are: Romanian (the official language of the state) and Russian. The birth rate is 9.8–11.8%, and mortality rate is 11.0%. Cardiovascular diseases are responsible for 57.5% of deaths; tumours cause 14.5% of deaths; diseases of the digestive system cause 9.1% of deaths; accidents, intoxications, and trauma 7.8%; and diseases of the respiratory system cause 4.8% of deaths. Life expectancy in Moldova is 70.97 years, 67.1 years for men and 75.0 years for women. The average life expectancy of people from urban areas is 73.55 years, which is 4.05 years more compared to rural areas (National Bureau of Statistics of the Republic of Moldova). For the past 24 years, the state has faced an imposing emigration (370,000 people—official data; 800,000—unofficial data), caused by the low quality of life, and by corruption. Remittances constitute 37% of the GDP. The average monthly salary is €241.5 (2015 figures).

Healthcare system

The healthcare system in the Republic of Moldova has started by the Semashko model that consisted of total state control. The Bismarck model was adopted after the reform of the medical system. In 2004, the system of Mandatory Medical Insurance was introduced (managed by the National House of Medical Insurance), based on mandatory contributions of employees (4.5% of the income) and employers (4.5% as well). People who do not have a place of work must buy the mandatory insurance card (4,056 MDL, approx. €185); if the card is bought before 31 March, a 50–75% discount if offered.

From 1998 to 2009, the number of hospitals was reduced from 276 (42,000 beds) to 82 hospitals (20,500 beds). In 2010, the healthcare system consisted of 34 regional hospitals, 10 municipal hospitals (in Chisinau and Balti), 18 republican hospitals, and

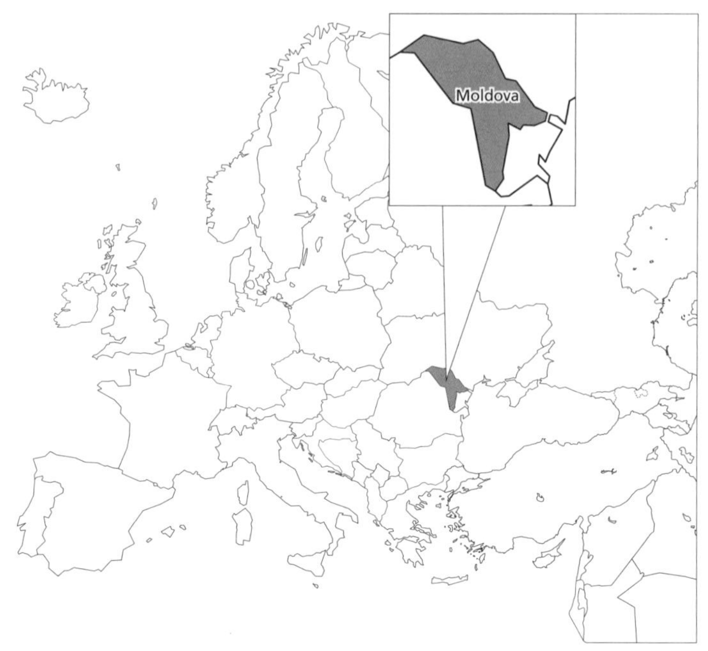

Fig. 2.21.1 Map of Moldova.

10 private hospitals. Other parallel health services continue to exist and are organized by other ministries—Ministry of Defence, Ministry of Internal Affairs, Ministry of Justice, Ministry of Transportation, and Border Police—including 10 hospitals in total and 91 ambulatory institutions. Bed provision for the population is 5.6 per 1,000 residents. Over 50% of hospitals (10 republican hospitals, 9 municipal hospitals, 8 departmental hospitals, and 8 private hospitals) with a capacity of 9,369 beds (46.8% of the total number of beds) are situated in Chisinau (National Bureau of Statistics of the Republic of Moldova).

The network of primary medical assistance consists of four types of providers: family doctors' centres (former policlinics); rural health centres; family doctors' offices (former rural medical points); and medical units for family doctors' assistants, that cover villages/regions with a population less than 1,000.

Emergency medical assistance is coordinated by the Institute of Urgent Medicine and is divided into five autonomous zones: Chisinau, central zone, north zone, south zone, and Autonomous Region Gagauzia. Besides four zonal stations of urgent medicine, there are 41 substations and 84 units of urgent medical assistance.

Current pain workforce

No statistics regarding pain epidemiology in the Republic of Moldova are available. Roughly, the prevalence of pain in the population can be estimated based on official public statistics for certain categories of diseases/patients, associated with the highest rates of pain. All statistical data refer to 2014. During 2014, in Moldova, 8,860 new cases of malignant tumours were registered (249 cases in 100,000 inhabitants), 48,764 patients have or had an oncological pathology (1,371 cases in 100,000 inhabitants). Around 105,600 patients suffered from traumas of different severity (29.7 cases in 100,000 inhabitants). Each year, over 150,000 surgeries are performed in the Republic of Moldova that require anaesthesiologic assistance. In 2014, 44,500 deliveries were registered. There are 182,500 patients with central nervous system (CNS) diseases; out of them, 72,000 were diagnosed in 2014. During the same period of time, six diagnoses of AIDS were made and 64 new cases of HIV were identified (National Bureau of Statistics of the Republic of Moldova). It is likely that the real number is higher.

Unfortunately, in the Republic of Moldova, there is no specialization or competence in the evaluation and of treatment of acute and chronic pain. Also there is no specialized organization regarding this matter. Traditionally, acute intense pain is treated by anesthesiologists (especially in big hospitals); migraines and neuropathic pain are treated by neurologists based on the usual theory and practice of their specialty. In 2014, in the Republic of Moldova there were 411 neurologists and 450 anesthesiologists (including residents). An intense Western migration of anesthesiologists is noted, the deficit being 70 doctors. Competence in pain treatment, in most of the cases, is autodidactic and acquired in courses and short traineeships abroad. It was possible to create an optional course of Evaluation and Treatment of Pain (5 days, 35 didactical hours) for the students in the fifth year of the Medicine Faculty of the Nicolae Testemitanu State Medical University of Medicine and Pharmacy.

Starting in autumn 2016, a new course of palliative medicine will be taught, and will be adapted and delivered to students, residents in family medicine, family doctors who pass courses of Continuous Medical Education, and administrators of medical institutions. Members of the Moldovan Society for the Study and Management of Pain contribute substantially in elaborating the curriculum and writing the manual for this course. In conclusion, the existing workforce is sufficient to offer qualified medical assistance regarding chronic pain only for 10% of the patients.

Challenges and opportunities to the future development of pain services

Education in the field of pain

Education is one of the biggest challenges in the field of evaluation and treatment of pain in the Republic of Moldova, because the medical folklore, personal beliefs, and myths are deeply buried in individual and social conscience.

The most frequent myths regarding pain related by population are:

- my doctor wants me to stop complaining;
- I don't want to be stung for the cost, I would rather endure the pain;
- pain relief will blur the eventual important symptoms;
- talking about pain will distract the doctor's attention from other symptoms;
- surgery means pain, I have to resign;

- pain during labour is given by God, analgesia during childbirth is dangerous both for the mother and child;
- the doctor knows better how painful it is and how much painkiller to prescribe;
- opioids cause dependency, it's better to suffer.

Many of the myths mentioned above are supported by the medical community.

A theoretical and practical knowledge deficit in the domain of pain is characteristic for countries in transition. For example, only two students of year 5 of the Faculty of Medicine (out of 150 students tested) could report the correct definition of pain according to IASP; only one patient out of five is treated according to the World Health Organization (WHO) Pain Ladder; only each third patient is prescribed a correct analgesic regimen.

Another thing that causes the knowledge deficit is the level of the medical personnel—empirical treatment, non-documented results, and resistance to new discoveries in the domain. Domestic studies have revealed that 72% of patients are not satisfied by the pain treatment in hospitals. One-third of patients took available analgesics as self-medication to calm postoperative pain, besides the medication prescribed by the doctor. Almost 80% of the respondents saluted the idea of an information point in the hospital regarding pain. More than two-thirds of patients suffered intense or unbearable pain during their hospital stay. In every hospital, each doctor has a method or cocktail of analgesics that he/she prescribes. Pain treatment is given on demand or when it becomes unbearable for the patients.

Accessibility of opioid analgesics and legislative barriers

Non-steroidal anti-inflammatory drugs (NSAIDs) and paracetamol are the most prescribed drugs. Usually, injectable solutions are preferred (IM), because it is thought that it is more 'effective' that way. In rare cases, oral medication is prescribed; in exceptional cases, the risk factors, treatment duration, or drug interactions of NSAIDs are taken into consideration.

Opioid analgesics are very limited in usage in the Republic of Moldova. Even though national standardized clinical protocols exist, which stipulate oral versions or transdermal medication, only the injectable forms are being used due to the complicated procedure to obtain a prescription (and exclusively for oncological patients), drastic evidence measures, and the limited dosages allowed. Yet only morphine, fentanyl, promedol (trimeperidine), and omnopon (contains morphine, papaverine, and codeine) are available in injectable forms. In hospitals, access to opioid drugs is limited to the operating rooms (ORs), intensive care units (ICUs), and rarely to surgical departments.

According to the Pain and Policy Studies Group in 2013, in the medical sphere, 10,4359 grams of opioids were used. Taking into consideration that most of that amount is represented by fentanyl used during surgeries, and methadone used in rehabilitation, we can conclude that only a small amount (especially morphine) is used to treat pain outside the hospital (to help cancer patients endure the pain) (Pain and Policy Studies Group, 2015).

Even if all medical forms of tramadol are available, injectable and oral forms are important due to their fast onset. It is the strongest analgesic available for the population, but obtaining a prescription is very difficult from an administrative point of view (the prescription has to have the institution stamp, the doctor's stamp, the special stamp 'for prescriptions', and the stamp of the medical director of the institution). Regarding neuropathic pain, gabapentin, pregabalin, amitriptyline, and the majority of modern antidepressants are available.

Structures and processes

Creation of specialized structures in the evaluation and treatment of pain (like acute pain services or (multidisciplinary) pain clinics), is some way off, at least for state hospitals. There are no quality indicators for the field of pain management in the medical system. Also, because of the economic situation of the country, the main goal of the medical system is patient survival and avoidance of vital and major complications. The notion of comfort, and of being pain-free remain at present a desideratum for the future.

Innovations

In 2008, the Moldovan Society for the Study and Management of Pain elaborated the concept of the *Pain Free Hospital.* It was inspired from the Fight against Pain national programme from France, as well as documentation workshops held at Centres of Evaluation and Treatment of Pain from St. Antoine (Paris), Ambroise Paré (Boulogne-Billancourt), CHU de Rennes, and mutualist clinic La Sagèsse (Rennes). The concept has the aim to improve the quality of pain management in hospitals and offers references, a set of standardized operational procedures, a protocol manual, elements of risk stratification, and patient safety, as well as a series of quality indicators and afferent action plans. A 'green point' was provided regarding pain, methods of declaration, evaluation, and treatment. Unfortunately this concept did not interest the Ministry of Health or any other hospital from Moldova in order to test its practical utility. The concept is available online at https://www.neverpain.org.

In September 2014, the Moldovan Society for the Study and Management of Pain started the project 'Inter-Professional, Simulation Based Training in Pain Assessment and Treatment of Chronic Pain in Family Medicine Practice', financed by the IASP grant *Developing Countries Project: Initiative for Improving Pain Education.* The aims of the programme were: (i) to update of theoretical knowledge about mechanisms, diagnostic and treatment principles, and organizational principles in acute and chronic pain; (ii) skills training to use different tools for pain assessment and pain relief (acute and chronic situations); (iii) practical application of knowledge acquired on standardized patients (via high-fidelity simulated scenarios, e.g. of a family doctor's office); (iv) and to provide specimens of pain assessment tools (VAS/NRD scales, and specific pain assessment questionnaires). During one month, 267 participants benefited from this programme (specialists in anaesthesia, intensive care, emergency medicine, family medicine, neurology, surgery, obstetrics and gynaecology, orthopedia, psychiatry, palliative care, clinical pharmacology; also nurses, social assistants, specialists in rehabilitation and kinesiotherapy). All participants attended a theoretical course for two full days regarding pain, five workshops, and four high-fidelity simulation scenarios with patient-actors.

Members of the Moldovan Society for the Study and Management of Pain, together with other colleagues from 21 hospitals from 11 European countries, participated during 2011–2012 in the PAIN OUT CPSP project (European Observational study on Chronic Post-Surgical Pain) under the auspices of the Clinical Trial Network of European Society of Anesthesiology. As a result, the prevalence of persistent postoperative pain was established in Moldova and Europe, several risk factors associated with persistence of pain 6–12 months postoperatively were identified.

Innovation in clinical practice

The Moldovan Society for the Study and Management of *Pain* distributes, with every occasion, rulers with the visual analogic score (VAS) to doctors and nurses during events that it organizes or participates in. VASs were implemented as a unidimensional autoevaluation of pain in the Institute of Urgent Medicine, N1 Municipal Clinical Hospital, Medpark International Hospital; multimodal postoperative pain therapy is applied in these hospitals, including strategies for risk reduction of postoperative pain persistence. Beginning in 2013, in the Institute of Urgent Medicine, postoperative analgesia by transversus abdominis plane block (done with ultrasound guidance) was implemented.

Conclusion

Pain is a global transnational problem, an integrated indicator which shows the level of development and maturation of a society; the level of democracy of the state; the status of fundamental human rights; the quality of medical services; the level of education and culture of the population. Doubtlessly, under the pressure of society and mass media as well, pain management will soon become a very important subject in the Republic of Moldova.

References

National Bureau of Statistics of the Republic of Moldova (2014). Population and Housing Census. The official report. Available at: http://www.statistica.md/newsview.php?l=en&id=5582&idc=30 [Online].

National Bureau of Statistics of the Republic of Moldova (n.d.). Social statistics. Health protection. Available at: statbank.statistica.md [Online].

Pain and Policy Studies Group, University of Wisconsin/WHO Collaborating Center, 2015. Available at: http://www.painpolicy.wisc.edu/country/profile/republic-moldova [Online].

Chapter 2.22

Norway

Petter Borchgrevink and Astrid Woodhouse

Background information

Norway has a population of 5.2 million people, 84% of whom are native born. Of these, some are Sami (ethnic background is not a census item so total numbers are not available) (Statistics Norway, 2017). Immigration, in descending order of the population, is from Poland, Lithuania, Somalia, Syria, and Pakistan. Children of immigrants constitute 3% of the Norwegian population. Official languages are Norwegian, New-Norwegian, and Sami (Fig. 2.22.1).

The Norwegian Pain Society (NPS) was founded in 2004 as a part of EFIC and as a Chapter of the International Association for the Study of Pain (IASP). Previously, there was a Scandinavian Association for the Study of Pain (SASP) that was an inclusive Chapter of IASP for the five Nordic countries. SASP now exists as a forum to promote and coordinate pain research in the Nordic countries, each of which has now established its own IASP Chapter. The NPS has 356 members: ~33% physicians, ~33% nurses, ~25% physiotherapists, and ~10% psychologists.

Healthcare system

The Norwegian healthcare system (National Insurance Scheme) is based on the principle of universal access, decentralization, and free choice of primary care provider (GP). This is managed by the Norwegian Health Economics Administration at the national level. Funding comes from general tax, from employee/employer contributions at source, and from co-payments of users of the healthcare system (160 NOK per GP visit, 200 NOK per specialist visit). While healthcare policy is controlled centrally, responsibility for the provision of services is decentralized although managerial and financial responsibility for the hospital sector is centralized. Norway has four regional health authorities with a medical school in each and these are responsible for specialized medical care in the country's 27 separate healthcare regions. The majority of the system is public, although there are some private practices and a small number of private hospitals. The private activity is mostly 'self-pay'. All Norwegian inhabitants are free to choose their own general practitioner and 99% are enrolled in a GP practice. The GPs are the gatekeepers to specialist care.

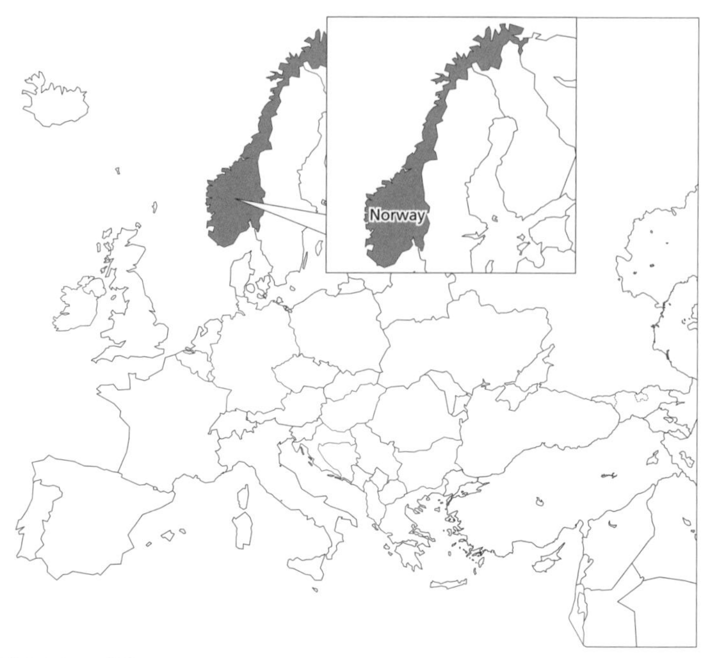

Fig. 2.22.1 Map of Norway.

Current pain workforce

There is no national registration of physicians in Norway that describes pain specialists. There is a Scandinavian Society of Anaesthesiology and Intensive Care course in Advanced Pain Medicine for physician specialists and to date, 30 specialists from Norway, primarily anaesthetists, have completed the course. The Health Ministry completed a hospital survey that identified 16 pain clinics, one of which now lacks a physician and is not functioning. More data from that survey is presently unavailable. The NPS convened a committee with representatives from the 40 programmes at institutions of higher learning that educate physicians (4), nurses (28), physiotherapists (4), and psychologists (4). Appropriate curricula were produced and are in use in the respective departments in all of Norway. The curricula are also available on the NPS website. The same committee is actively engaged in planning a curriculum for postgraduate pain education and pain specialty for physicians as well.

Challenges and opportunities to the future development of pain services

The NPS has been instrumental in organizing a pain centre network involving the four Norwegian multidisciplinary pain centres in the four University Hospitals (Oslo, Bergen, Trondheim, and Tromsø). They have a common, structured, physician–physiotherapist–psychologist evaluation for each new patient that is entered into a common database for the four centres. The challenge is the implementation of this programme and use of the database for research. It is now determined that this database will become a national quality register for all multidisiplinary pain clinics, which shall also be available for research.

The four pain programmes, in cooperation with the Norwegian Health Directorate and the NPS, have also developed guidelines for the organization and management of multidisciplinary pain clinics in Norway. The goal is to establish 12 secondary multidisciplinary pain clinics to better serve the population. These will be supervised by the university-based pain centres who will monitor their development in line with IASP guidelines. The challenge is to complete this task so that specialized multidisciplinary pain evaluation and treatment can become a reality throughout Norway.

Innovations

The coordination of comprehensive pain evaluation and treatment on a national basis is unique for pain to our knowledge. Norway is a relatively small nation which has helped this idea to evolve along with the centralized structure and oversight of the Norwegian healthcare system, and it seems that the goal is within the grasp of the system. The NPS has been instrumental in this process, and without its initiative and contacts within the Health Ministry this would not have been possible.

The NPS also has had a goal of creating a high-calibre yearly multidisciplinary meeting with invited international experts as speakers. The second goal for these meetings was to do this without commercial support, which the NPS feels flavours the meetings negatively. These goals have now been reached, with attendance reaching almost 400 individuals from many disciplines at the last meeting.

Reference

Statistics Norway (2017). **Available at:** https://www.ssb.no/en/ [Online].

Chapter 2.23

Poland

Jan Dobrogowski and Magdalena Kocot-Kępska

Background information

Poland sits in the centre of Europe, bordered by Russia, Lithuania, Belarus, Ukraine, Slovakia, Czech Republic, and Germany. It is approximately the ninth largest country in Europe with a population of 38,454,576 people, of whom 60.7% live in the cities, 1,748,916 in the main city of Warszawa. The population is shrinking. At present the average life expectancy is 73.5 years for men and 81.5 for women. The official language is Polish, but also spoken are Silesian, German, Kashubian, Lithuanian, and Belarusian. The Ethnic mix of the population is 97.1% Polish, 2.2% Silesian, 0.5% Kashubian, and 0.3% German (see Fig. 2.23.1) (Budzyński *et al.*, 2015).

The Polish Association for the Study of Pain was established in 1991, with the founding president Professor Jerzy Garstka. It became an IASP Chapter in 1991 and joined the EFIC in 1993. Currently there are 573 regular members and 12 honorary members. The core membership consists of anesthesiologists (279), dentists (104), neurologists (31), physicians (65), internal medicine specialists (25), as well as physiotherapists, general practitioners, and psychologists. As part of the Polish Association for the Study of Pain (PASP), there are the two following sections: the Orofacial Pain Chapter of PASP and the Interventional Chapter of PASP.

Healthcare system

According to Article 68 of the Polish Constitution, everyone is entitled to access to healthcare. Healthcare in Poland is delivered through a public healthcare system that is managed, funded, and supervised by the Ministry of Health, the National Health Fund, the Polish Ombudsman, local governments, and heads of the voivodships.

The healthcare system was reformed in 1999 when a new 'insurance treasury' model of funding was introduced. The system was founded on the principles of social solidarity, population-based health insurance, and equal access to public healthcare services.

The major source of funding in the system is health insurance paid to the National Health Fund (NHF). Citizens are obliged to pay to the NHF salary-based contributions amounting to 9% of their income. Patients who are uninsured have to pay the full cost of medical services.

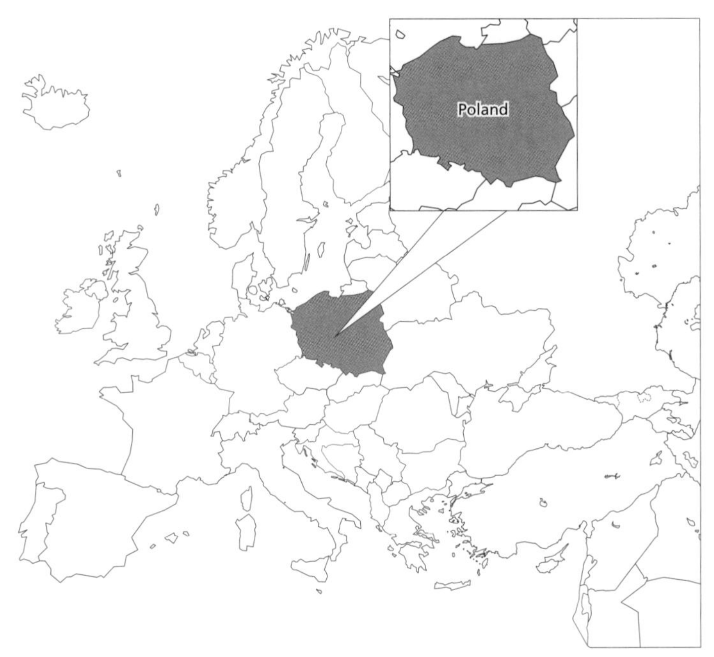

Fig. 2.23.1 Map of Poland.

The National Health Fund is responsible for the management and distribution of the collected funds. It pays for healthcare services provided to the insured and reimburses the cost of medications. The National Health Fund puts up health services for sale by public tender and signs contracts with the healthcare providers with the best offers.

However, private healthcare use is also well-established in Poland. According to a study conducted by the Public Opinion Research Center CBOS in 2012, 49% of Polish citizens use private healthcare (Hipsz, 2012).

Moreover, there are healthcare programmes that are financed directly from the treasury and are supervised by the Ministry of Health. These include, for instance, prevention programmes (e.g. vaccinations), highly specialized medical services (e.g. transplantations), public health programmes, teaching of medical professionals, medical research, central investments, blood donation centres, and centres for epidemiology.

Current pain workforce

Medical specializations in Poland are acquired in a one-step process during 3–6 year programmes, depending on a given specialty. The programmes include mandatory internships and courses. Participants are required to pass a national specialty examination at the end of each programme, which consists of both theoretical and practical parts. Since 2015, most specialty programmes include a five-day course of pain management. However, a specific specialty of pain medicine has not been established, but pain management constitutes an important part of the specialties of anesthesiology and intensive therapy, as well as palliative medicine.

According to an online survey carried out on the TacyJakJa.pl website, patients with chronic pain in Poland are managed primarily by family physicians, rheumatologists, and neurologists, whereas only 6% of them are referred to dedicated pain clinics (Kocot-Kępska *et al.*, 2015). The number of family physicians in Poland is approximately 22,000, which amounts to 2.2 physicians per one thousand patients (this ratio is lower by a half in comparison to the countries of 'Old EU').

The first pain clinic in Poland was founded in 1973 by Doctor Boleslaw Rutkowski in Gliwice. Subsequent pain clinics opened in academic centres in Warsaw, Katowice, Cracow, Lodz, and Poznan (Garstka, 2000). Pain clinics in Poland employ primarily anesthesiologists, but also neurologists and specialists in palliative medicine. Currently, there are approximately 200 pain clinics in Poland but most of them employ only a single physician and use a limited number of treatment strategies. Pain clinics that provide comprehensive services for chronic pain management are much less common.

In 2000, the Polish Association for the Study of Pain introduced a certificate that can be awarded to pain clinics that provide comprehensive pain management services. The criteria that have to be met in order for a given clinic to receive the certificate include comprehensive treatment of chronic pain with the use of pharmacotherapy, interventions, psychotherapy, physical therapy, and neuromodulation. Moreover, certified pain clinics have to be able to work with consultants in neurology, orthopaedic surgery, neurosurgery, psychology, and physical therapy. Currently, only 26 of the 200 existing pain clinics have a valid certificate and this number has not changed significantly for the last 10 years. The certificate is awarded for three years. Of the 26 certified pain clinics, only 10 are involved in research and graduate and postgraduate training of medical specialists.

In 2007, the Polish Association for the Study of Pain together with the Polish Society of Anesthesiology and Intensive Therapy, the Polish Society of Obstetrics and Gynaecology, and the Polish Society of Orthopaedic Surgery and Traumatology introduced a certification programme for hospitals and hospital wards, called the 'Pain Free Hospital'. As of today, the certificate has been awarded to 145 hospitals and 32 intervention wards, which comprises approximately 25% of all hospitals. The criteria for obtaining the 'Pain Free Hospital' certificate include evaluation and recording of postoperative pain, treatment of acute pain according to the principles of evidence-based medicine (EBM), and annual training of physicians and nurses in acute pain management. The certificate is awarded for three years.

As part of graduate training, courses in pain management are taught to six-year medical students, which include a three-hour seminar and a three-hour workshop as part of the courses in anesthesiology and intensive therapy or palliative medicine.

In 2007 the Polish Association for the Study of Pain, in cooperation with the Medical Center for Postgraduate Education of the Jagiellonian University, introduced two-semester studies, called 'Pain Medicine', for specialist physicians. The studies are designed for medical doctors—clinical specialists—and were created with a financial award from IASP. As of today, 600 physicians, mostly anesthesiologists, have graduated.

Since 2000, the Polish Association for the Study of Pain has published the *Pain* quarterly with original research and review articles in pain medicine. The quarterly is free of charge for members of the PASP. Moreover, the PASP has also published 15 handbooks and monographs in the field of pain diagnosis and management.

PASP experts also create national guidelines for specific issues in pain management. In 2014, PASP published the Polish guidelines for the diagnosis and management of neuropathic pain (Szczudlik *et al.*, 2014a, 2014b) and acute pain (Misiołek *et al.*, 2014). In 2015, PASP published the Polish guidelines for the use of strong opioids in patients with non-cancer-related chronic pain (Dobrogowski *et al.*, 2015).

Every three years, PASP organizes a national congress with foreign guest speakers. The first congress took place in 1994 in Krakow. Moreover, every two to three years PASP organizes international symposia, called 'Progress in Pain Treatment', and conferences of the PASP sections.

In 2015, the first EFIC Krakow Pain School 'Translational Pain Research, From Lab to Clinic' was organized in cooperation with the Department of Pain Pharmacology, Polish Academy of Sciences in Cracow. Professor Barbara Przewlocka was the initiator and head of the event.

Since 2015, an e-learning course 'LeczBol.pl' has been organized for physicians and nurses interested in pain medicine. The course on acute and chronic pain management is completed with an examination and continuing medical education (CME) credit awarded.

Challenges and opportunities to the future development of pain services

Because the current graduate pain medicine programme for medical students is not sufficient, PASP wrote a new programme based on the Core Curriculum EFIC and IASP. This new programme has been introduced as a pilot course for medical students of the Jagiellonian University.

The main goal of PASP in the nearest future is to create a subspecialization or a new module in pain medicine for specialist physicians. Experts of the PASP have already created an appropriate curriculum that has been presented to the Ministry of Health and the Supreme Medical Council.

Introducing a new specialization in pain medicine will increase the interest of physicians, and consequently the number of pain clinics.

The programme of certifying hospitals and pain clinics will continue as the certificate awarded by PASP documents high-quality services provided in accordance with guidelines of the IASP and EFIC. Moreover, the certificate is taken into account by the National Health Fund when signing contracts.

Hospitals and intervention wards are interested in obtaining the 'Pain Free Hospital' certificate and this programme will be extended to non-intervention wards (e.g. internal medicine, geriatric, and rheumatologic wards).

The teaching activities of PASP will also continue, including the e-learning course and postgraduate studies of 'Pain Medicine' as they help improve the quality and availability of pain treatment in Poland. So far, there exist no specific pain treatment wards in Poland onto which patients with severe non-cancer pain could be admitted. Therefore, there are plans to open five such wards (20 beds in total) in the academic centres. On such wards, intervention procedures will be carried out and subsequent hospitalization of patients with pain crises will be possible.

Innovations

According to epidemiological studies, 27% of adults in Poland suffer from chronic pain (Breivik *et al.*, 2006; Kocot-Kępska and Dobrogowski, 2004). This is higher than the European average, but the reasons behind it are not known. Patients with pain will increasingly require medical help, but the current state of knowledge of healthcare regulators, medical professionals, and patients lags behind.

PASP puts an emphasis on the education of students, physicians, and nurses in Poland in order to increase awareness of chronic pain as a stand-alone disease, and of the necessity of multidirectional treatment in accordance with the biopsychosocial model of chronic pain.

Introducing a comprehensive curriculum for medical and dentistry students is a difficult task which requires close cooperation between the deans of medical universities.

The postgraduate studies of 'Pain Medicine', based on the Core Curriculum of IASP, is an absolute innovation as there are currently no similar teaching programmes in Europe. The studies last two semesters and are held in Polish. The theoretical part consists of nine sessions—140 hours per year. The practical part is organized by the Department of Pain Research and Treatment of the Collegium Medicum, Jagiellonian University, and lasts 40 hours. The studies are completed by an examination that entitles participants to receive a diploma.

Because of the popularity of the Internet, all online teaching methods are very useful and convenient. The preparation of the e-learning course by PASP required a lot of time and effort from experts in the respective fields of pain medicine, as well as the cooperation with an agency specializing in organizing Internet platforms for medical teaching. It has been noted that e-learning courses should be completed by examinations with a possibility to obtain CME credit. This applies to physicians, nurses, and other healthcare professionals.

References

Breivik, H., Collett, B., Ventfridda, V., Cohen, R., Gallacher, D. (2006). Survey of chronic pain in Europe: prevalence, impact on daily life, and treatment. *Eur J Pain*, **10**, 287–333.

Budzyński, I., Kacperczyk, E., Korczak-Żydaczewska, K., *et al.* (2015). Area and population in the territorial profile in 2015. Warsawzawa, Poland: Central Statistical Office (CSO), Methodology, Standards, and Registers Department.

Dobrogowski, J., Wordliczek, J., Szczudlik, A., *et al.* (2015). Long-term strong opioid use in noncancer pain: A review of the literature and recommendation of the Polish Association for the Study of Pain, Polish Neurological Society, and Polish Society of Family Medicine. *Ból*, **16**, 9–29.

Garstka, J. (2000). A history of pain management in Poland. *Ból*, **1, 3**, 34–6.

Hipsz, N. (2012). Use of health services and health insurances. Korzystanie ze świadczeń i ubezpieczeń zdrowotnych. Bulletin BS/35/2012. Warsaw, Poland: Public Opinion Research Center (CBOS).

Kocot-Kępska, M., Dobrogowski, J., Zdziechowska, K., & **Czyżak, I.** (2015). Evaluation of the results of a survey among persons suffering from chronic pain. *Ból*, **16**, 9–19.

Kocot-Kępska, M. & **Dobrogowski, J.** (2004). The assessment of epidemiological survey of chronic non-malignant pain conducted across Europe in 2002 by Mundipharma Purdue. *Ból*, **3**, 18–24.

Misiołek, H., Cettler, M., Woroń, J., Wordliczek, J., Dobrogowski, J., & **Mayzner-Zawadzka E.** (2014). Recommendations for acute post-operative pain management AD 2014. *Ból*, **14**, 19–47.

Szczudlik, A., Dobrogowski, J., Wordliczek, J., *et al.* (2014a). Diagnosis and management of neuropathic pain: review of literature and recommendations of the Polish Association for the Study of Pain and the Polish Neurological Society—Part One. *Ból*, **15**, 8–18.

Szczudlik, A., Dobrogowski, J., Wordliczek, J., *et al.* (2014b). Diagnosis and management of neuropathic pain: review of literature and recommendations of the Polish Association for the Study of Pain and the Polish Neurological Society—Part Two. *Ból*, **15**, 18–21.

Chapter 2.24

Portugal

Ana Valentim and Pedro Ferreira

Background information

According to statistics from Portugal's 2011 Census (INE, 2012) and information provided by the Directorate-General of Health (DGS, 2016), Portugal has 10,562,178 inhabitants, of whom 52.2% are women, 19% older than 65 years of age and 2.25% older than 85. In May 2016, it was ascertained that older people's dependency ratio was 28.8 and life expectancy at birth was 79.55 (Portugal is in the top third of OECD performers), with women living approximately six years longer than men. The infant mortality rate per 1,000 live births is 3.12.

Regarding ethnicity, the majority of Portuguese inhabitants are Mediterranean, one of the subraces of the Caucasian race. In addition to these, there are a significant number of citizens of black African descent (approximately 100,000) who emigrated to Portugal during the 1975 decolonization period and, since 1990, many Eastern Europeans have chosen to live in this country. In 2011, approximately 395,000 inhabitants were of foreign origin, corresponding to 3.7% of the total population (see Fig. 2.24.1).

The Portuguese Association for the Study of Pain (APED) was created on 4 June 1991 and is affiliated to the International Association for the Study of Pain (IASP) as the Portuguese Chapter. APED is located at the Institute of Histology and Embryology of the Faculty of Medicine of the University of Porto. It has 477 members and is the largest multidisciplinary professional organization in the field of pain in Portugal. APED brings together professionals of different specialties and categories, most of whom are doctors (anesthesiologists, physiatrists, oncologists, internists, and neurosurgeons), some of them with a competence in pain medicine. It also includes nurses, psychologists, pharmacologists, and researchers in pain.

Healthcare system

In the early 1970s, the Portuguese health system was mainly characterized by the following aspects (OPSS, 2001, 2002):

- Unfavourable socioeconomic and health indicators, when compared to other Western European countries.
- Fragmented health services without a common structure: there were very few public hospitals and charity hospitals, social health services, public health services (after 1971 called health centres), municipal doctors, and separated units dedicated to specific conditions, such as maternal and child care, tuberculosis, and mental health. Private healthcare was provided on an ambulatory basis.
- Very little financing of public services, with only 2.8% of GDP spent in 1970.

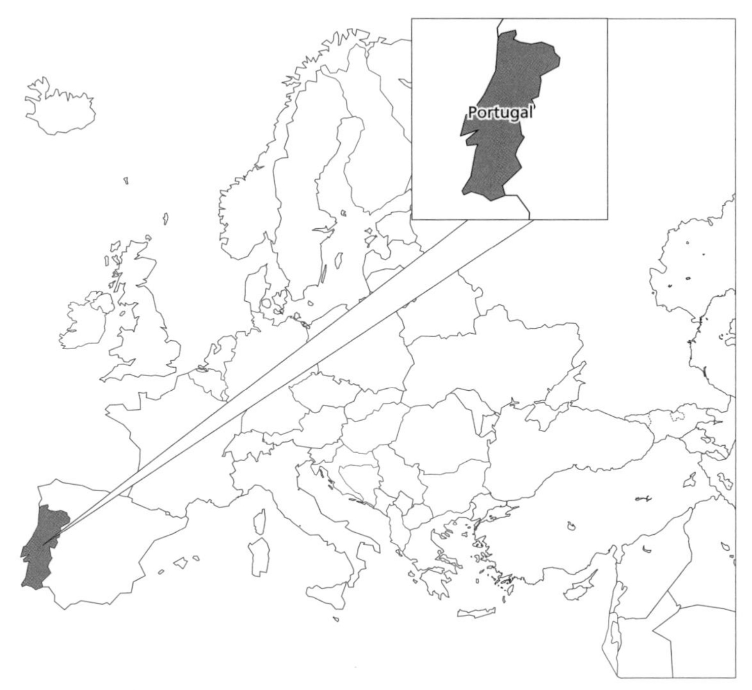

Fig. 2.24.1 Map of Portugal.

Health coverage was scarce and people's access to healthcare was very limited. However, after the 'Carnation' Revolution of 1974, a new Constitution of the Portuguese Republic was approved and the right to healthcare was granted. At the same time, equality of access to healthcare was promoted, irrespective of economic conditions and geographic location, as well as equity in the distribution of resources and use of healthcare services. In 1979, the creation of the Portuguese National Health Service (SNS) was an important component of the political and social democratization of the country. In a relatively short period of time, the SNS substantially increased the coverage of and citizens' access to healthcare. It also allowed for a real integration of the different healthcare resources. Portugal was moving from a classic Bismark health system to a Beveridge one. However, some health subsystems for certain population groups (e.g. civil servants, and the army) still persist in the new system. These subsystems are mainly financed through employee and employer contributions, including state contributions as an employer.

Portugal joined the European Economic Community in 1985. In 1990, the Portuguese Parliament approved the Basic Health Law and market mechanisms were introduced in the health system. The last two decades have been marked by a set of reforms, with particular emphasis on public–private partnerships for new hospitals, hospital emergency departments, and primary healthcare and long-term care networks.

Very substantial health improvements have occurred in recent years. Portugal is in the OECD's top-third of performers in terms of healthcare coverage (95% to 100%), but belongs to the middle-third concerning unmet medical care needs, especially due to waiting times and long distances to travel to access health services. Regarding the health workforce, according to the 2015 *Health at a Glance Report* (OECD, 2015), the number of doctors *per capita* in Portugal was 4.3 per 1,000 inhabitants (OECD: 3.3), while the number of nurses was 6.1 (OECD: 9.1), and hospital beds per 1,000 inhabitants, 3.4 (OECD: 4.8).

Concerning health system financing, in 2013 health expenditure was 9.1% of the Portuguese GDP, slightly higher than the OECD average (8.9%), and health expenditure per capita was 2,514 USD PPP, lower than the OECD (3,453). As a result of this, a large proportion of financing is private, mainly in the form of out-of-pocket payments: 26% of the health expenditure was spent on inpatient care; 48% on outpatient care; only 2% on long-term care; 20% on medical goods; and the remaining 4% on collective services. In terms of breadth of coverage, the Portuguese health system is predominantly financed through general taxation. The SNS covers all residents in the country; it is universal, comprehensive, and almost free at the point of use. Approximately 25% of the population is covered by health subsystems or voluntary health insurance. The service provision is mixed—public and private—and is centrally regulated, planned, and managed, although the delivery of healthcare services has been structured at the regional level. User charges are in place for most services. The depth of coverage is lowest for pharmaceuticals. The other situations in which user charges are most visible to the population are the use of emergency services, and visits to GPs and specialists.

Current pain workforce

Pain medicine does not exist as a specialty in Portugal; however, it is possible to obtain a certification in pain management through the Portuguese Medical Association (Competence in Pain Medicine). Currently, there are 123 doctors with certified skills in pain management but, due to the fact that many pain medicine physicians do not have the competence, it is impossible to estimate the exact number of professionals working in pain management. On the other hand, the number of general practitioners in Portugal is currently 8,201 (ACSS, 2015).

Several epidemiological pain studies have been carried out in Portugal. A Porto University Faculty of Medicine study (Azevedo *et al.*, 2012) between January 2007 and March 2008 is a landmark because it determined the prevalence and socioeconomic impact of chronic pain (CP) in Portugal. This cross-sectional nationwide epidemiological study was performed in a 5,094 random digit dialling sample of the Portuguese adult population. Based on the IASP definition, CP prevalence was 36.7% (95% confidence interval 35.3–38.2). Considering recurrent and continuous CP with moderate to severe intensity, the prevalence was 14.3%. The mean total annualized cost per CP subject was €1,883.30, amounting to €4,611.69 million nationally, with 42.7% direct and 57.3% indirect costs, and corresponding to 2.71% of the Portuguese annual GDP in 2010 (Azevedo *et al.*, 2016).

Another survey regarding pain education curricula across healthcare professions was conducted in Portugal by Observdor (2011). One hundred and sixteen health science courses were surveyed: medicine (7), dentistry (7), physiotherapy (16), psychology (33), nursing (42), and pharmacy (11). One of the main conclusions of this study was that pain is taught at undergraduate level in medicine, dentistry, physiotherapy, and nursing, and in most courses of psychology and pharmacy. However, this teaching is somewhat fragmented in terms of physiology and pharmacology with no discipline allowing for the integration of knowledge in the majority of cases. At postgraduate level the courses offered are diversified, allowing health professionals interested in this matter to bridge the gap between undergraduate and postgraduate courses (Observdor, 2011).

Challenges and opportunities for the future development of pain services

The major challenges facing the development of pain services in Portugal are the current structure, with services mostly concentrated in hospitals, the difficult access for many users, and a certain shortage of human resources. Creating more pain units with better connections between the different levels of care (hospital, primary, long-term) is one of the main challenges. It is also important to stress that Portugal has an ageing population living mostly in the interior of the country, which tends to visit the family doctor for pain treatment. These elderly patients have co-morbidities directly related to chronic pain (cardiovascular disease, cancer, and osteoarthritis, the prevalence of which increase with age). In this context, then, primary healthcare professionals need to receive better training in pain. Nevertheless, the new reality of an ageing population also represents an opportunity for the redesigning of healthcare, with greater involvement of the different entities, including civil society, solidarity institutions, professionals, and policymakers.

Innovations

In the last two decades several measures have been implemented. First, a working group dedicated to pain was created in 1999 by the DGS, working in close collaboration with APED to develop a National Programme for the Fight Against Pain (NPFAP), approved in March 2001 (Ministerial Dispatch, 2001). This plan, innovative at the national and international level, describes organizational models for pain management in hospitals, including several general guidelines for pain management. This programme was eventually replaced by the National Pain Management Plan (Prescriptive Law nº 11/DSCS/DPCD 2008) and the National Pain Management Strategic Plan, the latter having been approved in 2013. Furthermore, in June 2003 the DGS published a regulation (Prescriptive Law nº 09/DGCG 2003) declaring pain as the fifth vital sign. Since then, monitoring and recording pain intensity has become mandatory in all health services. In 2004, a pain medicine competence was created by the Portuguese Medical Association, promoting and recognizing the specialization of physicians dedicated to this field of medicine. In 2008 strong opioids were also reimbursed from 90% to 95%, depending on the patient profile (Order nº 10279/2008, Order nº 10280/2008). Another important step was the abolition of user charges for patients with chronic pain (Decree-Law nº 113/2011, 29 November). Finally, in 2013 new financing and descriptive codes for clinical procedures performed within pain medicine were established by ACSS (Official Journal, 1.ª série—n.º 80, 24 April 2013).

References

Administração Central dos Sistemas de Saúde (ACSS) (2015). Inventário de Pessoal do Sector da Saúde, 2014. Lisboa, Portugal: ACSS.

Azevedo, L., Costa-Pereira, A., Mendonça, L., Dias, C. C., Castro-Lopes, J. M. (2012). Epidemiology of chronic pain: a population-based nationwide study on its prevalence, characteristics and associated disability. *J Pain*, **13**, 773–83.

Azevedo, L., Costa-Pereira, A., Mendonça, L., Dias, C. C., Castro-Lopes, J. M. (2016). The economic impact of chronic pain: a nationwide population-based cost-of-illness study in Portugal. *Eur J Health Econ*, **17**, 87–98.

Direcção-Geral de Saúde (DGS) (2016). Circular Normativa da Direcção-Geral de Saúde nº 09/DGCG 14 June 2003. A dor como 5º Sinal vital. Registo sistemático da Intensidade da Dor 2003. Lisbon, Portugal: DGS. Available at: http://www.dgs.pt/ (accessed 25 June 2016) [Online].

Instituto Nacional de Estatística (INE) (2012). Portugal's 2011 Census. Lisbon, Portugal: INE. Available at: http://censos.ine.pt (accessed 10 April 2016) [Online].

Observdor (2011). Centro Nacional de Observação em Dor. Estado da Arte do Ensino da Dor em Portugal: Relatório Final May 2010. Lisboa, Portugal: CNOD. Available at: http://1nj5ms2lli5hdggbe3mm7ms5.wpengine.netdna-cdn.com/files/2015/08/Estado-da-Arte-do-Ensino-da-Dor-em-Portugal.pdf (accessed 21 April 2016) [Online].

Observatório Português dos Sistemas de Saúde (OPSS) (2001). *Conhecer os caminhos da saúde. Spring Report*. Lisbon, Portugal: OPSS. Available at: http://www.opss.pt (accessed 21 April 2016) [Online].

Observatório Português dos Sistemas de Saúde (OPSS) (2002). *O estado da saúde e a saúde do Estado. Spring Report*. Lisbon, Portugal: OPSS. Available at: http://www.opss.pt (accessed 21 April 2016) [Online].

Organisation for Economic Co-operation and Development (OECD) (2015). OECD Health Statistics 2015. Available at: http://www.oecd.org/els/health-systems/health-data.htm (accessed 19 May 2016) [Online].

Chapter 2.25

Romania

Adriana Sarah Nica

Background information

Romania is located in southeastern Central Europe, on the Lower Danube, north of the Balkan Peninsula and the northwestern coast of the Black Sea. On its territory is located almost the entire Delta and southern and central part of the Carpathian Mountains. It is bordered by Bulgaria to the south, southwest Serbia, Hungary to the northwest, north, and east Ukraine and Moldova to the east, and the Black Sea is to the southeast. Romania has been a nation state since 1918. According to National Institute of Statistics in 2013, Romania has a population of 21,790,479, which is gradually shrinking. The primary language is Romanian (see Fig. 2.25.1).

Healthcare system

The Romanian healthcare system is almost entirely owned by the state and consists of a series of networks of hospitals, clinics, and other medical institutions coordinated and managed by the Ministry of Health through its 42 County Directorates of Public Health. The Ministry of Health maintains the role of funding and coordination of national public health programmes. Primary care is currently provided by the family doctor, where there is an emphasis on providing a first filter and access to early problem-solving. Access to ambulatory care and hospital (outside emergencies) and free access to drugs is made through the family doctor. Today, doctors no longer have the status of employees of the state but are healthcare providers who enter into a contract with the health insurance companies. There is also a private system of providing medical services, adjacent to the extensive network of public and private pharmacies. In Romania a large segment of the population, although insured, cannot afford the extra costs of treatment, and do not have access to hospital services outside their town of residence.

In the Romanian Health Insurance System there is currently no specific specialty for pain management. Patients receive clinical assessment and pain treatment in the context of various diseases and medical addressability. The Romanian Association for the Study of Pain (known as the ARSD) is constantly involved in promoting specific health programmes; the only line that was successful was for palliative care. Given the growing number of potential beneficiaries with chronic pain (somatic or visceral) and the therapeutic strategy of the European platform, ARSD has made efforts to establish guidelines on the appropriate use of opioids in chronic non-oncological pain. So,

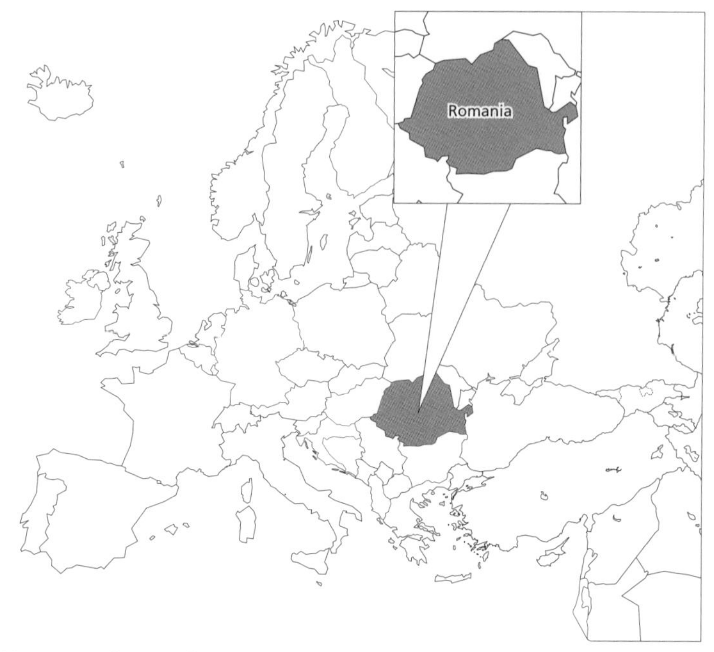

Fig. 2.25.1 Map of Romania.

ARSD representatives participated in 2002 at the Budapest Work Group and started a project in Romania with the Ministry of Health, and in 2005 a law was introduced: the 339 Law relates to the use of opioids in oncology and chronic non-oncological pain. Currently this law is partially applied in the medical therapeutics Romanian platform.

ARSD initiated under the aegis of excellence research programme CEEX 'Pro-Pain Control—Research on the developmental integrated network of national centres to optimize pain therapy in acute postoperative analgesia by patient self-managed application protocols'. There have been numerous requests to the Ministry of Health to initiate a project linked to a Romanian database on acute and chronic pain. Until now the project could not be initiated due to the rapid change of personnel at the Ministry of Health.

Current pain workforce

The Romanian Association for the Study of Pain was established in 1991 on the initiative of Doctor Lucian Sandu. It is Anaesthesia and Intensive Care focused, with 45 members from different specialties including: Anaesthesia and Intensive Care, Neurology, Internal Medicine, Psychiatry, Cardiology, and Rehabilitation Medicine. Over the years, the numbers of specialties interested in pain management has also included surgical specialties such as brain surgery, thoracic surgery, plastic surgery, and oncology. The annual general membership varies between 300 and 500. Analysing the number of specialties present at different times we can not only observe the constant interest of family physicians for the main subjects approached in pain management, but also an increase in members from family medicine and rehabilitation medicine. The association operates to (a) promote and encourage study, research, and scientific therapy in acute and chronic pain; (b) organize the teaching environment for training and improvement in pain management; (c) organize, support, and manage a place for the storage, processing, and distribution of support for pain management; (d) organize and support congresses, symposia, and specialized courses; (e) organize territorial centres for pain management; (f) organize and support an informational centre, including newspaper editing; collaboration, scientific exchange, and experience with similar national, regional, and international organizations; (g) sustain and promote patient specific interests; (h) protect the scientific and professional interests and rights of members; and (i) promote a human spirit of solidarity and benevolence. It is located in the University Hospital of Bucharest, Anaesthesia and Intensive Care Unit.

In 1994 a centre for pain at SUUB (Spitalul Universitar de Urgenta Bucuresti) was established, led by Lucian Sandu. A pain centre in Resita led by Dr Virgil Suru subsequently appeared, along with others in several locations offering pain therapy in private structures in Bucharest and other towns. From 1996 to the present, under the programme of Continuing Medical Education, ARSD organized annual courses (one or five days) with various topics related to the themes proposed by IASP and EFIC. This aimed to inform platform medical concerns in a multidisciplinary international context related to specific categories of evaluation, and the presentation of new techniques of investigation and treatment. In 2000, ARSD—in collaboration with Professor John Loeser (President of IASP)—organized an international Pain Management course lasting one week and attended by 75 students, which took place in University Hospital Bucharest. From 2002 to 2004 a new course was developed especially for community physicians (the target group being family physicians), for which classes took place for two days/week, and were attended by over 600 participants. The course was very well received.

Since 2001, ARDS has delivered competency based training in pain management. The courses are delivered by trainers and experts in pain management; the platform selected by ARSD from the University of Medicine and Pharmacy 'Carol Davila', from different experts involved in pain assessment and therapy (Anaesthesia and Intensive Care, Neurology, Neurosurgery, Internal Medicine, Psychiatry, Rehabilitation Medicine). The annual postgraduate training programme in pain management, held from 2001–2007, was attended by between 30–50 people each year. The syllabus included theoretical courses (one-third) and some practical (two-thirds) consisting of demonstrations, applications, and exercises, analysis, and case studies. The course was held over 12 months, and organized into several modules: current physiology and pathophysiology of acute and chronic pain; pain assessment; pharmacological therapy; non-pharmacological, non-invasive, or invasive interventions. Each module was assessed by a written test and a final clinical examination for each participant. At the end of training, participants perform a complex exam that contains all the theoretical and practical knowledge achieved, taking into account the basic specialty of each. Following successful examination, competence in pain management was achieved.

Although the course was a success, after six years the enrollments were not enough. Presently, there is a demand for this training competence, and ARSD is working on a new education programme following the curriculum of EFIC.

Between 1992–2004 each national congress was held with international participation. At the European Congress of Medical Rehabilitation (in Venice 2010) we discussed creating a special section, 'Recovery of Pain and ways to promote a working group between EFIC and ESPRM'. After four years in the interdisciplinary context at the European Society for Rehabilitation (ESPRM), it was proposed to organize a special section for management of pain in recovery, initiated by Professor Sarah Adriana Nica (Romania) and Professor Roberto Casale (Italy). Following these concerns, at the EFIC Congress in Florence (2013) ESPRM president Professor Dr Michaelis Xanti was invited together with EFIC President Professor Hans G. Kress to discuss the opportunities for the two societies to collaborate, in order to establish protocols between the European Society of Rehabilitation and the European Pain Federation.

Challenges and opportunities to the future development of pain services

There are challenges that emerge from the Societal Impact of Pain (SIP, 2011), an event attended by representatives of ARSD at both annual general meetings and in working group meetings. At the last meeting, Professor Adriana Sarah Nica, member of the EFIC Board for Romania, participated in the group discussing 'Pain—Rehabilitation and return to work'. There was important discussion on chronic pain within the programmes of rehabilitation therapy for professionally active people, collaboration between specialists in occupational medicine, and on recovery and return to work. In this context, ARSD representatives have tried in the past years to convince representatives from the Ministry of Health of the importance of this work in healthcare and of the social benefits of identifying various aspects of pain-related distress and disability.

Over the years, the conference themes were set according to the recommendations of IASP and EFIC. In the two to three days of the conference, ARSD held lectures on current pain-related or pain syndromes about various pathologies and involving clinical research from academic colleagues around the country. Meetings provided the opportunity to create a medical database on interdisciplinary pain management (e.g. pain in older people, neuropathic, paediatric, and dental pain).

In the past decade there have been many opportunities related to online medical education for pain management. The ARSD educational programme started the ability to select and send young doctors with different levels of experience to schools organized by EFIC European Pain Federation. This programme has been applied in Romania, including all disciplines of training, including: initiation in Pain Management at the School of Klagenfurt; continuous preparation for the Neuropathic Pain School in Montescano/Bergamo; and Palliative Care at the Liverpool School. In 2015, Professor Adriana Sarah Nica was invited to join the group of speakers at the School of Pain in Klagenfurt, where she presented the topic 'Equation Pain—Dysfunction in Pathologies of the Upper and Lower Limb'. During 2009–2016, 23 participants from Romania have benefited from the European Schools for Pain Management.

In the past two years, state hospitals began a process of evaluation and accreditation. Among existing procedures and protocols, pain assessment protocols are included with several categories of indicators, on pain characteristics, type of pain, pathological background, using pharmacological and non-pharmacological therapies. These steps could represent the initiation in Romania for a project to implement the database on acute and chronic pain, specific medical features, therapeutic, and socioeconomic factors.

In the context of higher education, in the past two years at the University of Medicine and Pharmacy 'Carol Davila' Bucharest, a course in Pain Management was introduced in the list of optional courses. It was received very well; the audience of 40 students in the first year later doubled. Meanwhile, ARSD, through subsidiaries in an academic promotion campaign, supported an optional course in other universities (Cluj, Iasi, and Timisoara). This will help students to better understand the pathogenic mechanisms, physiopathological manifestations, and therapeutic decisions regarding pain in a list of priorities. Finally, 10 years ago, the National Institute of Rehabilitation initiated a clinical research platform for pain management.

Innovations

ARSD applied an original research project designed for Pro-Pain Control, 'Research on the developmental integrated network of national centres for therapy of acute pain to optimize postoperative self-administered analgesia by the patient using application protocols' in the Program of Research Excellence 'CEEX'. The main objective of this project is to develop an integrated network designed to optimize postoperative analgesia controlled by the patient using intelligent systems for the controlled release of analgesic substances, based on clinical protocols developed in harmony with EU recommendations. The project was conceived in order to perform the following activities: creating a network of acute pain therapy for the development of methods for selecting patients by the study groups themselves; and to aid the study and development of analgesia protocols that will later be applied. The screening analysis methods currently used in the treatment of acute pain and analgesia were obtained through their application.

Protocols for postoperative analgesia and analgesia for birth were developed, based on initially informing and educating the patient on the most effective mode of administration, including the development of innovative therapies through smart pumps dispersing painkillers controlled by the patient. Through validation, review, and development of the postoperative analgesia protocols 'Final Guide to Acute Pain Therapy', these new methods of acute pain therapy were created and implemented throughout the network. The results were disseminated through roundtables, workshops, symposiums, and conferences, developing and publishing a guide for acute pain therapy (joint project ARSD-SRATI Romanian Society of Anaesthesia and Intensive Care), publications, and active dialogue between medical doctor and patients also.

Pain management in Romania is in development. Dimensions, knowledge, and therapeutic actions with a focus on pain are a large part of all medical specialties. There have been significant advances in pain management, but we currently face the major challenges of implementing the training programmes after EFIC recommendations were made to re-organize our infrastructure, and to grow interdisciplinary teams and patient education programmes.

References

National Institute of Statistics (2013). Available at: http://www.insse.ro/cms/en [Online].

Societal Impact of Pain (SIP) (2011). Pain in Europe VII—7th Congress of the European Federation of IASP Chapters (EFIC®). Available at: https://www.sip-platform.eu/events/archive/efic-2011 [Online].

Chapter 2.26

Russia

Nikilay N. Yakhno, Michael L. Kukushkin, and Maxim V. Churyukanov

Background information

Russia is the largest country in the world, located in the northern hemisphere of the planet, occupying a large part of Eurasia (Fig. 2.26.1). Russia has common borders with 18 countries, including the sea borders of the United States and Japan. From east to west, Russia stretches for 10,000 kilometres; from north to south, about 4,000 kilometres. Its total area is about 17 million square kilometres. Russia consists of 21 autonomous Republics, 6 territories (krai), 49 oblasts, 2 federal cities, 1 autonomic oblast, and 10 autonomic districts (Fig. 2.26.2). The Russian federation has 11 time zones. Moscow is its capital city, but there are 13 large metropolitan districts with a population of over a million people: Moscow, St. Petersburg, Nizhny Novgorod, Volgograd, Samara, Perm, Ufa, Kazan, Novosibirsk, Yekaterinburg, Omsk, Chelyabinsk, and Rostov-on-Don. There are also 1,030 cities, 2,153 towns, and countless villages. According to the report published by the Russian census in 2005, the total population of the country was 143 million people, the vast of the majority of whom occupy the European part, and around 20% living over the Urals (Population of Russia census data, 2005). Russia is one of the most multicultural countries in the world, accounting for about 160 nationalities. The national language is Russian.

Healthcare system

A budget-insurance healthcare system is provided by means of the state budget (federal and regional) and extrabudgetary funds of health insurance: compulsory health insurance (CBO) and voluntary health insurance (VHI).

The management and control of health institutions includes ministerial (federal), regional (large towns and cities), and local (municipal) levels. Government (federal, regional, municipal) health authorities have the right to control private medical institutions and private practitioners. In turn, the administrative structures of executive authority, responsible for the public health system, are under the jurisdiction of the legislature (the State Duma, the Federation Council). Supervision over the implementation of public health laws, in turn, is carried out by the judiciary structures and institutions. The Russian Federation Ministry of Health is in charge of the functions

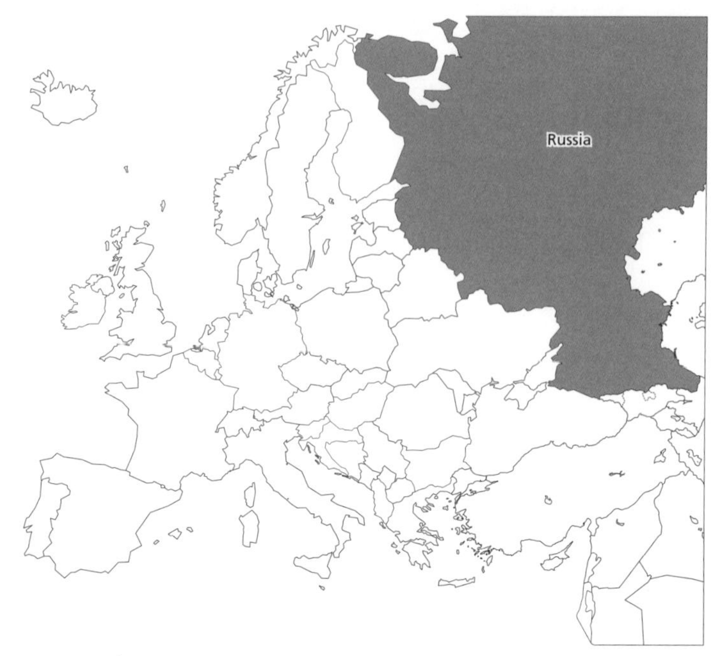

Fig. 2.26.1 Map of Russia.

of public policy and legal regulation in the sphere of healthcare, compulsory health insurance, and treatment drugs.

Structurally and organizationally, the public health system integrates various types of enterprises and institutions: (i) the federal and regional authorities and health institutions (public, budget healthcare system); (ii) structures and institutions of the state system CBO; (iii) private medical institutions and private practitioners (VHI authorities and institutions, and private health insurance); and (iv) social, religious, medical institutions, foundations, organizations, and institutions of charity.

Current pain workforce

The Russian Association for the Study of Pain (RASP) was established in 1989. In 1990 RASP became a collective member of International Association for the Study of Pain (IASP) and of the European Pain Federation (EFIC) in 1993. The RASP has a total of 465 members. Most of the members have a higher education. The largest specialty group is formed by the neurologists, anesthesiologists, rheumatologists, traumatologists, neurosurgeons, and physicians. Only a minority of these professionals work within a private setting or practice. The RASP is administered by an executive board including a president, two vice presidents, executive secretary, and 18 members. RASP members are elected at the general assembly of the members for a term of five years. According to the ongoing tasks the executive board organizes meetings once a

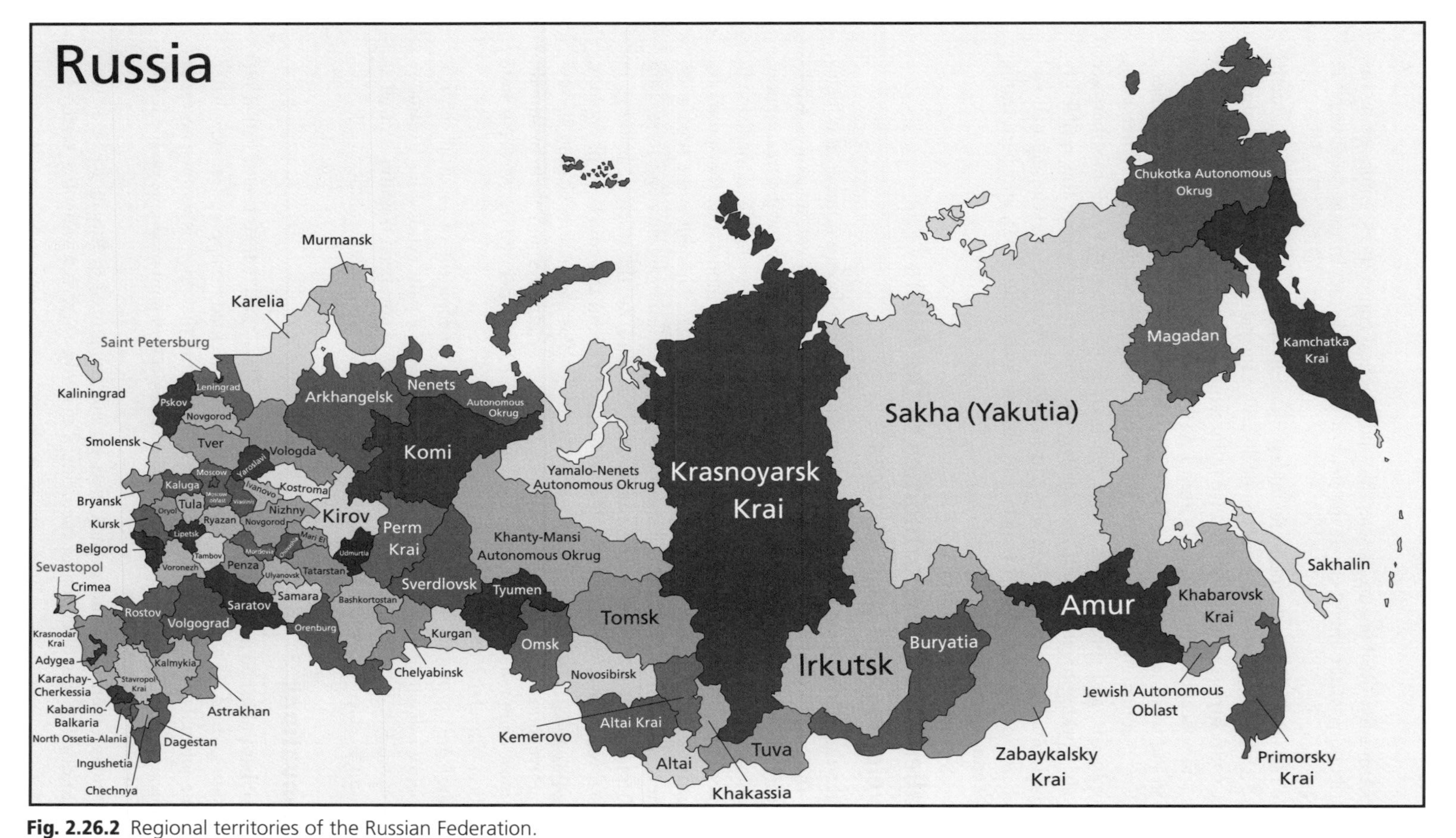

Fig. 2.26.2 Regional territories of the Russian Federation.

Adapted with permission from On The World Map, *Administrative divisions map of Russia*, Copyright © 2012–2017 Ontheworldmap.com. Available from http://ontheworldmap.com/russia/administrative-divisions-map-of-russia.html.

year. Annually RASP organizes scientific and practical conferences, emphasizing the contributions of the members in the field of pain medicine. In total there were 22 conferences.

We consider pain medicine to be underfunded in the Russian healthcare system. There is no specialized multilevel medical service for patients experiencing pain, so those with chronic pain do not receive full treatment. Analysing the existing experience and specialists' distribution within RASP, it can be assumed that an important role in the treatment of pain should be played not only by neurologists, anesthesiologists, rheumatologists, physicians (GPs), but also psychologists, psychotherapists, reflexologists, and specialists in motor rehabilitation. Currently RASP members are actively working together with the Russian government to improve the availability of opioid analgesics for patients with chronic pain syndromes, developing national standards for the treatment of acute and chronic pain syndromes, and performing active educational work.

Challenges and opportunities to the future development of pain services

The development of pain medicine as a new subdiscipline faces a number of difficulties. The main problem is that there are no standards of equipment, structures, workforce, or organization principles in medical institutions catering for the treatment of patients with various pain syndromes. The only nosological principle of medicine in terms of pain treatment is based on a dominant medical model, one that promotes singular causes. A significant limiting factor for their development is the separation of these clinics from Russian Federation Ministry of Healthcare nomenclature. Pain medicine is not included in the educational standard for the doctors' training in Russia. Nowadays, students study the problem of pain in the course of physiology, pathophysiology, neuroscience, and anesthesiology. Postgraduate education in several universities includes training courses on pain syndromes and their treatment. The most comprehensive training is conducted in I.M. Sechenov First Moscow State Medical University, but it is still not structured.

The RASP promotes the organization and the development of medical centres, specialized departments, laboratories, and surgeries for pain syndromes treatment. Moreover, RASP promotes the specialists' training and advanced training, as well as assisting in scientific research, inventions, and innovations implementation.

Innovations

RASP has published a quarterly scientific journal since 2004, which is now called the *Russian Journal of Pain*. The RASP executive board decided to supply a free newsletter with e-journal (pdf file) to RASP members. Apart from that, there is an open access to publications touching the scientific and clinical aspects of pain medicine on the RASP website: www.painrussia.ru.

Although pain medicine as such is as yet not recognized in Russia, RASP is trying to develop this direction of medicine. Currently, there is a widening search for organizational forms of Russian pain medicine system in many cities of the Russian Federation. Due to the efforts of doctors from many different specialties, there are now 40 units specializing in pain treatment in 17 Russian cities.

Today, there is a training system for specialists based on the course at I.M. Sechenov First Moscow State Medical University. The system involves an undergraduate stage, which includes the basic information considering pain medicine in terms of an elective course and a special 'pain school' for students; and a postgraduate stage, which includes interventional and multidisciplinary approachs in pain treatment.

Reference

Population of Russia census data (2005). Thirteenth Annual Demographic Report/Resp.

Chapter 2.27

San Marino

Daniele Battelli

Backgound information

San Marino Republic, formerly 'The Most Serene Republic of San Marino', is a small enclave in the centre-north of Italy, located between 'Emilia-Romagna' and 'Marche' regions. It is the third smallest country in Europe, but it is the most ancient still-living Republic in the world, since its foundation dates back to the year 301. It covers a landmass of only 61.19 sqaure kilometres and has a population of 33,086 (16,290 male; 16,796 female). Some 15.2% of the population is under the age of 14, 64% are between the ages of 14–65, and 18.8% are over 65. The dominant language spoke is Italian. San Marino has one of the world's highest life expectancies: 80.7 years for men and 86.1 years for women born in 2016 (CIA World Factbook, 2016) (see Fig. 2.27.1).

The San Marino Pain Society became a member of EFIC in 2009. Currently there are 41 members representing the core specialties of Anaesthesiology, Gerontology, Neurology, Rehabilitation, Internal Medicine, Orthopaedics, Ob-Gyn, Reumathology, Psychology, and Nursing.

Healthcare system

Healthcare in San Marino is provided by a public health agency, namely 'Istituto per la Sicurezza Sociale' (ISS), founded in 1955 and structured on a 'Beveridge' universalistic model. Healthcare is provided free of charge to all residents, regardless of age, sex, race, and social status, through three territorial primary care centres run by general practitioners and primary care nurses, and a state hospital. Home care is provided by primary care centres for general chronic ilnesses and fragile patients, and by a private association for cancer patients who require assistance and who do not need hospitalization. A national health authority, under the National Health Ministry, is appointed for private and public health accreditation and healthcare plan development. Since 1994, an electronic health record has been introduced for the whole healthcare system and drug distribution, with a single and interoperable software for both GPs and hospital physicians.

Current pain workforce

The rules for physician's registration in San Marino Republic resemble Italian ones. To work as a pain physician a five-year Diploma in Anaesthesia, Intensive Care, and Pain Medicine is required, since this discipline is included into the anaesthesiological field of activity of the country's healthcare system. The San Marino Pain Unit is the referral point for pain medicine and for central venous catheter (CVC) management, both for

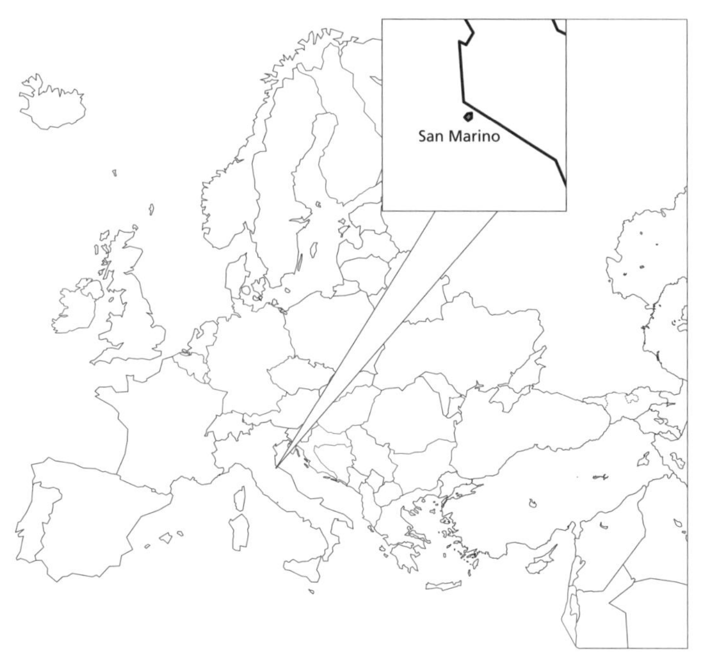

Fig. 2.27.1 Map of San Marino.

inpatients and outpatients, and consists of three anaesthesiology physicians and of five qualified nurses.

The pain unit also offers an ambulatory service for inpatients and outpatients, an operating room (OR) for interventional pain procedures, and a service for CVC and PICC (peripheral-inserted central catheter) insertion and management. Outpatient and inpatient pain pathways involves Rheumathology, Oncology, Orthopaedics, Neurology, Neurosurgery, Physical Medicine, and Psychology consultations, building a network with more than 20 physicians and 20 GPs who constantly interact for the management of acute and chronic pain patients.

Being a small country with a universal and highly digitized healthcare system, in the last 10 years a great emphasis has been put on drug prescription monitoring and retrospective analyses regarding analgesic drugs and their related clinical implications on the population. The results of that analyses have been presented to the Societal Impact of Pain Symposium in 2012 (SIP, 2012) and published on indexed papers (Battelli *et al.*, 2015).

Challenges and opportunities to the future development of pain services

Pain medicine in a small country setting poses peculiar challenges and opportunities. One of the main values for our healthcare system is to mantain an accessible and high-quality care to all citizens, and for that reason for the current year a performance indicator has been estabilished in our country, granting less than 15 days waiting time to obtain a first pain physician clinical evaluation for outpatients. One of the biggest issues for our country is to bring high-quality assistance for pain patients in the home care setting. A lot of work has been carried out with the local association of cancer patients, for pain and palliative care, in the past 10 years. Strong interaction between pain units and primary home care services will be directed to all non-cancer chronic pain patients in the future.

A third, but not less important, issue will be to manage the national supply of opioid medications. Opioid legal governance is under complex rulings between the local agencies and the Italian Ministry of Health.

Innovations

The San Marino Republic looked positively at the scientific interest surrounding the clinical uses of cannabinoid-derivative drugs. In 2016, a national plan for the establishment of a whole-cycle production of cannabinoid drugs was approved by the government, which will be put into practice in the coming years.

References

Battelli, D., Riccardi, R., Piscaglia, A. C., *et al.* (2015). Analgesic, antiulcer, antithrombotic drugs and organ damage: a population-based case-control study. *Minerva Med*, **106**, 323–31.

Central Intelligence Agency (CIA) World Factbook (2016). Available at: https://www.cia.gov/library/publications/the-world-factbook/geos/au.html [Online].

Societal Impact of Pain (SIP) (2012). Symposium: 6. Workshop 2012. Available at https://www.sip-platform.eu/events/sip-2012/programme/workshop-6.html [Online].

Chapter 2.28

Serbia

Miroslava Pjevic

Background information

Serbia is in the Balkan preninsula bordered by Albania, Bosnia and Herzegovina, Bulgaria, Croatia, Hungary, Macedonia, Montenegro, and Romania (see Fig. 2.28.1). It has a population of approximately seven million people. The population of Serbia is ageing and shrinking, and the average age is currently 41.1 years. The largest city in Serbia is Belgrade and the second largest is Novi Sad, with a population of about 300,000. Demographic transitioning to an older population is ongoing, with almost 17% of the Serbian population now above the age of 65 (Lukic, 2013). Novi Sad has always been a multiethnic town with a Serbian majority and Hungarian, Slovak, Croat, Rusyn, Romanian, Montenegrin, Muslim, Jewish, and other minorities. The history of this region is long and interesting, dating from before the Romans. On the Petrovaradin Hill, the Romans built a keep, which was later reconstructed by Hungarians, and maintained by the Turks. After the Turks were banished in the late seventeenth century, the Austrians erected a bridge-head, facing the fortress on the left bank of the Danube. The fortress was soon surrounded by a settlement populated by soldiers, craftsmen, and traders. When settlement expanded, its citizens, yearning for freedom, managed to buy it from the Empress Maria Theresa, who announced the proclamation of the 'free royal city' in 1748 and named it Novi Sad. In the nineteenth century, the city was the capital of Serbian culture, earning it the nickname 'Serbian Athens'. Today, Novi Sad is a modern European city, an industrial and financial centre, as well as a major cultural and educational hub.

Healthcare system

The healthcare system in Serbia is provided through a wide network of public healthcare institutions owned and controlled by the Ministry of Health. The system is founded on equity and solidarity with the idea of universal coverage for an extensive level of services (prevention, treatment, rehabilitation). The entire population has the right to use all services. Primary healthcare (level I) consists of healthcare centres (159), largely staffed by general practitioners, specialists (paediatricians, gynaecologists), nurses, and pharmacists. Secondary healthcare (level II) consists of general hospitals (41) and specialized hospitals (37). Tertiary healthcare (level III) includes clinical centres (4), medical centres (5), institutes, and clinics. Pain services in Serbian healthcare are insufficient and provided only through aproximately 30 outpatient pain units (levels II and III).

According to the Institute of Public Health of Serbia (2010), malignant disease occurences are growing by 3–5% per annum. This was a reason to establish the National Palliative Care Strategy, adopted by the Government in 2009. Palliative care

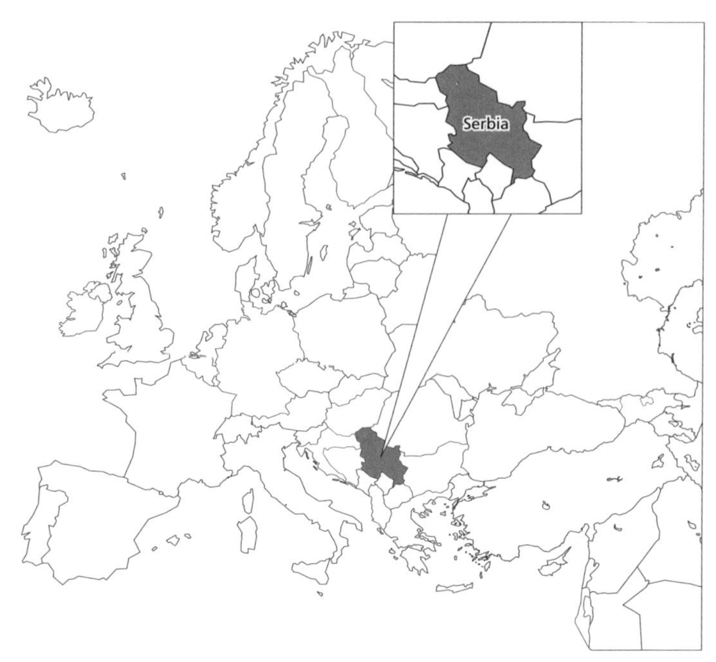

Fig. 2.28.1 Map of Serbia.

has been integrated into healthcare services, resulting with positive changes in cancer pain management. However, chronic non-cancer pain management is still not adequately incorporated into healthcare.

The health financing policy is an important and integral part of healthcare, but as a country in transition, Serbia faces difficulties in financing its health system. The most important source of public health system financing is the Republic Health Insurance Fund (RHIF). It collects revenues from obligatory insurance, various budgetary sources, funds from the national Pension Fund, and the Ministry of Finance Fund, among others (Stosic and Karanovic, 2014). The total health expenditure as a percentage of GDP was last measured at 10.60 in 2013.

The law also provides for private practice which, however, may be pursued exclusively by way of private funds. The private healthcare services are on the rise mainly employing consultants from the public sector on a temporary basis. The private healthcare sector is not included in the public funding scheme, but is more or less based on out-of-pocket payments, charitable donations, and direct service payments by private corporations. Within the context of European integration and public administration reforms, the introduction of the capitation system into primary healthcare in 2012 was a major payment reform recommended by the World Bank. Further, the concept of 'chosen doctors' esentially means that doctors should be paid relative to the number of patients, enabling possibly better coordination between different levels of care and better promotion of health and preventive services. Hospital payment reform is modelled by the diagnosis-related groups (DRGs) (Mathauer and Wittenbecher, 2012) as a kind of case-based payment (hospitals are basically paid the average cost for a case). The implementation of these two mechanisms should make the healthcare service more efficient, but needs an adequate monitoring system which imposes additional costs.

Current pain workforce

The primary care physician first encounters the chronic pain patient and makes an initial diagnosis and treatment within the primary care setting (Johnson *et al.*, 2013). Unfortunately, non-steroidal anti-inflammatory drugs (NSAIDs) are mostly the first therapeutic choice for all types of pain. Diclofenac is still one of the top 10 most prescribed drugs. Most primary pain care providers do not consider themselves prepared for practising pain management, owing to a lack of basic education. A gap in knowledge and reluctance to use opioids due to opiophobia, inadequate communication between physicians, nurses, and patients, are barriers of primary care settings. According to the International Narcotics Control Board, morphine consumption in Serbia in 2006 was 12.81 morphine equivalents per capita (mEq) relative to166 mEq as the adequate treatment of all pain conditions. Due to its low per capita morphine consumption, Serbia was selected as one of the countries to participate in the Access to Opioid Medication in Europe (ATOME) project. In 2010, the adequacy of opioid analgesic consumption had improved, increasing to 40.06 mEq per capita consumption of opioid analgesics, relative to 285.61 mEq per capita as the adequate amount (Radbruch *et al.*, 2014).

Primary care physicians collaborate with specialists by referring pain patients. Anaesthesiologists are the most skilled and dedicated specialists involved in pain treatment based on pharmacotherapy and anaesthetic techniques. Neurologists and Physical and Rehabilitation Medicine specialists are also involved in pain care in Serbia. Subspeciality and certification in pain medicine started from 2013/2014 school year at the Medical Faculty, University of Belgrade and 2014/2015 at the Medical Faculty, University of Novi Sad. Currently, there are only a few pain specialists. In addition, improving education is particularly important for primary care providers because of their key role in pain management, but a pain medicine subspeciality is not provided for them. Establishing Pain Medicine as a taught subject to the undergraduate medical school and nursing college curricula at the Faculty of Medicine, University of Novi Sad in 2010 was a good educational step towards change. Continuing medical education programmes, courses, symposiums, and workshops on chronic non-cancer and cancer pain have been launched by the Serbian Association of Pain Research and Treatment (SAPRT) from 2007. Additional resources for improvements in pain include: National Palliative Care Guidelines; National Cancer Pain Guidelines; Opioid Guidelines in Cancer Pain; *Pharmacotherapy of Cancer Pain* (textbook 2007); brochures on fear of opioids for healthcare professionals (HCPs), patients and families, supported by an IASP grant (2009); *Treatment of Chronic Pain in Adults* (e-learning publication-Interactive CD-R), supported by EFIC grant (2010) (Bošnjak, Beleslin, Vučković-Dekić 2007; Bošnjak, Šušnjar, Dimitrijević 2009; Milićević *et al.*, 2004; Nacionalni vodic dobre klinicke prakse za dijagnostikovanje i lecenje hronicnog bola maligne etiologije 2013; Pjevic 2010).

The Serbian Association of Pain Research and Treatment was established in Novi Sad in 2006 with a pioneering mission under the leadership of Professor Miroslava Pjevic, anaesthesiologist at the Clinical Center of Vojvodina in Novi Sad. SAPRT joined EFIC on 8 March 2007. There are over a hundred Chapter members with most specialists being anaesthesiologists and physical medicine and rehabilitation physicians.

Further to this, active cooperation is ongoing with international (EFIC, IASP) and EFIC Chapter organizations (SZZB, HDLB, APTBH, DGSS), and professional links have been made with global pain leaders (S. Erdine, Turkey; R. D. Treede, Germany; A. Kopf, Germany; N. Krcevski Skvarc, Slovenia; E. Kalso, Finland; B. Morlion, Belgium; C. Wells, United Kingdom; M. Schafer, Germany). Although the SAPRT recognizes the burden of pain on society in terms of individual suffering and social and economic costs, relieving pain is still not a national priority. A decade after SAPRT was established was not long enough to provide a national epidemiological study on chronic pain, so the true diagnosis of the chronic pain problem was not yet identified in Serbia. Two Serbian surveys on pain were conducted: a survey on pain intensity in cancer pain patients (2007, 2008) and a survey on cancer pain therapy (2012). In 2013, in a survey on fear of opioids, 88% of physicians were found to be reluctant to prescribe opioids and only 7% of patients did not object when morphine was suggested for pain relief. Physicians' reluctance was due to a fear of respiratory depression, and patients' fear related to concerns about tolerance, adverse effects, and dependence (Radbruch *et al.*, 2014). A survey on neuropathic pain treatment in primary care (SAPRT, 2010) and a survey on efficacy of chronic pain treatment in everyday practice (Boricic *et al.*, 2013) confirmed that NSAIDs are mostly used. Although the majority of co-analgesics are available, carbamazepine was mostly prescribed in neuropathic pain patients, because it is a fully reimbursed medication. Reimbursement restrictions and costs of other co-analgesics have been identified as a barrier to equal access and the right to access an appropriate management for neuropathic pain. Elimination of these barriers and optimization of healthcare outcomes are possible, not only by efforts of professional organizations such as SAPRT, but also by raising the government's awareness and actions on the behalf of governmental agencies and funders.

Challenges and opportunities to the future development of pain services

The SAPRT has been continuing efforts to adapt pain managament system to the national reality and overcome pain underdiagnosis and undertreatment. The SAPRT did much to increase awareness and education among HCPs, general public, healthcare authorities, and policymakers. In addition, SAPRT has endorsed the European platform 'Societal Impact of Pain' (SIP) created in 2010. However, SAPRT dedicated much time to opiophobia and elimination of the low morphine consumption problem, while recognizing that pain treatment has never been, nor should ever be, synonymous with opioid therapy. Today it is important to identify chronic pain as one of the national priorities and scope chronic pain by studying its epidemiology in Serbia. These data are needed to help shape ongoing efforts. Establishing the National Pain Strategy and following an action plan against pain would provide more training, pain services, pain specialists, and adequate monitoring. Pain medicine needs to be incorporated into national healthcare services. All these actions are health quality improvement measures and pain control is an important part of quality improvement.

Innovations

Significant progress has been made, but much work remains, as chronic pain is the most common reason people seek medical help, a major reason for taking medication, a major cause of disability, and a key factor in quality of life and productivity. The

National Pain Strategy would be a potential driver not only in pain care, but in pain prevention, education, and research. Interdisciplinary programmes for pain management through specialized centres such as an interdisciplinary centres with evidence-based, interdisciplinary management for individuals with complex chronic low back pain is a primer of innovative practice in the organization of pain care. Improving education is important for primary care physicians, although they are not covered by the pain medicine subspecialization. A further goal is to ensure all healthcare providers, including pharmacists, are enrolled in continuing pain education programmes, as well as the curricula of medical schools and nursing colleges. The Serbian economy is still developing and pain-related research is in short supply. Biological and psychological research need to be advanced to help transition effective treatments from research into practice.

References

Boricic, K., Vasic, M., & Grozdanov, M. (2013). *Rezultati istraživanja zdravlja stanovništva Srbije, 2013 godina*. Belgrade, Serbia.

Bošnjak, S., Beleslin, D., & Vučković-Dekić, Lj. (2007). *Farmakoterapija kancerskog bola. Monografije naučnih skupova AMN SLD. Serija B*, **1** (1), 1–245.

Bošnjak, S., Šušnjar, S., & Dimitrijević, J. (2009). *Institut za onkologiju i radiologiju Srbije: Centar za razvoj palijativnog zbrinjavanja. Opiofobija: Šta plaši zdravstvene radnike? Ministarstvo zdravlja Republike Srbije*. Beograd.

Institute of Public Health of Serbia (2010). 'Dr. Milan Jovanović—Batut'. Cancer incidence and mortality in Central Serbia 2008. Report, no. 10. Belgrade, Serbia: Cancer Registry of Central Serbia.

Johnson, M., Collet, B., & Castro-Lopes, J. M. (2013). The challenges of pain management in primary care: a pan-European survey. *J Pain Res*, **6**, 393–401.

Lukic, V. (2013). Population trends in Serbia and the implications for settlement system. *Forum Geografic*, **12**, 67–74.

Mathauer, I. & Wittenbecher, F. (2012). *DRG-based payment systems in low an middle-income countries: Implementation experiences and challenges*. Geneva, Switzerland: WHO.

Milićević, N., Bošnjak, S., Gutović, J., & Nalić, D. (eds) (2004). *Palijativno zbrinjavanje onkoloških bolesnika: nacionalni vodič za lekare u primarnoj zdravstvenoj zaštiti* (Palliative care of cancer patients: national clinical practice guideline) 1.izd. Beograd: Medicinski fakultet Univerziteta u Beogradu.

Nacionalni vodic dobre klinicke prakse za dijagnostikovanje i lecenje hronicnog bola maligne etiologije (2013). Klinicki vodic 22/13. Beograd, Republicka strucna komisija za izradu i implementaciju vodica dobre klinicke prakse, Ministarstvo zdravlja Republike Srbije.

Pjevic, M. urednik (2010). *Lecenje hronicnog bola kod odraslih (Interaktivni CD-R), edicija praktikum: 65*. Novi Sad: Medicinski fakultet Univerziteta u Novom Sadu (Supported by EFIC grant).

Radbruch, L., Junger, S., Payne, S., & Scholten, W. (2014). *Access to Opioid Medication in Europe (ATOME). Report and recommendations to the Ministry of Health*. Bonn, Germany: Pallia Med Verlag.

Serbian Pain Association of Pain Research and Treatment (SAPRT) (2010). *Results of a Survey on Physicians' Experiences in Treating Neuropathic Pain*. Novi Sad, Serbia: SAPRT.

Stosic, S. & Karanovic, N. (2014). Health care economics in Serbia: Current problems and changes. *Vojnosanit Pregl*, **71**, 1055–61.

Chapter 2.29

Slovakia

Marta Kulichová

Background information

The Slovak Republic is the geographical centre of Europe, and is usually known as Slovakia (see Fig. 2.29.1). The republic was established on 1 January 1993 after Czechoslovakia split into two countries: Czech Republic and Slovakia. The political system in both countries is a parliamentary democracy and the first day of the year is the national holiday of the new democracy.

Slovakia is a landlocked country and is surrounded by five neighbours: on the west lies the Czech Republic and Austria, to the north is Poland, east is the Ukraine, and in the south is Hungary. It has a territory of 49,000 square kilometres which is is divided into 8 large regions and 79 smaller counties. Slovakia has a population of 5.4 million (51% female) and an average population density of 110 people per square kilometre. The population growth rate is 0.01% (2016 est.). The life expectancy at birth in the total population is 77.1 years (73.5 years for men and 80.9 years for women). The birth rate is 1.4. Most inhabitants live in cities and towns (55%). The dominant ethnicity is Slovak (80.7%), others are Hungarian (8.5%), Roma (2%), and unspecified 8.8%. The official language is Slovak. Some 87% of the population have religious beliefs and most of them (69%) belong to the Roman Catholic Church. Other religions include: Lutherans (6.9%), Greek Catholics (4.1%), Protestant Reformers (2.0%), and Orthodox Church (0.9%).

Slovakia is a high-income advanced economy with a very high Human Development Index, a very high standard of living, and as a society it performs favourably in measures of civil liberties, press freedom, Internet freedom, democratic governance, and peacefulness. The country maintains a combination of market economy with universal healthcare and a comprehensive social security system. The country joined the European Union in 2004 and the Eurozone on 1 January 2009. Slovakia is also a member of the Schengen Area, NATO, the United Nations, the OECD, and the Council of Europe. The Slovak economy is one of the fastest growing economies in Europe and third fastest in the Eurozone. Although regional income inequality is high, 90% of citizens own their homes. In 2016, Slovak citizens had visa-free or visa-on-arrival access to 165 countries and territories, ranking the Slovak passport eleventh in the world. Slovakia is the world's biggest per-capita car producer with a total of 1,040,000 cars manufactured in the country in 2016 alone. The car industry represents 43% of Slovakia's industrial output, and a quarter of its exports (Slovak Republic, 2016; IndexMundi, 2016).

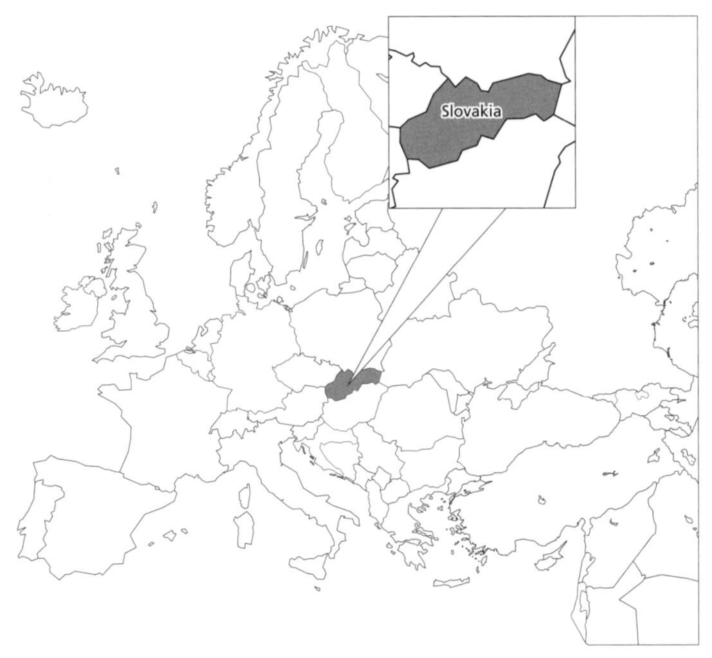

Fig. 2.29.1 Map of Slovakia.

Healthcare system

The healthcare system in Slovakia is administered by the Ministry of Health. There are state and private healthcare providers. Slovakia has 92 hospitals, of which 3 are university hospitals and 44 are state hospitals. The hospital bed density is 6 beds/1,000 people. There are five health insurance companies responsible for the collection of the health insurance contributions and for reimbursements. The General Health Insurance Company covers the majority of the population. Most medical services in Slovakia are free at the point of delivery for those who qualify, but some services are only subsidized and citizens must pay part of the cost. Co-payments exist for some prescription drugs, some dental treatment, and medical devices. An initial medical examination in case of an illness is provided by state or private practitioners. Every person has the right to choose a general practitioner who usually provides basic healthcare and can refer a patient to an appropriate specialist for futher medical examination or treatment. Appointments with a doctor and referrals to a consultant are free. Prescription medicine for those who suffer from chronic illness or those who belong to the medically vulnerable groups (e.g. pregnant women, war veterans, diabetics, and tuberculosis patients) are exempt from all charges. Drugs are divided into three groups, with the first category consisting of essential drugs, which are fully reimbursed by the insurance companies. The second category are partially subsidized, and the third group receives no subsidy at all.

Current pain workforce

The Slovak Society for the Study and Treatment of Pain (SSSTP) was founded in 1993, following the split of the Czechoslovak Federation. At this time, it became a member 'in formation' of IASP. The society did not become a full member of IASP until the Congress of IASP held in Vienna in 1999. SSSTP became a member of EFIC from its first meeting, held in Halle, in 1994. The SSSTP has 164 members, mostly anaethesiologists. SSSTP covers three sections: palliative medicine (36 members), interventional pain therapy (25 members), and section algesiological sisters, or pain nurses (36 members).

Doctor Stanislav Fabuš opened the first pain clinic in Martin, Slovakia on 1 March 1984. He was the first person to establish Slovakian pain therapy as an individual medical field. In Slovakia, Dr Fabuš is considered the equivalent to the United States pain specialist, J. J. Bonica, founder of IASP, and he is the doyen of Slovak pain therapy, standing behind every early development and propagation in the field. He was the head of the Department of Anaesthesiology at Martin Faculty Hospital. Starting this first pain clinic was an unprecedented step as there were no domestic examples, no experience, and no known consumer demand. Pain was regarded as a symptom of other diseases and as such was addressed by physicians of various specialties with a prescription of painkillers. The Slovak Society for Study and Treatment of Pain was established in Martin on 26 March 1993 following the split of the Czechoslovak Federation. At that time in Martin, the first Slovak meeting on pain was held, starting the tradition of annual national congresses on pain therapy entitled 'Slovak Dialogues on Pain'.

Slovak representatives attended the 5th World Congress of IASP held in Paris in August 1993, which initiated the establishment of EFIC. The SSSTP, represented by Marta Kulichová, became an associate member of this association on its meeting held in Halle in 1994. However, the society did not become a full member of IASP until the Congress of IASP held in Vienna in 1999. The 5th Slovak Dialogues on Pain were held in Prešov in 1997 and were attended by two of the most important representatives of World and European pain therapy—the then President of IASP Professor J. M. Besson from Paris and the President of EFIC, Professor M. Zimmermann from Heidelberg. To date, these have been the most prominent specialists that ever attended our congresses. Combined meetings have been held with the Czech IASP Chapter annually since 2000, known as the Czechoslovak Dialogues on Pain. This conference occurs alternately in the Czech and Slovak Republics and has become the leading and most prestigious scientific conference in the area.

Challenges and opportunities to the future development of pain services

Formalization of a specialty in pain therapy has been attempted since 1992. We have repeatedly asked the Ministry of Health to issue methodical guidelines on the development of the network of pain therapy centres. Our suggestions were regarded as interesting, but were initially unacceptable during this problematic period of time because pain specialization then did not exist anywhere in Europe. However, subsequently, we managed to gain support of the foremost specialist in Anaesthesiology and Intensive Medicine (AIM), Milan Májek, and thanks to his recommendation and support the concept of pain therapy was approved on 5 March 1998. The approval of the Specialty Order on Further Education of the Physician was delayed until 2003. This constituted pain therapy as an independent subspecialty of AIM, Neurology, Internal Medicine, and Paediatrics.

Official postgraduate education was organized in 1991 at the Department of AIM of the University Hospital in Martin. In December 2003, the AIM department of the Slovak Postgraduate University in Bratislava allowed the first physicians to complete their postgraduate education in pain therapy: Attestation in Pain Medicine. This was an unprecedented achievement even from a European perspective and education in pain treatment; more than 80 persons have now graduated in pain medicine. The requirement for enrolment in Pain Medicine is an attained specialization in the following branches of medicine: Anaesthesiology and Intensive Care, Paediatrics, Internal Medicine, Neurology, Clinical Oncology, or Orthopaedics. Length of training is a minimum of three years. The training consists of theoretical and practical parts, 36 months practice in the workplace for the treatment of pain, including 12 weeks' stay at accredited workplaces in pain treatment. Specialized study is completed after passing the specialized final exam.

Innovations

In 2005, we successfully managed to establish a subspecialty of Pain Therapy in Banska Bystrica and we now have two associated accredited educational facilities in Banska Bystrica and Martin. Medical student education in pain therapy has been difficult, because the deans of our medical schools were not interested in teaching pain therapy as an individual subject. Jessenius Faculty of Medicine in Martin offered 'Palliative Medicine and Pain Therapy' as an optional subject during the ninth semester of their Medical University from 1999 to 2013. Sadly, this has now ceased. Nevertheless, in Slovakia we have a well-functioning Slovak Society for the Study of Pain and are a regular member of EFIC and IASP. Every year we organize the international Czechoslovak Dialogues on Pain in the Slovak or Czech Republic—the last one was held this year in Bratislava with the attendance of the European Pain Federation president Dr Chris Wells. We have established a network of 43 pain clinics and have published two books in the Slovak language: *Algesiology*, by Marta Kulichová in 2005, and *The Pathophysiology of Pain* by Igor Martuliak in 2014, from which our doctors have gained information for their attestation.

There are many examples of innovative practice from both individual practitioners and from teams. One example of leadership in improving practice in pain management was the knowledge translation from the optimal acute pain services, developed at the University Hospital in Martin, and applied nationally across hospitals in Slovakia. Further, we have been investing in interventional pain treatments as part of the basic provision of pain treatment in Slovakia.

At present the SSSTP is active, dynamic, and ready to accept new challenges. We consider it a useful model with relevant learnings that could be extended to other pain societies, particularly from Eastern Europe, and we look forward to sharing our learning and also learning from others.

References

IndexMundi (2016). Slovakia Factbook Demographics. Available at: http://www.indexmundi.com/slovakia/#Demographics [Online].

Slovak Republic (2016). *Guide to Slovakia*. Available at: http://www.slovak-republic.org [Online].

Chapter 2.30

Slovenia

Marija Cesar Komar, Nevenka Krčevski-Škvarč, and Gorazd Požlep

Background information

Slovenia has a population of two million people. It has been an independent nation since 1991, and borders Italy, Austria, Hungary, and Croatia. The main language spoken is Slovenian. The majority of Slovenia's population is Slovene (83%) (Census, 2002) and predominantly Roman Catholic (Fig. 2.30.1). The country has been facing pronounced population ageing, ascribable to a low birth rate and increased life expectancy. In 2014 females can expect to live 83.5 years and males to 77.6 years (Republic of Slovenia Statistical Office RS, 2016). The total dependency ratio of population is 48.7% (CIA, 2015).

The Slovenian Association for Pain Management—Slovensko združenje za zdravljenje bolečine (SZZB)—was founded in 1996 on the initiative of Nevenka Krčevski Škvarč, who collected 41 pain medicine practitioners and supporters. SZZB became an IASP Chapter and a member of EFIC in 1997. This was announced at the EFIC Congress Pain in Europe II in Barcelona. Since then, membership has grown to 102 registered members. Members are mainly anesthesiologists (about three-quarters), followed by physical therapy specialists, neurologists, general surgeons, family physicians, psychologists, emergency medicine doctors, a neurosurgeon, and a paediatrician.

Healthcare system

The healthcare system in Slovenia is a public service provided through the public health service network. This network also includes other institutions, private physicians, and other private service providers on the basis of concession. The system of health insurance is divided into compulsory, voluntary, and additional coverage for health insurance, and insurance for services that are not a constituent part of compulsory insurance. Compulsory health insurance is mandatory for all citizens and does not cover all costs of treatment except for children, schoolchildren, and for certain illnesses and conditions.

Primary healthcare services are organized locally, such that they are equally accessible to all people without discrimination. Very few pain units are situated at primary healthcare services. Slovenia has organized secondary healthcare services at hospitals locally also and a few institutions of tertiary healthcare level. Each hospital and institution has organized pain units and centres.

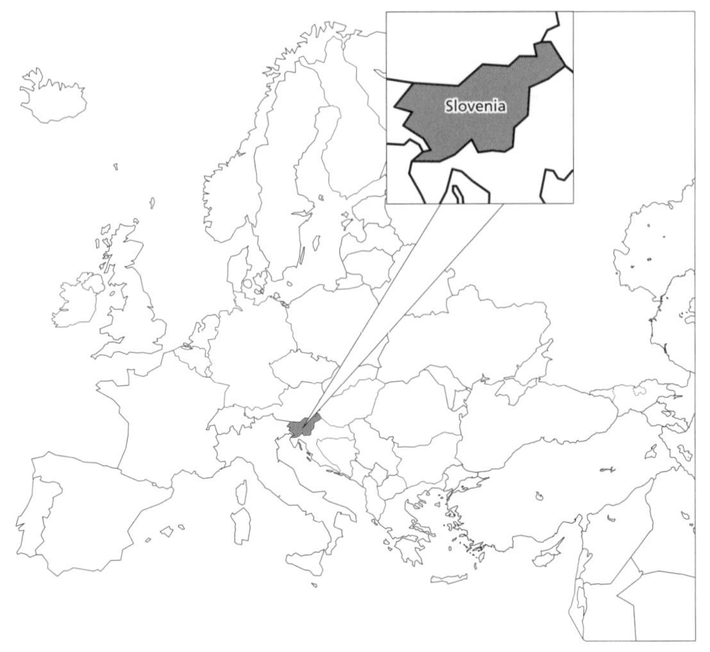

Fig. 2.30.1 Map of Slovenia.
Copyright © Pyty/Shutterstock.com.

Current pain workforce

Slovenia has about 5,700 active physicians; of them about 1,100 are family physicians. In the healthcare system there is no pain management specialism, but about 40 physicians have acquired knowledge in pain management and as many for palliative care. Pain management is traditionally practised by anesthesiologists, and by physical medicine and neurology specialists. The problem of chronic pain in Slovenia is well recognized. The main force in the development of pain medicine is the SZZB. The association takes responsibility for pain medicine education, and recognizes the need for a specialty in the field, as well as the need to share common knowledge in pain management. We organize the annual educational Seminars on Pain, and this year will be the nineteenth. Traditionally we also organize an interdisciplinary scientific meeting devoted to the field of pain medicine, which was recently dedicated to the European Year against Pain.

Areas of innovation and challenge

Our scientific meetings are aimed to meet the needs of all healthcare professionals working in pain, and are updated and enriched with the participation of prominent domestic and foreign lecturers from Europe and worldwide. We held our first Pain Congress in 2009. Written materials were published for all meetings; the bibliography consists of 28 publications. SZZB's very important achievements include the following publications (see Cesar-Komar 2006, 2007, 2008, 2009; Krčevski Škvarč *et al.*, 1997, 2007; Lahajnar *et al.*, 2008, 2009, 2015; Pirc *et al.*, 2007):

- Survey on postoperative pain (1997).
- Survey of chronic pain in Slovenia (2007).
- Guidelines for opioid use in patients with chronic non-malignant pain (2007 and will be renewed in 2017).
- Guidelines for cancer pain treatment (2008, 2010, 2015).
- The SZZB plays an active part in EFIC's initiative, 'Societal Impact of Pain'. We presented the problem and the proposals for improvement in Slovenian Parliament in the year 2011. The battle for national policy for pain management is still present.
- The experts from SZZB have been collaborating with the Slovenian Ministry of Health in the production of the National Plan for Palliative Care, which was accepted in 2010.
- In 2012 we succeeded in introducing pain medicine as a complementary subject to the undergraduate curriculum in our faculties of Medicine.

We have also translated the educational material for the 'Change Pain' courses and have provided lectures for general practitioners. It has been a great privilege and honour for the SZZB to organize the biannual European Pain Federation EFIC School for Cancer Pain and Palliative Care in Maribor since 2015, an event that is proving to be very well-received, providing much needed access to expertise, training, knowledge, and development.

Challenges and opportunities to the future development of pain services

The major challenges in the development of existing pain units are to establish centres with interdisciplinary staff. Further, we have three centres where invasive neuromodulation is taking place, yet have no one pain clinic in the country. It seems essential to establish two in the university settings in Slovenia, which also fit geographically to promote adequate and optimal management for the patients suffering with pain.

The next challenge is to introduce the subject of pain medicine as mandatory in all medical schools and for students to start in postgraduate education with the aim of reaching the level of Pain Medicine Specialist. In the near future, we will try to achieve a European Pain Federation EFIC Pain Diploma for junior colleagues.

Innovations

To date, we have been able to take part in international studies phase III treatment development and to perform our own clinical trial, and we will continue with our efforts to improve pain research.

We plan to produce more guidelines for pain management, to renew the existing ones, and to repeat and perform more epidemiological studies to better establish an accurate picture of the current burden of pain and treatment needs.

To achieve these goals, we understand the need to be more active in medical politics nationally. Finally, but importantly, we will continue to take every opportunity to promote pain medicine generally, to promote our pain association and grow its membership, and attract all specialties in the field of medicine and cooperating professions.

References

Census (2002). Population by ethnic affiliation, Slovenia, Census 1953, 1961, 1971, 1981, 1991, and 2002. Statistical Office of the Republic of Slovenia. Available at: http://www.stat.si/popis2002/en/rezultati/rezultati_red.asp?ter=SLO&st=7 [Online].

Cesar-Komar, M. (ur.) & Krčevski-Škvarč, N. (ur.) (2006). *Paliativna medicina: zbornik predavanj*, 10. Seminar o bolečini z mednarodno udeležbo, Maribor, 9. in 10. junij 2006. Maribor: SZZB—Slovensko združenje za zdravljenje bolečine, str. 11–16. Available at: https://plus.si.cobiss.net/opac7/bib/21465049?lang=sl [Online].

Cesar-Komar, M. (ur.), Pirc, J. (ur.), & Kožar, E. (ur.) (2007). *Akutna bolečina: zbornik predavanj*. Maribor: SZZB—Slovensko združenje za zdravljenje bolečine, 126 str., ilustr. ISBN 978-961-91825-1-2. Available at: https://plus.si.cobiss.net/opac7/bib/233128704?lang=sl [Online].

Cesar-Komar, M. (ur.) (2008). *Pooperacijska bolečina, Zbornik predavanj*. Maribor: SZZB—Slovensko Združenje za zdravljenje bolečine, 156 str. ISBN 978-961-91825-2-9. Available at: http://www.worldcat.org/title/pooperacijska-bolecina-zbornik/oclc/449403696 [Online].

Cesar-Komar, M. (ur.), Rodi, Z. (ur.), & Pirc, J. (ur.) (2009). 1. kongres Slovenskega združenja za zdravljenje bolečine z mednarodno udeležbo s pridruženim Simpozijem o klinični nevrofiziologiji bolečine in s 25. predavanjem v spomin dr. Janeza Faganela. *Program in zbornik prispevkov*. Ljubljana: Sekcija za klinično nevrofiziologijo Slovenskega zdravniškega društva, 172 str., ilustr. ISBN 978-961-6526-31-9. Available at: https://plus.si.cobiss.net/opac7/bib/247415040?lang=sl [Online].

Central Intelligence Agency (CIA) (2015). The World Factbook, Dependency Ratios Slovenia. Available at: https://www.cia.gov/library/publications/the-world-factbook/fields/2261.html [Online].

Krčevski Škvarč, N., Pečan, M., Godec, M., Stare, J., & Kamenik, M. (1997). Pacientova pričakovanja in izkušnje z akutno postoperativno bolečino: rezultati ankete "Bolečina po operaciji": The patient's expectations and experiences with acute postoperative pain: results of inquiry Pain after surgery. *Zdravniški Vestnik*, **66**(2), 61–4.

Krčevski Škvarč, N., Godec, M., Cesar Komar, M., Lahajnar, S., Pirc, J., Salihovič, M., Šarman, M., Vrabl, Ž., & Zupančič, M. (2007). Usmeritve za uporabo opioidov pri bolnikih s kronično bolečino, ki ni posledica rakave bolezni: Slovensko združenje za zdravljenje bolečine, delovna skupina = Guidance for opioid use in patients with chronic noncancer pain: Slovenian association for pain management working group. *Zdravniški Vestnik*, **76**(6), 381–7.

Lahajnar, S., Krčevski Škvarč, N., Stepanovič, A., & Čufer, T. (2008) Usmeritve za zdravljenje bolečine pri opdraslem bolniku z rakom = Guidance for cancer pain treatment in adult patients. *Zdravniški Vestnik*, **77**(1), 7–12.

Lahajnar, S., Krčevski Škvarč, N., Stepanovič, A., & Čufer, T. (2009). Priporočila za zdravljenje bolečine pri odraslem bolniku z rakom. 2. izdaja, Ljubljana. ISBN 9768-961-91470-4-7.

Lahajnar, S., Krčevski Škvarč, N., Stepanovič, A., & Čufar, T. (2015). Priporočoila za zdravljenje bolečine pri odraslem bolniku z rakom. 3 izdaja, Maribor. ISBN 978-961-91825-5-0.

Pirc, J., Cesar-Komar, M., & Bizilj, S. (2007). Kronična bolečine v Sloveniji: poročilo o prevalenci kronične bolečine in primerjava z evropskimi podatki. SZZB.

Republic of Slovenia Statistical Office RS, Population Demographics (2016). Available at: http://pxweb.stat.si/pxweb/Database/Demographics/Demographics.asp [Online].

Chapter 2.31

Spain

Rafael Galvez Mateos and
Juan Perez Cajaraville

Background information

Spain has a population of over 46 million people, 75% of whom live in the cities (Fig. 2.31.1). The population is growing, last year at 0.02%. The total population is currently 46,468,102, of which 51% are women. 4.39 million are foreign nationals. Most of the population (69%) are aged between 15–64 years, and 14.4% are aged 0–14 years, and 16.5% are over the age of 65. The infant mortality rate is currently 3.37 deaths per 1,000 live births, and life expectancy at birth in Spain is second in Europe and fourth worldwide (United Nations, 2015).

There are five co-official languages spoken in Spain (Catalan, Valencian, Galician, Basque, and Aranese) and four unofficial languages (Austrian, Aragonese, Arabic, and Berber). The most common language is Spanish (with 95% native).

Healthcare system

Healthcare in Spain is the responsibility of all of the 17 autonomous communities into which the nation is divided. Spain has a public and practically free national healthcare system, although patients co-finance part of the medication cost according to their purchasing power. The transfer of responsibilities to the autonomous communities means that each can enact its own legislation on healthcare. Thus, some communities are more advanced than others in the provision of technology for pain treatments, although patients can be referred to another community if the specific analgesic technology required is not available in their own.

Current pain workforce

There are around 191 pain units in Spain, including both the public and private healthcare system. The first unit was established in 1973 by Dr Madrid Arias in the Doce de Octubre Hospital in Madrid. Pain units are categorized as level 1, level 2, or level 3, in accordance with Ministry of Health standards and recommendations, considering the number of professionals, beds available, and analgesic technology. Most pain units in Spain are level 2, and very few are level 3. Almost all units are led by anaesthesiologists, with a few being run by neurosurgeons and the rest by other healthcare professionals. Alongside the public healthcare system, there is a network of private hospitals and clinics in most Spanish cities, where the higher level private centres have pain units.

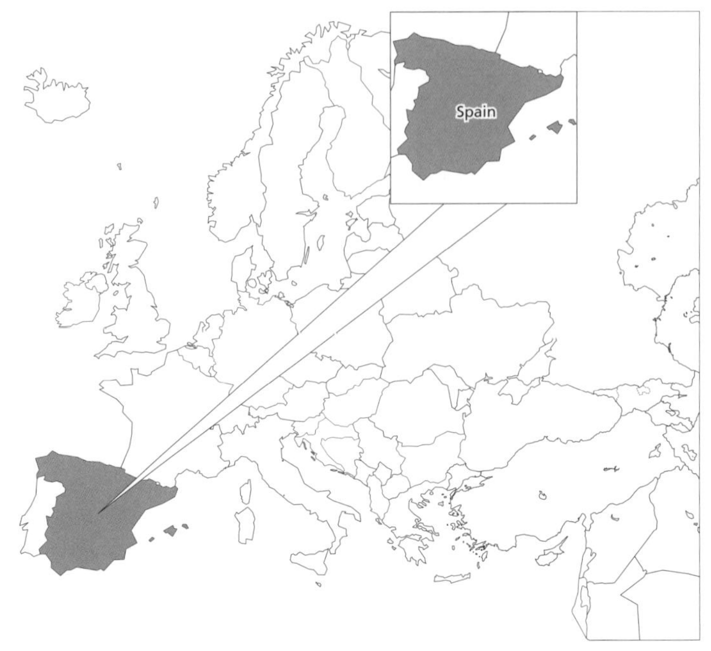

Fig. 2.31.1 Map of Spain.

Most professionals in pain units have completed a postgraduate Master's degree or specialist courses on pain diagnosis and treatment, besides attending courses/workshops on current analgesic techniques (radiofrequency, spinal cord stimulation, spinal infusion, and so on). Most invasive analgesic procedures are conducted in pain units using ultrasound. The Spanish Pain Society (SED) promotes, supports, and implements training courses on the applications of ultrasound in pain at the annual SED Congress and other regular workshops.

Challenges and opportunities for the future development of pain services

Spanish Pain Society

The Spanish Pain Society (Spanish initials, SED) is a professional, multidisciplinary non-profit association covering the whole of Spain, which was founded in Madrid in May 1990. Its original aims were to promote scientific research on the mechanisms and treatments of pain, to make society aware of this problem, and to encourage constant improvement in assessment techniques and therapies for patients in pain. The SED is a Chapter of the International Association for the Study of Pain (IASP), which is the reference body for the World Health Organization (WHO) on matters related to pain. The mission and values of the SED are to promote and facilitate research on the health outcomes of pain treatment under conditions of routine clinical practice in order to optimize therapeutic approaches and generate data for evidence-based therapeutic decision-making by professionals.

SED members are in turn incorporated within 11 pain societies in the Spanish autonomous regions of Andalusia, Aragon, Balearic Islands, Canary Islands, Castile-Leon, Castile-La Mancha, Catalonia, Galicia, Madrid, Murcia, and Valencia. New societies are being established at an increasing rate. The SED is formed by professionals from different specialties and disciplines, mainly physicians. Members also include pharmacologists, psychologists, qualified nurses, physiotherapists, and other healthcare-related professionals. According to the latest count (2016), our society has 1,027 members. The most common medical specialty is anaesthesiology, as in other European pain societies. The headquarters of our society have been in Madrid since 2012, at 241, Paseo de la Castellana. It is the meeting place for the board of directors and is open to all members. The full-time secretary of the SED is Maria Jose Moreno.

The organization structure follows IASP guidelines. It is governed by a board of directors that comprises the president, treasurer, secretary, past president, and eight representatives of SED members. The board is elected every four years by SED members and endorsed by the General Assembly. There have been seven presidents of the SED. None of the positions on the SED board of directors are remunerated. The SED currently has five advisory committees: executive committee, congress and finance committee, accreditation committee, scientific committee, and communications committee.

There are 11 study groups: orofacial pain and headaches, basic science, ethics, neuromodulation, acute pain, infant pain, neuropathic pain, oncologic pain, musculoskeletal pain, opioids, and radiofrequency. Every year, each group presents its training and work programmes (courses, meetings, workshops, clinical guidelines, and so on) and is represented at the national congress. The groups possess their own statutes and are periodically renewed, being formed by one member of the SED board of directors and four to six SED members, one of whom acts as the secretary. In June 2001, the SED created the Spanish Pain Foundation (Spanish initials, FED) in order to sensitize the general population to the problem of chronic pain and enhance basic and clinical research in our country. The Foundation has its own governing body.

International and national relationships

- IASP: Numerous SED members are affiliated to the IASP and register for its international congresses, and SED members have long figured among the highest number of registrations. In addition, one member of the SED board of directors maintains a direct relationship with the IASP for all purposes.
- The European Federation of IASP Chapters (EFIC): A close relationship is maintained, with the active participation of SED members in all EFIC events. As in the case of the IASP, one of the members of the SED board of directors is in regular contact with the EFIC.
- FEDELAT (Latin American Federation of Pain, comprising different Latin American Pain Societies): The SED is one of the societies with the closest and longest-lasting links to this federation, lasting over several decades. This relationship, facilitated

by the language, is coordinated by an active SED member. The SED and FEDELAT exchange speakers and organize joint round tables at their congresses in a biannual and alternating manner. The SED also has numerous Latin American affiliates.

- The SED has close relationships with other Spanish scientific societies, including (initials in Spanish) the SEOM (Spanish Society of Medical Oncology), SEOR (Spanish Society of Radiotherapy Oncology), SECPAL (Spanish Society of Palliative Care), SER (Spanish Society of Rheumatology), SEGG (Spanish Society of Geriatrics and Gerontology), Spanish Fibromyalgia Association, and primary healthcare societies (SEMFYC, SEMERGEN, and SEMG), among others.
- The SED also has important relationships with healthcare administrations, especially the Ministry of Health, and its active participation has resulted in multiple interventions, including the following documents:
  - '*Estándares y Recomendacionesen las Unidades del Dolor*' (Standards and Recommendations in Pain Units), 2009: http://www.msc.es/organizacion/sns/planCalidadSNS/docs/EERR/Unidad_de_tratamiento_del_dolor.pdf
  - '*Marco para la Mejora del Abordaje del Dolor en el SNS*' (Framework to Improve the Approach to Pain in the SNS [Spanish National Health System]), 2014: http://www.msssi.gob.es/organizacion/sns/planCalidadSNS/pdf/excelencia/CISNS_DocumentoMarcoDolor.pdf
  - '*Estrategia de Seguridad en el paciente del Sistema Nacional de Salud*' (Safety Strategy in the National Health System Patient), 2015: http://www.seguridaddelpaciente.es/resources/documentos/2015/Estrategia%20Seguridad%20del%20Paciente%202015-2020.pdf

In addition, the creation of an Expert Diploma in Pain Medicine is currently under way.

Publications and scientific activities of the Spanish Pain Society

The Spanish Pain Society Journal *(Revista de la Sociedad Española del Dolor)* was first published in 1994 to give voice to the SED and as a written communications medium. Since then, it has gradually become the most widely distributed international journal on pain in the Spanish language. It is included in international Spanish-language databases and will be translated into English in the future, establishing its place in English-language reference indexes. The journal is considered an important source of information on pain throughout Latin America. It comprises different sections for original papers, reviews, clinical notes, and letters to the editor, and also features a news bulletin for members on SED matters. The journal is published on paper and online.

Since 2010, the SED has offered its own Master's degree (http://portal.sedolor.es/master/) on the study and treatment of pain. It lasts for two years and comprises 120 credits, divided into eight theory sections on a single interactive platform, with an additional period of clinical practice in a pain unit. The director of the course is supported by a coordinator for each section. The SED has published a series of books on different pain-related topics, including: opioids, post-herpetic neuralgia, postoperative pain, recommendations on neuropathic pain, and ziconotide guidelines. In 2016, the SED first published its *Pain Medicine Manual*, written with the participation of around 100 SED members (Manual de Medicina del Dolor, 2016). It contains 500 pages divided into 50 chapters all on pain-related issues and is the main national work of reference on pain.

Innovation

- The SED is the reference national scientific society on pain and is constantly consolidating this solid knowledge base through its scientific contributions, economic solvency, and institutional support.
- The SED strives for the implementation of pain units in all relevant hospitals in all Spanish healthcare areas.
- The SED will continue to pursue and develop a specific Spanish Diploma on Pain in cooperation with the Ministry of Health and the Ministry of Education and Culture.
- The SED will also direct a campaign for members to participate in the examination for the European Pain Diploma, ensuring the adequate accreditation of pain unit professionals in pain management. All members of the Society are recommended to obtain this diploma.
- The SED will persist in its continuous basic and advanced training on pain and analgesic technology in order to enhance the knowledge and abilities of its members.
- The SED will continue to work alongside the Ministry of Education to promote undergraduate training on pain in medicine and nursing degree courses.
- The SED supports the EFIC and IASP in highlighting the importance of training in safety issues related to different analgesic treatments.
- The SED will continue to encourage the relationship with the FEDELAT, signing new accords on conferences, training, and the rotation of professionals.
- Increased promotion of research is gradually being undertaken by the SED, providing more grants for its members and planning round tables and workshops at SED congresses.
- Paediatric care has also been targeted by the SED, with the creation of a specific work group to improve the hospital and out-of-hospital treatment of infant pain throughout Spain.
- The SED considers it to be important for pain units to unify the recommended criteria for pain assessment and to facilitate the sharing of analgesic treatment protocols. One future goal must be the standardization of clinical data gathering on pain.

References

Manual de Medicina del Dolor (2016). *Sociedad Española del Dolor*. Madrid, Spain: Ed Panamericana.

United Nations (UN) (2015). The 2015 Revision of World Population Prospects. Department of Economic and Social Affairs of the United Nations Secretariat. Available at: https://esa.un.org/unpd/wpp/publications/files/key_findings_wpp_2015.pdf [Online].

Chapter 2.32

Sweden

Anna Bjarnegård, Carina Carlsson, Eva Gåve, Rolf Karlsten, Malin Lindbäck, Elisabeth Persson, and Malin Ernberg

Background information

Sweden is located in Scandinavia in the north of Europe (see Fig. 2.32.1). It has been a kingdom for more than 750 years, which makes it one of the older states in Europe. Sweden is one of the smaller European countries with a population of approximately 10 million. Although considered a homogeneous country there has always been immigration, and since the 1960s immigration has increased. At present, 21.5% of its inhabitants were either born abroad or one of their parents was born abroad. Swedish is the official language, with Finnish, Sami, Meänkieli, Romany, and Yiddish as recognized minority languages. Life expectancy in 2015 was 84 years for women and 80 years for men (Statistics Sweden, 2017).

Healthcare system

The Swedish healthcare system has, since the mid-1950s, been mainly government-funded and decentralized, although private healthcare has increased in recent years. Healthcare is financed mainly through taxes levied by county councils and municipalities and is organized and managed on three levels: national, regional, and local. At the national level, the Ministry of Health and Social Affairs establishes principles and guidelines for care and also sets the political agenda for health and medical care.

A county council is a political body whose representatives are elected by the public every four years. The executive boards of a county council exercise authority over hospital structure and management, and ensure efficient healthcare delivery. County councils also regulate prices and the level of service offered by private providers. According to the Swedish healthcare policy, every county council must provide residents with good-quality healthcare services and work towards promoting good health in the entire population.

Sweden is, put simply, divided into 21 county councils, each with 60,000–1,900,000 inhabitants. Around 90% of the Swedish county councils' work involves healthcare but they are also involved in other areas, such as culture and infrastructure. The county councils have considerable leeway in deciding how care should be planned and delivered. This explains the wide regional variations throughout Sweden.

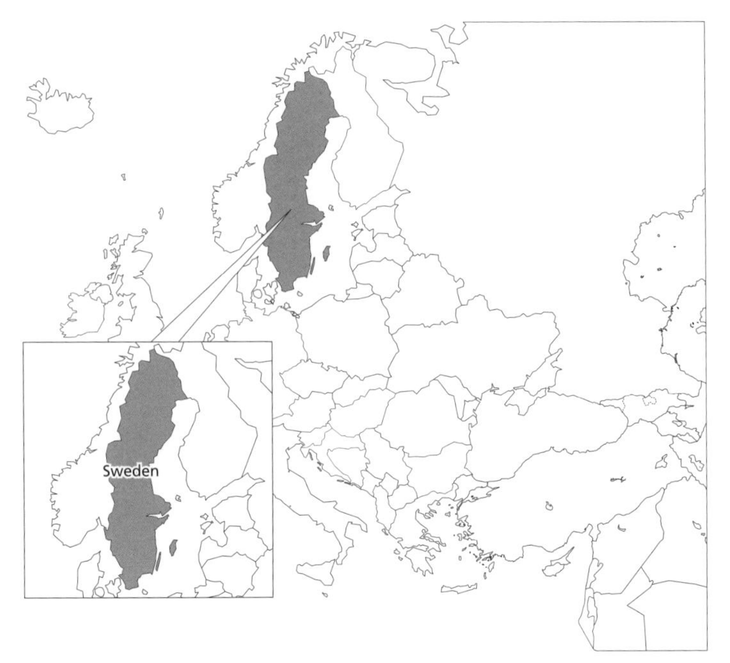

Fig. 2.32.1 Map of Sweden.
Copyright © Pyty/Shutterstock.com.

The Swedish National Board of Health and Welfare (SoS) published recommendations for the national care of people with chronic non-malignant pain conditions in 1994 (SoS, 1994). Patients with persistent pain are firstly taken care of by local primary care, then by special pain teams in primary care, and afterwards by multimodal tertiary specialist rehabilitation clinics.

Current pain workforce

The majority of patients with long-term pain are managed within primary care. Persons seeking care for their pain in primary care can see a physician, district nurse, occupational therapist, or physiotherapist for a first visit. Healthcare providers can then refer to each other when necessary. Referral may also be written to a psychologist or a social worker, a multidisciplinary team, or to a specialist clinic.

In the beginning of 2016, a group of experts received an assignment from the National Coordination Group for Knowledge Dissemination (NSK) to identify prerequisites for the diagnosis, treatment, and rehabilitation of patients with chronic pain around Sweden. The survey shows how pain care is organized, which treatments are recommended and implemented, and the status of education and research in different regions of Sweden (NSK, 2016). The results of the survey indicate great differences across the country. There is a lack of specialists in most regions and the survey shows that specialists within pain are very unevenly distributed in relation to the population and expected demands. Half of the regions in Sweden report that they have multidisciplinary pain clinics at their county hospitals. However, very few of the clinics meet the international criteria according to IASP. Often a specialized physician is the sole representative, and access to psychiatrist, nurse, psychologist, and physiotherapist is lacking. Access to an occupational therapist and social worker is even more rare. The number of multidisciplinary teams per region varies greatly and does not meet expected demands.

In Sweden physicians (since 1992), dentists (since 1993), and physiotherapists (since 1995) have been able to specialize in pain. For all three professions, the education takes place under supervision in permanent employment. For physicians, pain medicine is an add-on specialty in pain management. Quality control rests on the supervisor who certifies that the objectives have been achieved. Orofacial pain and jaw function (stomatognathic physiology) is a recognized dental specialty with a three-year education. An external reviewer examines the candidate. Both for specialists in pain medicine and orofacial pain, a certificate is issued by SoS. There are about 180 specialists in pain medicine in Sweden and about 6,600 specialists in general medicine, and presently about 50 orofacial pain specialists. Physiotherapists can obtain a specialist degree in pain and pain rehabilitation in a minimum of three years. The certificate is issued by the Scientific Council of the Swedish Association of Registered Physiotherapists (www.fysioterapeuterna.se). There are about 70 certified physiotherapists in pain and pain rehabilitation. For other professions, there are recommended courses and educational pathways within pain.

The Swedish Pain Society

The Swedish Pain Society (SPS; n.d.) aims to promote cooperation, development, and training related to pain diagnostics, pain management, pain rehabilitation, and pain-clinical-related activities in Sweden; and to promote advocacy regarding pain and pain-clinical problems. SPS was founded in 1995 (with the former name the Swedish Pain Forum) based on the need for a multidisciplinary forum with discussions on pain research and its application in clinical practice in Sweden. The association involves members from seven different professional pain associations (i.e. physicians, nurses, physiotherapists, psychologists and social workers, occupational therapists, and caregivers specialized in paediatric pain and in orofacial pain). The number of members is approximately 2,050; 1,000 physical therapists, 500 nurses, 220 paediatric pain specialists, 170 physicians, 100 dentists, 30 occupational therapists, and 30 psychologists/social workers. Since 2010 SPS is a member of IASP and EFIC.

SPS's annual meeting in October, the Swedish Pain Forum, has grown from an informal meeting with about 50–60 participants to a large conference with 400–500 delegates from across the country. Most lectures from the conference are available on the website: http://smartinformation.se/videoforelasningar/.

National reviews or surveys on pain and pain training

The Swedish Agency for Health Technology Assessment and Assessment of Social Services (SBU) is an independent national authority that evaluates healthcare interventions from a broader perspective, covering medical, economic, ethical, and social aspects. The assessments are based on systematic literature reviews of published research and are thorough and rigorous.

SBU evaluated the scientific support for rehabilitation in 2006 and 2010 (SBU, 2010). An important finding was the support for multimodal rehabilitation for chronic back pain regarding return to work and sick leave. Such multidisciplinary rehabilitation programmes can include a combination of psychological interventions, physical activity/exercise, manual and physical methods, and patient education. The report emphasizes the lack of knowledge regarding the evaluation of the different components in multimodal rehabilitation, health economic aspects, and long-term effects.

Challenges and opportunities facing the development of pain services

Treating pain has been a challenge for medicine for a long time. With the introduction of anaesthesia in 1846 came the possibility to control pain during surgery. The need for pain control also after surgical procedures started a development with 'nerve block clinics' around the Second World War, mainly managed by anaesthesiologists and surgeons. Since the 1970s, pain rehabilitation has been conducted at rehabilitation clinics in Sweden.

Despite the reports on pain services and suggested actions from SoS and SBU, it is obvious that the expansion of pain clinics has not reached the goals that were set. Seven years after the first report, a survey showed that 67% of secondary care hospitals did not have a pain clinic as suggested by SoS in 1994 (Lidbeck 2001). This situation has only marginally improved and is currently under investigation.

The number of physicians certified in pain medicine is slowly increasing, but not at a speed that matches the need. In 2001, only 58% of the physicians working with chronic pain patients in secondary care were specialized in pain medicine (Lidbeck 2001). There is also a problem that many of the active physicians are approaching retirement. Again, this is subject to current investigation by the expert group assigned by NSK.

The situation is similar for orofacial pain specialists; there are too few specialists and not even all counties have orofacial pain clinics. Another challenge is the need for better collaboration between medicine and dentistry regarding orofacial pain patients. Many of these patients are seen independently at the hospitals pain clinics and at orofacial pain clinics. Preferably orofacial pain specialists should also be part of multidisciplinary pain rehabilitation teams.

Even though there is a national registry for rehabilitation of chronic pain (see section 'Innovations'), Sweden still lacks national registries for large groups of pain patients. There is a need for a more extended national register (e.g. for outpatient clinics, neuromodulation, postoperative pain, and orofacial pain). An open register that can compare sites and methods is of substantial importance in developing high-quality care for the patient.

Pain needs more recognition in education and training. Pain management is in many ways a multidisciplinary challenge and there is a need for this aspect to be part of the education and training of future students and healthcare professionals. Pain and pain treatment must be an important part of the training at universities for future dentists, nurses, physiotherapists, physicians, psychologists, social workers, and occupational therapists. There is an opportunity to integrate training for several of these students to emphasize the importance of team efforts in the treatment of both acute and chronic pain.

Opportunities for growth and development

The growing evidence regarding the impact of acute pain treatment on mobilization and outcome, as well as the high prevalence and very high societal costs for chronic pain, have raised the interest for pain treatment and rehabilitation in Swedish society. Numerous reports from national boards and the introduction of financial support for pain rehabilitation are clear indicators of this (SKL 2016).

The experiences when successfully introducing and developing the national registry for chronic pain rehabilitation (see section 'Innovations') will be of great value in the ongoing discussions for developing national registers to include larger groups of pain patients. The general interest for pain and pain research is high among healthcare givers, nurses, physiotherapists, psychologists, occupational therapists, social workers, and researchers. This is shown for example by the high and growing interest in participating in national congresses organized by the SPS. There is hope for the future.

Innovations

In order to reduce sick leave numbers for persistent diffuse pain in back, neck, and shoulders, to prevent long-term sick leave, and to get patients into treatment and back to work as quickly as possible, in 2008 a political plan for guaranteed rehabilitation of pain and moderate mental health problems was launched. The goal was to facilitate access to healthcare for these patient groups and provide a qualified and effective rehabilitation. This initiative increased the number of pain rehabilitation clinics over Sweden and also promoted a primary care level of pain care based on multidisciplinary teams. The project was evaluated and few positive results were shown in terms of early return to work. But the access to treatment and the health of patients suffering from long-term pain improved. Therefore, some political stimulation for the continuation of these treatment programmes continues (Swedish Association of Local Authorities and Regions, 2016).

The Swedish Quality Registry for Pain Rehabilitation (SQRP) was introduced in 1998 by the Swedish Society of Rehabilitation Medicine, which aims to increase quality within pain care, facilitate evaluation and evidence-based treatment, and motivate development within each unit. This national registry is now used by a majority of the facilities involved in specialist pain rehabilitation. The registry offers access to standardized questionnaires and a database with pre- and post-measures of pain rehabilitation treatment, using the same measures, which enables follow-up of patient-reported outcomes and comparison between clinics. There is a growing number of scientific publications based on data from the registry (e.g. Gustavsson *et al.*, 2012; Stålnacke *et al.*, 2015). Work is currently ongoing to also create a similar registry for primary care pain rehabilitation (SQRP, 2017).

Following the introduction of pain medicine as an add-on specialty for physicians, the Scandinavian countries have joined forces in the education of future specialists. The Scandinavian Society of Anaesthesiology and Intensive Care (SSAI) have introduced a two-year course in advanced pain treatment for pain specialists under training, which covers an important part of the theoretical learning. The role of this course in promoting networking in and between the Scandinavian countries cannot be underestimated. Since its start in 2000, more than 200 physicians from the Nordic countries have been trained. Not only physicians can take the course (e.g. in the beginning of 2016 the first orofacial pain specialist received a diploma).

There are examples of improved collaboration between orofacial pain clinics and ordinary pain clinics (e.g. in 2016 the pain clinic at Karolinska University Hospital in Huddinge employed an orofacial pain specialist). For many years there has been a similar collaboration between the orofacial pain clinic at Malmö University and the clinic for rehabilitation medicine in Lund.

In 2014 members of the SPS and the Swedish College for Pain Medicine initiated a task force towards a National Plan for Swedish Pain Care. The objective was to increase awareness in decision-makers about the importance to take steps towards improving Swedish pain care through creating competence centres, education, guidelines, routines, and developments within the pain field. A dialogue with politicians and practitioners within the pain field throughout Sweden has developed from this initiative and resulted in the assignment of the expert group previously described (see section 'Current pain workforce').

Pain is a diverse field and a complex problem. Therefore, pain care faces many challenges and requires continual development and improvement. In the view of SPS, the most important steps towards improved pain treatment have been encouraging a multidisciplinary view in the management of chronic pain, and aiming at national guidelines and pain care models. This has not yet been achieved, and to succeed, many different steps have to be taken towards these goals.

References

Gustavsson, A., Bjorkman, J., Ljungcrantz, C., *et al.* (2012). Socio-economic burden of patients with a diagnosis related to chronic pain-register data of 840,000 Swedish patients. *Eur J Pain*, **16**, 289–99.

Lidbeck, J. (2001). Despondent voices on Swedish pain care: 'Situation feels depressing, I have considered to quit my work as pain specialist'. *Läkartidningen*, **98**, 2024–30 (in Swedish).

National Board of Health and Welfare (SoS) (1994). *Treatment of chronic pain.* SoS-report 4 (in Swedish, abstract in English).

National Coordination Group of Knowledge Dissemination (NSK) (2016). National Assignment—Pain. Available at: webbutik.skl.se/sv/artiklar/nationellt-uppdrag-smarta.html (accessed 11 August 2017) [Online].

Statistics Sweden (SCB) (2017). *Population*. Available at: http://www.scb.se (accessed 12 March 2017) [Online].

Stålnacke, B. M., Haukenes, I., Lehti, A., Wiklund, A. F., Wiklund, M., & Hammarström, A. (2015). Is there a gender bias in recommendations for further rehabilitation in primary care of patients with chronic pain after an interdisciplinary team assessment? *J Rehabil Med*, **47**, 365–71.

Swedish Association of Local Authorities and Regions (SKL) (2016). *Rehabilitation guarantee*. Available at: http://skl.se/halsasjukvard/sjukskrivningochrehabilitering/smartaochpsykiskohalsa.1002.html (accessed 12 March 2017) [Online].

Swedish Council on Health Technology Assessment (SBU) (2010). *Rehabilitation of patients with chronic pain conditions*. Stockholm, Sweden. SBU report no. 198 (in Swedish).

Swedish Pain Society (n.d.). Official website. Available at: http://swedishpainsociety.com (accessed 12 March 2017) [Online].

Swedish Quality Registry for Pain Rehabilitation (SQRP) (2017). Official website. Available at: http://www.ucr.uu.se/nrs/ (accessed 12 March 2017) [Online].

Chapter 2.33

Switzerland

André Ljutow and Christine Cedraschi

Background information

The Swiss Association for the Study of Pain (SASP) was established in 1990 as the Swiss Chapter of the international Association for the Study of Pain (IASP) and of the European Pain Federation (EFIC).

Although located in the very heart of Western Europe, Switzerland is not a member of the European Union (Fig. 2.33.1). Switzerland is a federal republic consisting of 26 cantons, with Bern as the seat of the federal authorities. A country of slightly more than eight million inhabitants, Switzerland has four official languages and cultural regions: German (spoken by two-thirds of the population), French (spoken by about a quarter), Italian (spoken by less than 10%), and Romansh (hardly 1% of a very specific region). Residents are almost equally distributed between men and women; slightly more than a fifth of them are less than 20 years old, more than half are between 21–60, and another fifth are 61 and over.

The SASP has a total of 348 members. More than half have German as their main spoken language, less than a fifth of them work in French, and a very small proportion use Italian as their work language. The majority of SASP members are men (60%) and have a medical training (80%). The largest specialty group is formed by anaesthesiologists (56%), followed by general practitioners (12%), psychologists (10%), neurologists (8%), and rheumatologists (7%). Only a minority (about 25%) of these professionals work within a private setting or practice. The SASP is administered by an executive board including a president, vice president, past president, a treasurer, and two bystanders. Since 2000, five councillors have been elected to help the executive board in the various commissions and work groups that have been implemented over the course of the years. The members of the board are elected by the general assembly of the members for a term of three years that can be renewed once. The board meets three to five times, according to the necessities of the ongoing tasks. An annual scientific congress is organized, emphasizing the contributions of the members via a poster session, where members are asked to participate with the contributions they may have made to their 'main' specialty meetings.

Healthcare system

In Switzerland every person has to be affiliated to a health insurance (there are more than 200 companies), whatever their working status or age. Persons with small family

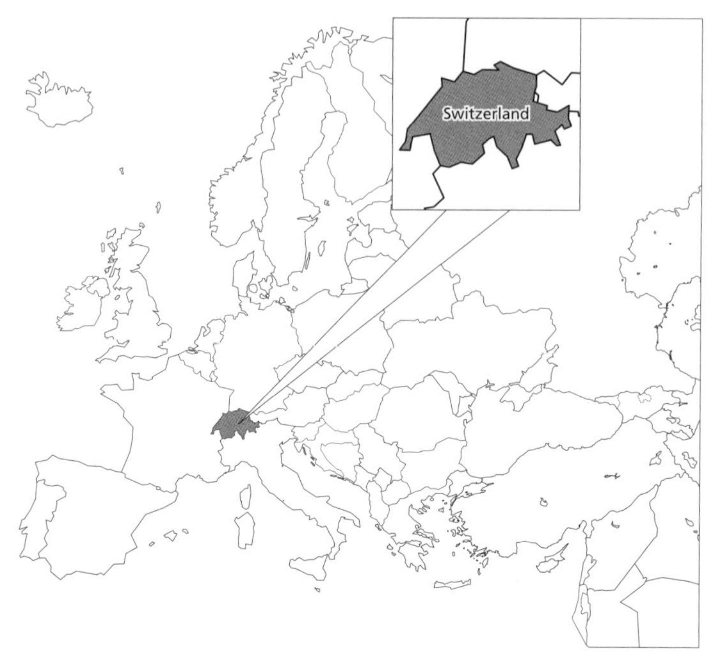

Fig. 2.33.1 Map of Switzerland.

income can apply for support for the fees to pay at their hometown or community. The minimum health insurance pays for non-accident-related healthcare costs. The patient always has to pay a franchise, at the minimum 300 Swiss francs a year (about €270). Furthermore, all medical costs include a 10% contribution of the patient. Accidents are covered by a specific insurance, which is supplied by the employer to working people. Almost half of accident insurances are covered by the Suva, the Swiss National Accident Insurance Fund, an organization under public law. Suva has a big influence on what is accepted as an accident and has a wide range of possibilities to accept costs, even for rehabilitation and social integration. Treatment in a hospital not due to accident is covered by the health insurance by almost half, while the other half is paid by the district. In each of the 26 districts, prices for hospital stays are defined separately. For a few years, most hospital treatments are paid according to the system known as the diagnoses-related group, which also includes payment for stationary multidisciplinary pain assessment and one to three week multimodal pain treatment.

Pain medicine has no official title in Switzerland. The SASP is once again working on that problem, striving to reach recognition.

Hospitals are partly in public ownership (district hospital), and partly in private ownership. There are five universities with their university hospitals in Geneva, Lausanne, Bern, Basel, and Zurich. All of them offer special pain units. But only at the Geneva University Hospitals, at the district hospital St. Gallen, and at the Swiss Paraplegic Centre in Nottwil have truly interdisciplinary pain centres been created. As there is no official recognition, these developments depend on the personal initiatives of medical professionals committed to the treatment of patients suffering from pain and its consequences.

Current pain workforce

As described below, there is at present no clear path or official recognition for pain medicine in Switzerland. It is thus quite difficult to provide statistics regarding the specialists and generalists working in the field of pain treatment. However, drawing from the membership of SASP, anaesthesiologists, neurologists, rheumatologists, general practitioners, and also psychologists, physiotherapists, and chiropractors seem to be an important part of the pain workforce.

This is an important point as studies such as the one on Pain in Europe (Breivik *et al.*, 2006) have shown that the prevalence of pain problems, including chronic pain, is at least as high in Switzerland as it is in other countries that have a certified pain curriculum. A survey is currently being performed regarding pain sites and severity, interferences with function, and health-related quality of life in community-dwelling older adults. The first results show that pain tends to increase with age and that back pain in particular appears to be a more permanent condition in the older groups. In this sense, low back pain may be part of the definition of a subgroup of older people at risk of becoming frail in relation with higher levels of functional limitations, psychological difficulties, and social restrictions, hence globally impaired health-related quality of life (Luthy *et al.*, 2015; Cedraschi *et al.*, 2016).

Challenges and opportunities to the future development of pain services

Up to now, only interventional pain treatment has received an official recognition with special pay scale consequences. As there is up to now no official recognition or certification for pain education, the SASP has formulated a specific standard for pain education. Briefly, members who are certified health professionals (psychologists, medical doctors, and so on) and have attended an 80-hour education course and successfully completed the final exam can apply for the title 'Schmerzspezialist SGSS®/Spécialiste Douleur SSED®'. For the time being, about a quarter of SASP members have gained the title. Activities are ongoing to establish an official recognition by the Swiss Federation of medical doctors regarding pain medicine, which certainly will further promote and value the need for pain education. A conference of university pain physicians, mostly anesthesiologists, is discussing pain education of medical students. Meanwhile, in Zurich a pain curriculum has been established for 12 years now in the form of an elective course, which includes 36 hours of pain-related medical education.

Innovations

Although pain medicine as such is as yet not recognized in Switzerland, there are a number of ongoing clinical and scientific activities dealing with pain. Pain research is not only performed at the university centres, but also in specialized pain units. The centre for pain medicine at the Swiss Paraplegic Centre in Nottwil/Lucerne is a beacon example for a true multidisciplinary pain centre, following the IASP criteria.

- The team currently includes clinicians from a variety of medical and other healthcare disciplines (anaesthesiologists, occupational therapists, neurologists, neurosurgeons, neuropsychologists, orthopaedic surgeons, rheumatologists, psychiatrists, psychologists, physical therapists, and sports therapists).
- All physicians and therapists are qualified and licensed in their specialty, and have expertise in pain management.
- The clinical director has a large expertise in pain management, with a Master's degree in Interdisciplinary Pain Medicine from the Vienna Medical University and is presently president of the SASP.
- The centre works on a multidisciplinary basis, both for assessment and treatment. Indeed, the initial evaluation considers the information coming from the various members of the team and multidisciplinary coordination of treatment is emphasized from the very start.
- Data are collected and summarized, allowing for evaluation and continuous quality improvement efforts. In this regard, the team devotes many efforts to disseminate relevant information to patients, other healthcare providers and organizations, and the public at large, and to provide educational activities and training in multidisciplinary pain management for clinicians from multiple disciplines (e.g. physicians of different specialties, clinical psychologists, nurses, physical therapists). The members of the team are also actively engaged in research, in cooperation with national or international universities or research institutes.

The Multidisciplinary Pain Centre at the Geneva University Hospital works along the same lines both in terms of clinical work and of research activities.

References

Breivik, H., Collett, B., Ventafridda, V., Cohen, R., & Gallacher, D. (2006). Survey of chronic pain in Europe: prevalence, impact on daily life, and treatment. *Eur J Pain*, **10**, 287–333.

Cedraschi, C., Luthy, C., Allaz, A. F., Herrmann, F. R., & Ludwig, C. (2016). Low back pain and health-related quality of life in community-dwelling older adults. *Eur Spine J*, **25**, 2822–32.

Luthy, C., Cedraschi, C., Allaz, A. F., Herrmann, F. R., & Ludwig, C. (2015). Health status and quality of life: results from a national survey in a community-dwelling sample of elderly people. *Qual Life Res*, **24**, 1687–96.

Chapter 2.34

The Netherlands

Gertie Filippini, Kris Vissers, and Michiel Reneman

Background information

In Europe, the geography of the Netherlands is unusual in that most of its land has been reclaimed from the sea and is situated below sea level, strongly protected by dikes (Fig. 2.34.1). Considering the density of its population, the country is among the most densely populated on Earth: in 2016 it counted 503 inhabitants per square kilometre. Consequently, the Netherlands is highly urbanized; it has a population of 17,000,000. The age structure is as follows: 0–14 years (17.4%), 15–64 years (67.7%), 65 and over (14.9%), and life expectancy is 79.55 years (male 76.9 years, female 82.3 years). The major ethnicity and language is Dutch; according to Eurostat, in 2010 there were 1.8 million foreign-born residents in the Netherlands, corresponding to 11.1% of the total population (Statistics Netherlands (CBS), 2016). The Dutch population is progressively ageing because of a good health status and growing because of immigration, resulting in an increasing life expectancy. This demographic development has consequences for healthcare and social security policies. As the Dutch population ages, the proportion of people of working age, as a percentage of the entire population, decreases. Important policy advisers like the Central Bureau for Statistics (CBS: https://www.cbs.nl/en-gb) and the Central Bureau for Economic Policy Analysis (CPB: https://www.cpb.nl/en) indicate that this will cause problems with the current system of old age retirement programmes: fewer people will work to pay for old age retirement, while more people will need retirement. Furthermore, the overall healthcare costs increase each year like in most European countries.

Altogether, governmental offices reform the system of healthcare and social security with a focus on:

- an increase in work participation of each citizen in the job market;
- opening the healthcare market towards more competitive healthcare insurance companies, hoping this policy will result in reduced healthcare costs per capita.

Healthcare system

The healthcare system in the Netherlands is based on the principle of solidarity and egalitarianism. Healthcare insurance in the Netherlands is mandatory for each citizen. Funding of healthcare has several key players: civilians, insurance companies,

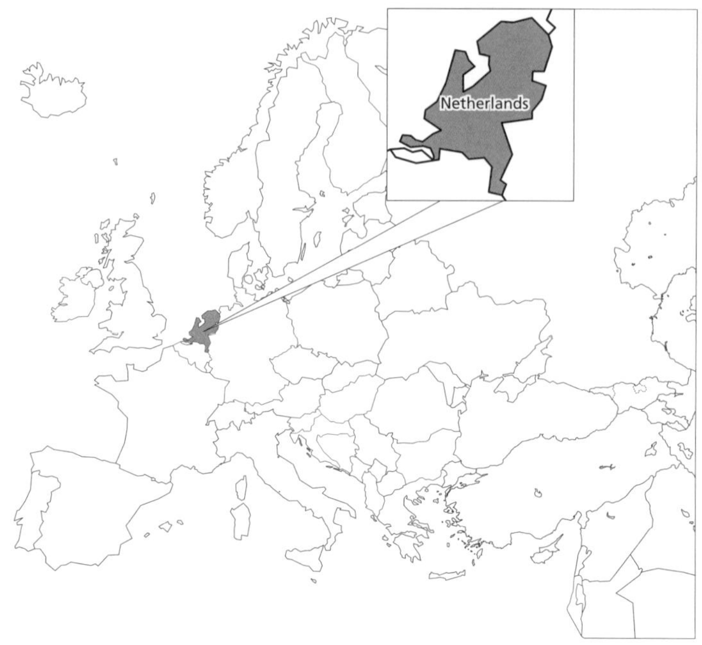

Fig. 2.34.1 Map of the Netherlands.

purchasers, and providers of care as well as the government. Civilians aged over 18 years pay mandatory health insurance fees, depending on income. Healthcare is covered by two statutory forms of insurance: basic insurance and long-term care. Healthcare regulations are determined by the Ministry of Health, Welfare and Sport in consultation with patient rights, healthcare providers, and health insurers. The healthcare authority supervises this system and the healthcare inspection supervises the quality of the healthcare providers (Fig. 2.34.2) (Brochure Ministry of Health Welfare and Sport, 2016).

Current pain workforce

Chronic pain is a large medical problem and is a universal affliction of mankind. Even though there is a huge number of new scientific insights, the pathophysiology of chronic pain is not yet fully understood, current treatments are moderately effective or effective for a limited number of patients and clinical practice, and patients only have very limited access to effective treatment strategies. The salience of pain as a disease on its own has grown since the Second Word War, when new ideas about pain were generated. The founder of the International Association for the Study of Pain (IASP), John Bonica, devoted his career to the study of pain and introduced the multidisciplinary approach of pain diagnosis and management. In the 1950s, William Noordenbos, professor of neurosurgery in Amsterdam, studied the anatomy and physiology of the

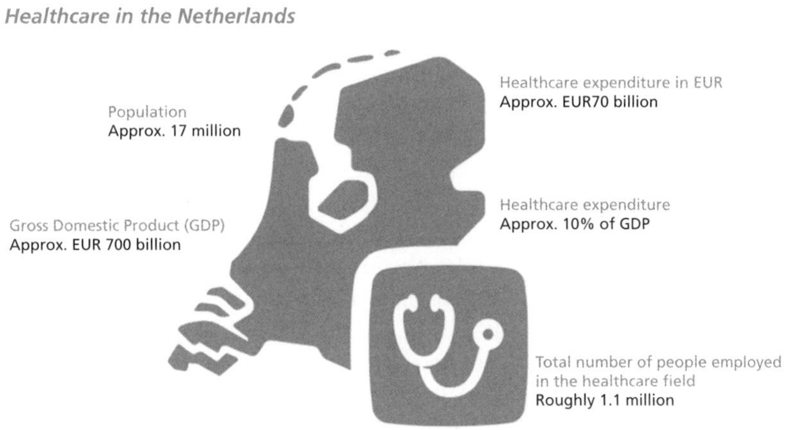

Fig. 2.34.2 Healthcare in the Netherlands.
Reproduced with permission from the Ministry of Public Health, Welfare and Sport, the Netherlands, January 2016.

spinal cord extensively and became one of the founding fathers of modern pain medicine in the Netherlands. His studies about pain (Noordenbos, 1959) inspired Ronald Melzack and Patrick Wall to describe the 'gate control theory of pain' and his contributions to the field of pain helped inaugurate the current era of research in central and peripheral pain mechanisms.

In the 1960s, the internal and surgical medical specialties in our country had different opinions about pain, reasoning between conservative or invasive treatment for pain. Since 1975, different medical specialties started to collaborate and founded the multidisciplinary Dutch Pain Society, as the second Chapter of IASP. An important motivation for the members of Dutch Pain Society (DPS) was the launch of the biopsychosocial model of Professor Engel (Engel, 1977) inducing a first report on the organization of chronic pain of the Ministry of Health in 1986 (Voorhoeve, 1986). In 1993, the DPS was playing an active part in the creation of EFIC. At that time, the Ministry of Health together with the Netherlands Organization for Health Research and Development (ZonMw) started a national programme on pain in academic centres. This induced the start of six multidisciplinary expertise centres for the study of pain and the inauguration of the first professors in pain and palliative care, namely Menno Sluijter (Maastricht University Medical Centre), Ben Crul (Radboudumc, Nijmegen), and Wouter Zuurmond (Vrije Universiteit, Amsterdam).

In 2011, under the inspiration of EFIC and the Societal Impact of Pain (SIP) programmes, a second National Health Care Institute report on pain was published initiating the next phase of implementation of the improved prevention, diagnosis, and management of chronic pain in the Netherlands (Huygen, 2011).

Since 2011, DPS has been collaborating with Pain Alliance Europe. Nowadays patient-centred care supports the active involvement of patients and their families in the design of new care models and in decision-making about individual options for treatment of chronic pain in the Netherlands.

Until 2017, the Dutch Pain Society consisted of 350 individual members, mostly healthcare professionals from different core specialties. To induce and facilitate further developments and improved pain management for the individual patient, the DPS was transformed into Pijn Alliantie in Nederland (PAiN). in April 2017. This pain alliance is a cooperation of most scientific societies of medical specialties, allied health professionals, nursing and paramedic professionals, governmental and public institutions, the patient organizations for chronic pain, and relevant stakeholders in the field of pain. The scientific medical journal '*Nederlandstalig Tijdschrift voor Pijn en Pijnbestrijding*' will be incorporated and continued in the Pijn Alliantie.

Chronic pain is associated with substantial healthcare consumption, reduced work capacity, high costs, and poor treatment efficacy. The lifeblood of multidisciplinary pain care in the Netherlands is the Pijn Alliantie. There is no national registry for specialists working in pain, but various healthcare professionals are trained and qualified in the field of pain of their own discipline. In 2011, population research was done and a national review was written about epidemiology and treatment of chronic pain in the Netherlands (Bala, 2011). In response to this national picture, as in international findings, a national report was written in which fundamental conclusions and implications to increase the recognition of pain as a significant public health problem in the Netherlands were made (Huygen, 2011).

Much of the responsibility for front-line pain care relies on general practitioners, who are not sufficiently trained in pain assessment and comprehensive, evidence-based treatment approaches for pain. Therefore, more collaboration is needed between primary care physicians and pain specialists in different clinical disciplines and settings, including multidisciplinary pain clinics. People with chronic pain can be referred by their general practitioner to attend a specialist pain clinic or multidisciplinary pain centre for assessment and optimal pain management and/or integrated (ambulatory) rehabilitation programmes and centres.

Challenges and opportunities facing the development of pain services

The improvement of pain care in the Netherlands faces different challenges:

- Insufficient evidence-based diagnosis and treatment programmes for pain: most pain management strategies formulated in national and international guidelines only have weak to no evidence. Since reimbursement for healthcare programmes in the Netherlands is directly related to proven evidence, most of the (multidisciplinary) pain management programmes are not reimbursed impeding a better organized pain care programme. Effectiveness for multidisciplinary pain rehabilitation is robust, although mean effect sizes are modest, and these programmes are reimbursed.
- Insufficient national targeted collaboration between institutions for healthcare, employment policies, and reimbursement of healthcare. This hinders optimal care for patients whose work participation is temporarily or structurally decreased by pain, and eventually affects society. The issue of work participation of patients with pain is one of the four spearpoints of EFICs efforts to schedule the forum on the Societal Impact of Pain.

- Insufficient societal attention for the prevention of acute and chronic pain, including cancer pain.
- Absence of a National Pain Strategy Plan for the Dutch population under guidance of the Ministries of Health and of Economics, endorsing a population-based, 'biopsychosocial' approach to pain care that is grounded in scientific and interdisciplinary aspects and tailored to individual needs at the patient level based on recent evidence-based paradigms of a stepwise integrated approach.
- Absence of a national quality and patient outcome monitoring programme inducing evidence of the reality and impact of pain in society and for the individual patient.
- Absence of structured education on pain in the schools for nurses and allied health professionals, and in the university-based programmes for medical professionals.
- Insufficient possibilities and budget for the initiation of research programmes.

However, the Dutch Pain Society has been very active in gaining influence and partnership at various levels of healthcare in the Netherlands:

- A common consensus-based national report on chronic pain (Huygen 2011; Bala 2011) in which demography and specific opportunities, challenges and limitations of various problems of pain in our country are described is generally accepted and can be the start of a national programme for pain for the Ministries of Health and Economics, together with the Pijn Alliantie.
- As a product of this report, the Pijn Alliantie, together with the national patient organizations for pain and the National Health Care Institute (Zorginstituut Nederland) launched the National Standard of Care for Chronic Pain (Multidisciplinary Standard of Care on Chronic Pain, 2017) which is a consensus-based programme from a patient's perspective proposing strategies to improve the prevention, diagnosis, and management of pain at a national level, involving most stakeholders.
- The Ministry of Health launched a dedicated implementation programme on pain called the 'Health Deal on Chronic Pain'. This deal should guarantee that more patients should be better managed concerning their chronic pain for the same healthcare costs.
- A national week against pain to launch the international themes of IASP and EFIC.
- International collaborative initiatives by expertise centres.
- Participation in national and international scientific societies of pain specialists and experts.
- Supporting and collaborating with the patient alliance for pain: '*Samenwerkingsverband pijnpatiënten naar één stem*' (http://www.pijnpatientennaar1stem.nl/).

Innovations

The Dutch Pain Society and united pain patient's organizations have collaborated with healthcare authorities in a combined effort to develop a multidisciplinary standard of care on chronic pain (Multidisciplinary Standard of Care on Chronic Pain, 2017), based on a patient's perspective. This standard describes current optimal pain care from a patient perspective, based on professional (evidence-based) guidelines. It also describes where evidence-based care is available or if there is a shortcoming; the final product has been delivered in the first quarter of 2016. At Q2 2016, the standard was in the authorization phase. The steering group aims to have this standard of care authorized by a large variety of organizations, representing professionals, patients, and insurers. Both the pain patient alliance and a multidisciplinary representation of the former Dutch Pain Society members were responsible for the development of this standard of care and will together be responsible for the further implementation and future organization of pain care.

The Dutch Pain Society is one of the oldest pain societies in the world. DPS induced different strategies to raise awareness about chronic pain as a disease in the Netherlands and abroad. In 2017, the DPS was transformed to Pijn Alliantie, a collaborative cooperation of medical specialists, nurses, allied healthcare professionals, the patient alliance for pain, consultants in pain, and different stakeholders. The Pijn Alliantie will take the lead in inducing a national plan for the further development and implementation of the national standard of care on pain including educational and research programmes. Pijn Alliantie will fulfil and comply with all standards and guidelines of IASP and EFIC, hence meeting all criteria to remain a full Chapter of IASP. The Pijn Alliantie will further support and take leadership in the future developments and innovation of pain care for people with pain.

References

Bala, M. (2011). Epidemiology of chronic pain and its treatment in the Netherlands. *Neth J Med*, **69**, 141–53.

Brochure Ministry of Health Welfare and Sport (2016). Healthcare in the Netherlands. Available at: https://www.government.nl/binaries/government/documents/leaflets/2016/02/09/healthcare-in-the-netherlands/healthcare-in-the-netherlands.pdf [Online].

Engel, G. (1977). The need for a new medical model: a change for biomedicine. *Science*, **196**, 129–36.

Huygen, F. (2011). Rapport Chronische Pijn, Regieraad (National Health Care Institute, taskforce chaired by professor Huygen). Available at: http://www.dutchpainsociety.nl/files/rapport-regieraad-chronischepijn-2011.pdf [Online].

Multidisciplinary Standard of Care on Chronic Pain/Zorgstandaard Chronisch Pijn (2017). Available at: http://www.dutchpainsociety.nl/files/ZorgStandaard_Chronische_Pijn_versie_2017_03_28.pdf [Online].

Noordenbos, W. (1959). *Pain*. Amsterdam, the Netherlands: Elsevier

Statistics Netherlands (CBS) (2016). Available at: https://www.cbs.nl/en-gbc [Online].

Voorhoeve, P. W. (1986). Rapport Pijnbehandeling, Gezondheidsraad. National Health Care Institute and Ministry of Health, Welfare and Sport, taskforce chaired by professor Voorhoeve. The Netherlands.

Chapter 2.35

Turkey

Nuri Süleyman Ozyalcin

Background information

Turkey is a democratic parliamentary country that geographically spans both Europe and Asia. To the west it borders Greece and Bulgaria, to the east Georgia and Armenia, and to the south Iraq and Syria (see Fig. 2.35.1). The total population of Turkey in 2016 was 79,814, 871 (Turkish Statistical Institute, 2016). The country's official language is Turkish. Life expectancy at birth is 75 years (Turkish Statistical Institute, 2012a). Infant mortality is 12.20 per 1,000 live births (Turkish Statistical Institute, 2012b).

The first Algology department was founded in Istanbul University, School of Medicine in 1986. The Turkish Society of Algology was founded in 1987, and in 1991, the IASP Turkish Chapter was founded. The name of Chapter is the Turkish Society of Algology. Currently there are 212 members in the chapter, including the core specialties of: anesthesiology (101), physical therapy and rehabilitation (78), and neurology (33). The Turkish Chapter was one of the first established among all chapters and there have always been close relations and communications with the EFIC.

Turkey hosted the congress of 7th World Society of Pain Clinicians (WSPC) in 1996, the 18th European Society of Regional Anaesthesia (ESRA) in 1999, the Second World Institute of Pain (WIP) in 2001, and Pain in Europe V—European Federation of IASP Chapters—EFIC in 2006.

Healthcare system

Turkey operates a national healthcare level system, regulated by the Ministry of Health. Primary care is provided by general practitioners or family physicians. A tertiary healthcare service in pain is provided by algologists in university and training hospitals. Healthcare in Turkey consists of a mix of public and private health services, with the Ministry of Health as the main provider. There are 27,954 medical institutions, which equates to 1.7 doctors for every 1,000 people and 2.54 beds for every 1,000 people. Turkey has universal healthcare under its Universal Health Insurance system. Under this system, all residents registered with the Social Security Institute (SGK) can receive medical treatment free of charge in hospitals contracted to the SGK. The public healthcare system covers nearly everything except admissions to private hospitals. The social health security system covers some part of private health security system expenses. Some 76.3 billion liras are being spent on healthcare annually, with 79.6%

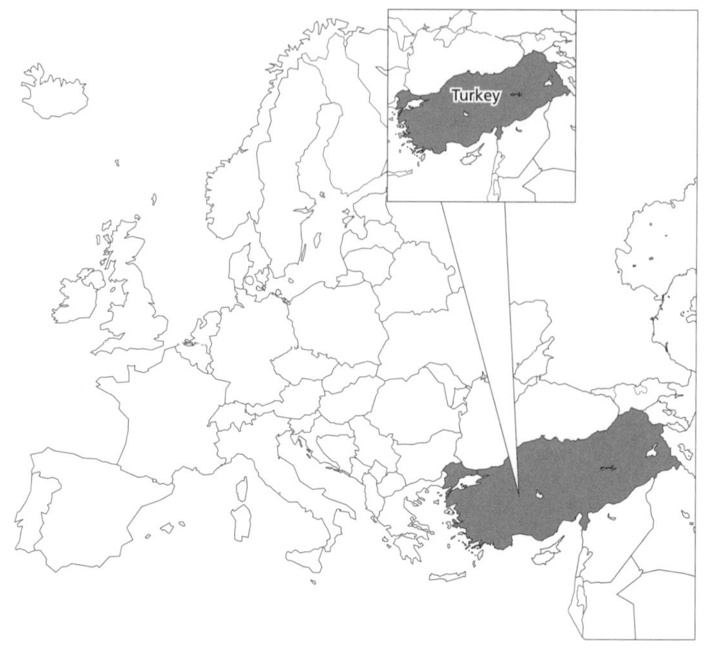

Fig. 2.35.1 Map of Turkey.

of funding coming from the SGK and most of the remainder (15.4%) coming from out-of-pocket payments.

Current pain workforce

Algology is a subspecialty lasting two years after a five-year anaesthesiology residency, or four years' physical therapy and rehabilitation, or four years' neurology residency in Turkey. The Turkish subspecialist examination is conducted as a national standardized multiple choice test provided once a year since 2012.

In Turkey, there are nearly 250 certified pain specialists who are working in the field of pain. The distribution for core specialties is approximately 60% anesthesiology, 25% physical therapy and rehabilitation, and 15% neurology. A small number of neurosurgeons and radiologists who are not certified perform interventional pain therapy.

The Turkish Society of Algology regularly organizes postgraduate education by courses and cadaver workshops for algology fellows targeted at standardizing basic and advanced knowledge, and increasing skills and practice in using diagnostic methods. Our association is organizing a national congress every two years. The 14th and the last of these congresses took place last November 2016 in Antalya with the participation of 307 doctors. During the congress, cadaver and ultrasonography courses were also held with intense participation. In addition, national board certification exam of algology for pain specialists (algologists) is available in Turkey once a year. The last exam was held in Ankara in June last year and six pain specialist qualified to take board certification successfully in this exam. *Ağrı-Pain* is the official journal of the Turkish Society of Pain and has been published quarterly since 1988. The languages of the journal are Turkish and English. It has been included and indexed in Index Medicus-Medline, EMBASE/Excerpta Medica, Index Copernicus, Gale/Cengage Learning and TÜBİTAK-ULAKBIM Turkish Medical Index. It has recently been submitted to SCI/SCI-E.

Challenges and opportunities to the future development of pain services

The main challenges we face are in the inadequate awareness of pain medicine in the general community and healthcare providers, the excessive and unnecessary use of interventional procedures, and the need for three different core specialists.

By contrast, there are many opportunities for development in pain medicine in Turkey. There is a strong historical background of pain medicine in Turkey, and its technological and pharmacological developments for pain therapy are growing rapidly. Yet there is still an increased need for pain services due to the needs of society and increased admission to pain clinics. The main goal of the Turkish associations will be to standardize the basic knowledge of pain education in pain clinics.

Innovations

All anaesthesiology, physical therapy, and rehabilitation and neurology specialists' communication must be increased with the algology subspecialty. National projects on the subject of algology are founded by research centres at the universities: the Scientific and Technological Research Council of Turkey (TÜBİTAK) and the Prime Ministry State Planning Organization of the Turkish Republic (DPT). The Turkish Society of Algology regularly organizes training courses for algology, although we recognize that training courses must be improved.

Our society and its board collaborated with the Turkish Medical Association Coordination Committee of Specialist Societies afresh to begin the accreditation of pain clinics. Ankara University Pain department was the first clinic to be accredited by our national pain board.

Although a limited number of centres are active in the field of algology in the country, these centres are capable of many of the procedures required for the proper diagnosis and treatment of pain. However, an increase in the number of pain specialists is urgently needed to improve algology practice. A national network in especially cancer pain is needed in Turkey, which may be helpful for the effective management of cancer patients.

References

Turkish Statistical Institute (2012a). Demographic Structure of Turkey and its Future, 2010–2050, Table 8: Countries and Turkey ranked by expectation of life at birth, 2010–2015 and

2045–2050, 2012. Available at: http://www.turkstat.gov.tr/PreHaberBultenleri.do?id=13140 [Online].

Turkish Statistical Institute (2012b). Demographic Structure of Turkey and its Future, 2010–2050, Table 7: Countries and Turkey ranked by infant mortality rate, 2010–2015 and 2045–2050, 2012. Available at: http://www.turkstat.gov.tr/PreHaberBultenleri.do?id=13140 [Online].

Turkish Statistical Institute (2016). Population and Demography, Population by years, age group and sex, 1935–2016, 2016. Available at: http://www.turkstat.gov.tr/UstMenu.do?metod=temelist [Online].

Chapter 2.36

Ukraine

Vladimir Romanenko

Background information

Ukraine has a population of 42.5 million people, 7 million of whom live in the main cities of Kyiv, Kharkiv, Odesa, Dnipro, and Lviv (see Fig. 2.36.1). The population has been decreasing during the last 25 years (CIA World Factbook, 2002). Some 69% are aged 15–64 years, 15% aged 0–14, and 16% are over 65 (State Statistics Service of Ukraine, 2016). Most people speak Ukranian but other languages spoken are Russian, Armenian, Azerbaijani, Belarusian, Bulgarian, Crimean Tatar, Gagauz, German, Greek, Hungarian, Karaim, Krymchak, Moldovan, Polish, Romani, Romanian, Rusyn, Slovak, and Yiddish. Some 77.8% of the population are Ukranian, but 17% identify as Russian (Ukrainian Office of Statistics, 2001). Ukraine has an area of 603,628 square kilometres, making it the largest country entirely within Europe (UN, 2016). Ukraine is a unitary republic under a semi-presidential system. Its capital and largest city is Kiev (Kyiv). Ukraine maintains the second-largest military in Europe after that of Russia. Ukraine has long been a global breadbasket because of its extensive, fertile farmlands, and it remains one of the world's largest grain exporters. The diversified economy of Ukraine includes a large heavy industry sector, particularly in aerospace and industrial equipment. Ukrainian is the official language of Ukraine; its alphabet is Cyrillic. The dominant religion in the country is Eastern Orthodoxy.

The Ukrainian Association for the Study of Pain (UASP) was established in 2009, under the leadership of Prof. Igor Romanenko. It joined EFIC in 2010. Currently there are 271 members, with the core specialities being neurologists, anaesthesiologists, orthopaedists, neurosurgeons, gynaecologists, oncologists, endocrinologists, and general practitioners (GPs).

Healthcare system

Ukraine's healthcare system is state subsidized and freely available to all Ukrainian citizens and registered residents. However, it is not compulsory to be treated in a state-run hospital as a number of private medical complexes exists nationwide. The public sector employs most healthcare professionals, and those working for private medical centres typically also retain their state employment.

Hospitals in Ukraine are organized along the same lines as most European nations, according to the regional administrative structure; as a result, most towns have their own city hospitals and many also have district hospitals. Larger and more specialized

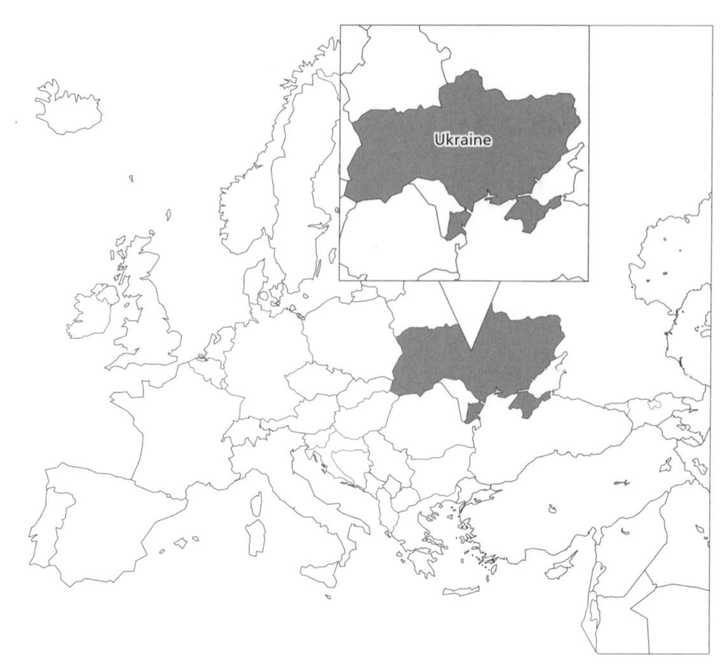

Fig. 2.36.1 Map of Ukraine.

medical complexes tend only to be found in major cities, with some even more specialized units located only in the capital of Ukraine, Kyiv city. However, all regions have their own network of general hospitals, which is typically well-equipped and able to deal with almost all medical problems.

In March 2009, the Ukrainian government started the reform of the healthcare system by creating a national network of family doctors and improving medical emergency services. In September 2016, a new team at the Ministry of Health introduced a vision of the public healthcare system as being based on updated health insurance and individual physician's licences, starting from 2017.

Current pain workforce

At present there is no pain specialty in Ukraine. Different specialists manage patients with pain in their everyday practice. There are about 23,000 general practitioners in Ukraine and development of the family medicine network is currently proclaimed as a healthcare system priority for the coming years.

In this scope, UASP has established one-day intensive seminars for general practitioners on 'must-know' issues in acute and chronic pain management. More than 2,500 physicians have so far participated in such seminars since 2015.

Another educational initiative of UASP are winter and summer pain schools. They feature more comprehensive programmes, based on the EFIC core curriculum for postgraduate medical education and cover a wide range of topics in the form of lectures and hands-on workshops.

The *Ukrainian Journal of Pain* is published quarterly and has been since 2012. It is the official journal of UASP, presenting to its readership original articles, lectures, topical reviews, proceedings of meetings and other materials.

Challenges and opportunities to the further development of pain services

The biggest challenge today in pain medicine is inadequate awareness of the problem of pain in the general and professional medical community. Another challenge is related to opioids. Currently overly complicated opioid prescription procedures are in force, a very limited number of molecules and forms are available on the market, no oral morphine or transdermal opioid delivery systems are available, and 'opioid-phobia' is common among doctors. Another challenge is the low number of interventional pain procedures and neurostimulations that are made to pain patients.

The opportunities and further steps for development of pain services include: the adaptation and introduction of the EFIC and IASP core curricula for undergraduate and postgraduate medical education in all medical schools of Ukraine; implementation of all points of the Societal Impact on Pain (SIP) strategy in Ukraine; and the establishment of algology as a new and separate medical specialty in Ukraine. Collaborative work with Ministry of Health officials is also planned in terms of improving legislation towards easing the politics of opioid prescription and turnover.

Another important issue to work on is the establishment of a national pain service that will feature a network of multidisciplinary pain centres, multidisciplinary pain clinics, pain clinics, and pain practices to provide easy access to pain management for all citizens.

Innovations

As of now, UASP has implemented a core programme of postgraduate continuous medical education on pain that consists of small local symposia in different cities, big national conferences, and a distance-learning programme. This system enables doctors to keep up-to-date with the latest news in pain management (including Global and European Year Against Pain materials). It also allows one to keep track of activity each particular doctor was involved in and may be a basis for a pain certification platform in future. In the past few years, the UASP has managed to establish a truly interdisciplinary community that shares common views on the problem of pain and has a huge potential to grow and develop.

References

Central Intelligence Agency (CIA) World Factbook (2002). Available at: https://www.cia.gov/library/publications/the-world-factbook/fields/2002.html [Online].

State Statistics Service of Ukraine (2016). Databank *0204.* Distribution of permanent population by gender, age groups and settlement type. Available at: http://database.ukrcensus.gov.ua/MULT/Dialog/statfile.asp?lang=2 [Online].

Ukrainian Office of Statistics (2001). Population by ethnic nationality, 1 January, year. ukrcensus.gov.ua. Kyiv, Ukraine: Ukrainian Office of Statistics. http://2001.ukrcensus.gov.ua/eng/results/general/nationality/ [Online].

United Nations (UN) (2016). Ukraine—United Nations Statistics Division. Kyiv, Ukraine: Ukrainian Office of Statistics. Available at: http://data.un.org/CountryProfile.aspx?crname=Ukraine [Online].

Chapter 2.37

United Kingdom

Ann Taylor

Background information

The United Kingdom (UK) incorporates Scotland, England, Wales, and Northern Ireland (see Fig. 2.37.1). The population of the UK is approximately 63,742,977, of which 17.3% are 0–14 years of age, 12.6% 15–24, 41% 25–54, 11.5% 55–64, and 17.5% are 65 years and over. More than two-thirds of men and almost 6 in 10 women are overweight or obese. In 2014, 9.89% of GDP was on health expenditure (no more recent figures) and the hospital bed density was 3 beds per 1,000 population, physician density was 2.77 physicians/1,000 population. Seventy-nine per cent (79%) of the population are urbanized and there is a 0.99 male/female sex ratio. The life expectancy is 78 years of age for men and 82 years of age for women. Eighty-seven per cent (87%) of the population are white; 3% black/African/Caribbean/black British; Asian/Asian British: Indian 2.3%, Pakistani 1.9%; 2% are mixed; and 3.7% other (IndexMundi, 2016). The official language of the UK is English; however, other indigenous languages are recognized: Scots, Scottish Gaelic, Welsh, Irish, and Cornish.

Healthcare system

The National Health Service (NHS) was launched in 1948 and is the world's largest publicly funded health service. It emerged because of the belief that good healthcare should be available to all, regardless of wealth, and one of the central components was that the NHS should be funded from people's tax contributions, ergo, means tested. Aneurin Bevan, the Welsh Health Secretary, is seen as the founder of the NHS. Park Hospital in Manchester was the first NHS hospital to be opened, bringing together health professions to provide services that were free to all at the point of delivery.

Heathcare in the UK is now devolved with the component countries (i.e England, Northern Ireland, Scotland, and Wales) each having their own systems of publically funded healthcare. Each is funded by and accountable to separate governments and parliaments and also includes smaller, private sector, and voluntary provisions. A variety of differences now exist as a result of this devolution.

The total expenditure on healthcare as a proportion of GDP in 2013 was 8.5%. This figure is below the Organisation for Economic Cooperation and Development's average of 8.9% and considerably less than comparable economies such as France (10.9%), Germany (11.0%), Netherlands (11.1%), and Switzerland (11.1%). The percentage of healthcare provided directly by the state is higher than most European countries,

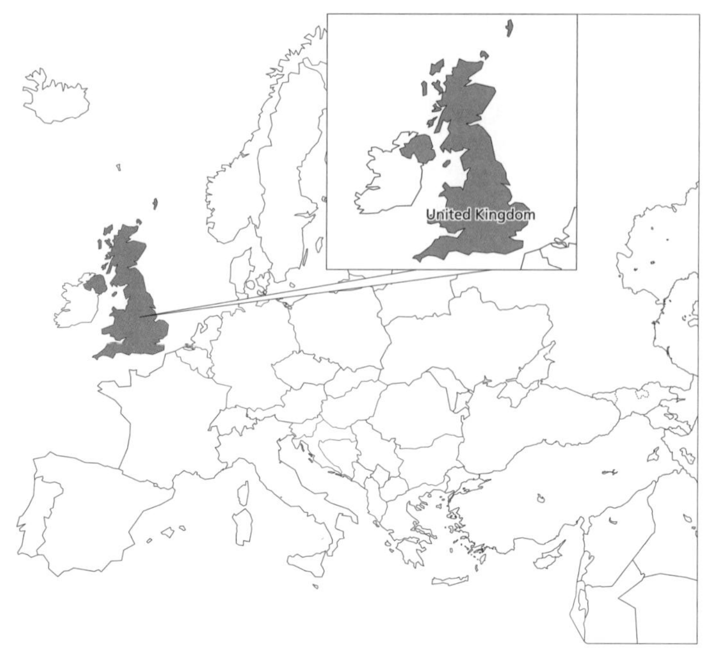

Fig. 2.37.1 Map of the United Kingdom.
Copyright © Pyty/Shutterstock.com.

which have insurance-based healthcare with the state providing for those who cannot afford insurance.

There are many differences now between the devolved nations in terms of healthcare and include how patients access non-emergency support, best practice and cost-effectiveness guidance, planning and delivering services, hospital parking and prescription charges, use of polyclinics, the role of the private sector in public health, and the funding and performance of healthcare. Similarities exist with the use of general practitioners, role of hospitals, community pharmacies, and those seeking private healthcare.

In England, in 2013, a reorganization of the NHS took place leading to the development of Clinical Commissioning Groups (CCGs). CCGs now commission most hospital and community NHS services in the local areas for which they are responsible and are overseen by NHS England, which also has the responsibility for commissioning primary care services. Within England, there is a clear delineation between specialist and specialized pain services which has been clearly described by Collett (2014), and those leading pain services will need to be at the heart of the debate in terms of which services are to be commissioned.

In Northern Ireland, the publically funded service responsible for the administration of public health and other social care services is Health and Social Care in Northern Ireland (HSC). The funding of the service is by the Northern Ireland Executive through its Health Department. Care is free of charge to all UK citizens and while the services provided are sometimes referred to as the NHS, it differs from

England and Wales in that, like Scotland, it also includes social care. NHS Scotland provides the majority of healthcare and it is publically funded. Health and social care policy and funding are the responsibility of the Health and Social Care Directorates of the Scottish Government. Local NHS Boards are responsible for health and well-being in their locality and these are supported by a number of non-geographical special health boards providing national services. NHS Wales provides the majority of healthcare and is the responsibility of the Welsh Government. Local health boards deliver all NHS services within local geographical areas and are supported by three All Wales Trusts, which operate nationwide agencies and services. Unlike Scotland and Ireland, social services are provided by local authorities (councils) in both Wales and England.

For further information on the impact on pain services due to the differences in how the NHS is configured across the UK, to which members of the British Pain Society (BPS) made a significant contribution, please see the Faculty of Pain Medicine's (FPM) 2015 publication *Core Standards for Pain Management Services in the UK* (FPM, 2015).

Current pain workforce

The British Pain Society provides support for health professionals across these four countries, with its head office situated in London. It is the largest multiprofessional organization in the field of pain within the UK and is the oldest such Society in the world, being first registered as a charity in 1979. The BPS became part of EFIC in 1993. Membership of the BPS comprises health professionals and scientists. While the majority of the society is represented by those working in the field of pain, membership also includes those working in other settings where patients commonly present with painful conditions and therefore there is a mix of specialist and generalists. Currently, the largest professional membership group is Anaesthesia (592 members), followed by Nursing (170), Psychology (107), Physiotherapy (92), General Practice (20), and others. To ensure that we have a patient voice, the BPS has a patient liaison committee, of which there are currently 1,217 members.

The United Kingdom also has a Faculty of Pain Medicine, which is responsible for pain training and specialty registration for anaesthetists. While there are profession-specific pain interest groups, no other professional body operates pain specialty registration.

Currently, there are no figures on the number of specialists working in pain across professional groups, but there are figures for pain medicine specialists. The FPM is looking at identifying data sources and establishing sustainable collection methods to facilitate workforce planning. In the Spring Edition 2014 of *Transmitter*, the following information was presented (FPM, 2014) (see Table 2.37.1).

In terms of generalists, there are no data available and indeed it is unclear how a 'generalist' would be defined, although it is a term commonly used. The GP with Special Interest in Pain title is recognized and documentation does outline the expectation of this role (PwSI Stakeholder Group, 2009). A similar role is recognized for pharmacists. However, for both, it is not a registerable qualification and therefore gaining information about how many exist within the UK is problematic. The UK has recognized the specialty of palliative medicine since 1987, which includes pain management training as a core activity, although this is mainly confined to pain in advanced cancer.

Table 2.37.1 Pain medicine specialists

Country	Chronic pain specialists per 100,000 population	Reported rate as % of total population	Average new referrals per specialist annually
Scotland	1.0	0.29	285
Northern Ireland	0.9	0.31	329
Wales	0.8	0.27	351
England	0.8	0.25	317

Reproduced with permission from McGhie, J., Workforce Update, Faculty of Pain Medicine of the Royal College of Anaesthetists, *Transmitter: Newsletter of the Faculty of Pain Medicine*, Spring 2014, Copyright © 2014 the Faculty of Pain Medicine, available from http://www.rcoa.ac.uk/system/files/FPM-Transmitter-Spring-2014.pdf

There have been a number of recent national reviews and surveys undertaken, itemized as follows:

- *National Pain Audit. National Pain Audit: Final report.* Available at: http://www.nationalpainaudit.org/media/files/NationalPainAudit-2012.pdf (London 2010–2012, endorsed by BPS)
- *Health Survey for England 2011: Chronic pain.* NHS Health and Social Care Information Centre. Available at: https://catalogue.ic.nhs.uk/publications/public-health/surveys/heal-surv-eng-2011/HSE2011-Ch9-Chronic-Pain.pdf
- Fayaz, A., Croft, P., Langford, R. M., *et al.* Prevalence of chronic pain in the UK: a systematic review and meta-analysis of population studies. *BMJ Open* 2016; 6:e010364 (doi:10.1136/bmjopen-2015-010364)

Challenges and opportunities to the future development of pain services

There are a number of challenges facing pain services:

- Currently NHS services are reactive rather than proactive in managing people with pain. There is not enough emphasis on identifying those with acute pain who are at risk of developing chronicity (pain-related disability) or people who have chronic pain and are not, or are no longer, coping with their pain.
- The National Institute for Health and Care Excellence (NICE) has produced evidence-based national guidance and advice to improve health and social care. However, there is a dichotomy between the pain-related evidence-based guidelines that NICE produce and the complexity of care that may be required by those living with complex persistent pain. There are challenges in developing pathways that reflect NICE, but also promote individualized care planning. NICE also produce quality standards which set out the priority areas for quality improvement (NICE, 2017). At present, there is no quality standard for persistent pain and coding of those living with pain is complex and currently inadequate.

- Education about pain among clinicians needs to be improved (Ellis *et al.*, 2012) and healthcare professionals experience inadequate pain education as undergraduates (Briggs *et al.*, 2011). Anaesthesia is the only medical specialty that has recognized postgraduate pain training in medicine, although, as mentioned above, palliative medicine also includes training in cancer pain.

Opportunities include:

- The Faculty of Pain Medicine , with significant contribution from the BPS, has produced core standards for pain services within the UK and has provided an opportunity to protect pain services from being underresourced and diluted.
- The English Pain Summit has produced a number of work streams which are (or have been) tasked with addressing issues within pain and its management, and has provided an opportunity for raising the profile of pain and actions in regard of it (Price, 2012).
- An online pain education initiative, jointly conceived and written by the Faculty of Pain Management and BPS provides opportunities for health professionals to learn about pain management through an evidence-based e-learning platform, e-PAIN (e-PAIN, 2015).

Innovations

A number of important documents have been published supporting innovation in practice and these include:

- *Intrathecal drug delivery for the management of pain and spasticity in adults; recommendations for best clinical practice* (2015), BPS (Eldabe *et al.*, 2015).
- *Opioids Aware: A resource for patients and healthcare professionals to support prescribing of opioid medicines for pain*, funded by Public Health England, hosted online by the FPM (2014), contributions by BPS (Faculty of Pain Medicine, 2014).
- FPM's *Core Standards for Pain Management Services in the UK* (2015), contribution by BPS (Faculty of Pain Medicine, 2015).
- Royal College of Nursing's *Pain Knowledge and Skills Framework for the Nursing Team* (2015), endorsed by BPS (Cox *et al.*, 2015).
- *Standards of good practice on spinal interventional procedures in pain medicine* (2015), joint FPM and BPS publication (Collighan *et al.*, 2015).
- *The use of drugs beyond licence in palliative care and pain management* (2012), joint BPS and Association for Palliative Medicine (Bennett *et al.*, 2012).
- Royal College of General Practitioners' *Pain Management Services: Planning for the future guiding clinicians in their engagement with commissioners* (2013), endorsed by BPS (Johnson *et al.*, 2013).
- BPS's *Cancer Pain Management* (2010), supported by the Association for Palliative Medicine and the Royal College of General Practitioners (Raphael *et al.*, 2010).

In addition, the BPS is examining its role and on how to raise the profile of pain within the UK with the formation of a task force and strategy: 'PAIN:LESS Campaign'.

References

Bennett, M., Simpson, K. H., Ahmedzai, S., *et al.* (2012). The use of drugs beyond licence in palliative care and pain management. British Pain Society and Association for Palliative Medicine. Available: https://www.rcoa.ac.uk/system/files/FPM-DrugsBeyondLicense.pdf [Online].

Briggs, E. V., Carr, E. C., & Whittaker, M. S. (2011). Survey of undergraduate pain curricula for healthcare professionals in the United Kingdom. *Eur J Pain*, **15**, 789–95.

Collett, B. (2014). Commissioning of Pain Services, Faculty of Pain Medicine, the Royal College of Anaesthetists. Available at: https://www.rcoa.ac.uk/system/files/FPM-PAIN-SERV-COMM.pdf [Online].

Collighan, N., Gupta, S., Balasubramanian, S., *et al.* (2015). Standards of good practice on spinal interventional procedures in pain medicine. Faculty of Pain Medicine and British Pain Society. Available: https://www.britishpainsociety.org/static/uploads/resources/files/spinal_intervention_A5_Final_April_2015_1.pdf [Online].

Cox, F., Cannons, K., & Lewis, S. (2015). Pain Knowledge and Skills Framework for the Nursing Team. Royal College of Nursing. Available: https://www.rcn.org.uk/-/media/royal-college-of-nursing/documents/publications/2015/august/pub-004984.pdf [Online].

Eldabe, S., Duarte, R., Raphael, J., Thomson, S., & Bojanic, S. (2015). Intrathecal drug delivery for the management of pain and spasticity in adults; recommendations for best clinical practice. British Pain Society. Available: https://www.britishpainsociety.org/static/uploads/resources/files/itdd_2015_pro_v3.pdf [Online].

Ellis, B., Johnson, M., & Taylor, A. (2012). Education as part of wider health policy and improvement strategies. *Brit J Pain*, **6**, 54–8.

e-PAIN (2015). eLearning for Pain management, e-PAIN Modules & Sessions Update, 2015. Available at: https://www.rcoa.ac.uk/system/files/FPM-ePAIN-Session-Update-Feb2015_0.pdf [Online].

Faculty of Pain Medicine (FPM) (2014). Opioids Aware: A resource for patients and healthcare professionals to support prescribing of opioid medicines for pain. Faculty of Pain Medicine. Available: http://www.rcoa.ac.uk/faculty-of-pain-medicine/opioids-aware [Online].

Faculty of Pain Medicine (FPM) (2015). Core Standards for Pain Management Services in the UK. Faculty of Pain Medicine. Available: http://www.rcoa.ac.uk/system/files/CSPMS-UK-2015-v2-white.pdf [Online].

IndexMundi (2016). United Kingdom Demographics Profile 2016. Available at: http://www.indexmundi.com/united_kingdom/demographics_profile.html [Online].

Johnson, M., Hart, O., Taylor, A. M., *et al.* (2013). Pain Management Services: Planning for the future guiding clinicians in their engagement with commissioners. Royal College of General Practitioners. Available: http://www.rcoa.ac.uk/system/files/FPM-Pain-Management-Services.pdf [Online].

Price, C. (2012). Report: Putting pain on the Agenda: The Report of the First English Pain Summit, Policy Connect, 2012. Available at: http://www.policyconnect.org.uk/cppc/research/report-putting-pain-agenda [Online].

PwSI Stakeholder Group (2009). Guidance and competences for the provision of services using practitioners with special interests (PwSIs): Pain Management. Available at: http://www.rcgp.org.uk/clinical-and-research/clinicalresources/~/media/7739CDCC2D164910A66D9F5596577C2D.ashx [Online].

Raphael, J., Ahmedzai, S. H., & Barrie, J. (2010). Cancer Pain Management. British Pain Society. Available: https://www.britishpainsociety.org/static/uploads/resources/files/book_cancer_pain.pdf [Online].

The National Institute for Health and Care Excellence (NICE) (2017). Quality standards set out the priority areas for quality improvement in health and social care. Available at: https://www.nice.org.uk/standards-and-indicators [Online].

Section 3

Special issues

Chapter 3.1

Pain in later life

Gisèle Pickering

Introduction

Worldwide population ageing is unprecedented and enduring (EC, 2012), and the European Union (EU) as a whole is, in particular, confronted with an ageing population. The proportion of persons aged 65 or over is 19% today and projected to increase to almost 30% by 2080; and those aged 80 or over represent 5% today, but this will rise to more than 12% by 2080. This demographic trend confronts the EU with major health challenges, notably regarding the burden of pain and its societal consequences. The 2012 EFIC report on healthy ageing (EC, 2012) stressed that chronic pain is associated with reduced quality of life and that chronic pain intervention can reduce pain and improve quality of life. Strategies have been outlined (Breivik *et al.*, 2013) from a public health perspective to help overcome barriers to effective pain care, resulting in particular from deficiencies in education and access to interdisciplinary pain management services. Building on these and on the recurring observation that pain in older people is still undermanaged, we focus here on how clinical practice and research could pave the way to better management of pain in older persons.

From education to customized geriatric pain management

Pre and postgraduate education in pain medicine for healthcare professionals is pivotal, but there are large differences in structure, healthcare services, and training facilities between EU member states. Pain medicine may be recognized as a specialty, subspecialty, 'add-on' specialty, or competency-based training, and the same applies sometimes to general practice and geriatrics. Since the launch of 'Pain in the Elderly' year in Istanbul in 2005, geriatric pain medicine has gained a place in most EFIC Chapter societies and in European and national geriatric societies and associations. The state of the art in pain medicine in geriatrics in Europe is, however, poorly documented and will need to be explored in order to develop a real work force of pain management at a European level: this applies not only to education but also to geriatric clinical management as a whole.

Older persons have needs that change with ageing, live often in different settings, and have varied physical and mental status. Most older persons live at home and are encouraged to remain as long as possible in their own environment, for both economic and affective reasons. Healthcare costs are largely due to hospitalization. Prevention strategies to limit hospital admission of older people appear to be the most useful means to achieve cost savings (Lazkani *et al.*, 2015), but the home care provided must be of good quality.

Elderly patients often have a fatalistic attitude and believe that pain with ageing is normal (Roy, 2004). Some patients are proactive in seeking treatment, while others simply tolerate the pain, seeking treatment too late, or merely as a pretext for social contact. The community physician (general practitioner: GP) is often their first regular port of call, and referral to a pain clinic or pain specialist usually occurs when GPs have exhausted the treatments at their disposal and pain has become unbearable for the patient. Between 18–20% of older people live in long-term care settings and nursing homes, and a variable percentage is transiently present in hospital, palliative care units, and accident and emergency departments. Obstacles to effective pain management in older persons are numerous, including patient beliefs and attitudes towards pain, impaired cognition and communication, dementia, and frailty. Treatment must be finely customized, according to pain evaluation, co-morbidity, and multiple medication. Education programmes, the development and use of observational behavioural scales, and stepwise pain management have addressed some of these barriers and tend to improve outcome. There are, however, often limitations in terms of financial resources, facilities, and appropriately trained healthcare professionals.

Initiatives, although embryonic in some countries, have been developed in recent years and need to be continued. For older persons living in the community, pain management interventions, often included in palliative care programmes, have been developed to train medical and non-medical healthcare providers to detect and evaluate pain, especially in patients with cognitive disorders or dementia, and to manage drug compliance in order to prevent and anticipate drug interactions.

In hospital, retrospective studies in medical and surgical wards reported a considerable delay, of several days, before specialized pain consultation. Evidence indicates that 30% of older patients were not seen for comprehensive pain evaluation prior to discharge from hospital and 30% had no individual consultation for pain management while in the ward. This was attributed to the often heavy workload of doctors and nurses in acute care, and to other medical issues taking priority. Mobile teams specialized in acute and chronic pain management in older persons have been developed in some European hospitals, with activities ranging from organizing the management of 'patient-controlled analgesia' equipment, to providing information and training. Mobile multidisciplinary teams could also optimize pain management in wards with elderly patients who are difficult to transfer from one setting to another, especially in rural and remote regions.

Older persons are admitted to emergency departments more often than younger patients: those aged ≥85 years are four times as likely to present in emergency departments as those aged 35–59 years (Lowthian *et al.*, 2011). Between 21–40% of older persons admitted to hospital have cognitive impairment or communication disorders, and many of these present with suspected pain. Nationally accepted pain assessment tools for persons with cognitive impairment vary from country to country. Older persons are less likely than younger ones to receive an analgesic or opioid, regardless of pain severity (Todd *et al.*, 2007; Platts-Mills *et al.*, 2012). Emergency department staff report feeling burdened by patients with cognitive impairment, which is seen as the greatest barrier to providing the optimal emergency care (Fry *et al.*, 2014). Emergency department admissions are continuously rising, and specific actions should be undertaken to improve care management in this setting (Moustafa *et al.*, 2017).

In residential care facilities for the aged, where pain is an everyday phenomenon, a number of obstacles have been identified as recurring barriers to adequate pain management (Pickering *et al.*, 2001; Savvas and Gibson 2015). Implementation of sustainable evidence-based practice for the assessment and management of pain has been shown to improve staff self-assessed efficacy and practice, with improved analgesic practice and pain outcomes (Savvas *et al.*, 2014). Structured educational interventions for nurses concerning pain assessment and management in older people in hospital or residential care facilities may enable changes in practice, alleviating pain intensity and improving the assessment and management of pain (Manias *et al.*, 2011). Studies addressing the implementation of standards and evaluating outcomes should be further developed.

Very few pain clinics in Europe are specifically designed to cater for the needs of older people with persistent pain. A multifaceted multidisciplinary approach has been recommended for a number of years. Multidisciplinary pain programmes, clinics, and centres have been developed and are important tools in the treatment of chronic pain (Kaiser *et al.*, 2013). Very few, however, specifically target elderly people, who have different expectations, pharmacology, co-morbidities, and associated treatments than younger adults. Older persons who attend a multidisciplinary pain clinic are not representative of older persons with chronic pain in the community (Kung *et al.*, 2000), and the specificities of each setting need to be highlighted for appropriate pain management. Setting up specific geriatric pain medicine clinics, however, is very difficult today, with health systems under severe threat from lack of financial resources.

The challenge of pain evaluation

Self-reporting is the most reliable indicator of the presence and intensity of pain, and should always be tried, even in older patients with cognitive impairment. More than 30 observational pain assessment tools have been developed and validated for use when self-report is not possible (Hadjistavropoulos *et al.*, 2014). The European COST programme 'Pain assessment in patients with impaired cognition, especially dementia' has brought together researchers and clinicians from a wide range of scientific disciplines. It aims to develop a comprehensive and internationally agreed assessment toolkit for older adults. It also presents the possibility of organizing annual training schools for doctoral and postdoctoral students, giving them a unique opportunity to make known their own research on pain in geriatrics. A number of papers were produced and are solid milestones in the construction of a European action programme for Pain in Geriatrics (de Tommaso *et al.*, 2016).

Despite the large number of available scales, very few have been translated and validated in foreign languages or compared between each other (Pickering *et al.*, 2010; Martin *et al.*, 2016). It is thus essential to use observational scales adequately in the pathology, setting, and population in which they were first validated or revalidated (Martin *et al.*, 2016). It is important that scales should be validated in, rather than extrapolated to, any new clinical setting (Moustafa *et al.*, 2017). Future research is needed on interventions implemented by multidisciplinary teams of health professionals, to provide recommendations on situations in which a given scale should be used and not used. Observational scales help to decipher pain, but a principle of precaution must always be applied if they seem to suggest that pain is not present, as they are discriminatory rather than diagnostic tools. For example, a scale such as Algoplus®, designed for acute pain evaluation, needs supplementing with a chronic pain evaluation tool such as Doloplus®, as Algoplus® is liable to 'overlook' pain in 17% of older patients (Pickering *et al.*, 2013; Martin *et al.*, 2016). Further research should focus on the metrology and limitations of available scales and on a transverse approach, testing the scales in a wide range of situations.

Pain assessment as such is just one aspect of evaluation in older people. A full geriatric assessment should complement pain assessment. Full geriatric evaluation, including cognitive and emotional status, mobility, and quality of life, must be made, and requires good knowledge not only of pain medicine but also of the specificities of the older person. In older people, there is a strong bidirectional link between functional decline and decreased ability to perform activities of daily life due to decreased physical and/or cognitive performance associated with age and disability (Consortium, 2015) and chronic disease.

Chronic pain is frequent in older people; it affects more than 50% of older persons living in the community and more than 80% of nursing home residents. Rheumatologic disease, alongside osteoarthritis, is the most common pathology in older people. Pain, ranging from mild to severe, is a frequent symptom of osteoarthritis and impacts quality of life, activities of daily life, is associated with depression, and disrupts sleep (Parmelee *et al.*, 2015; Pickering *et al.*, 2014).

One type of chronic pain, neuropathic pain, shows higher prevalence than in the general population (over 10%), and is particularly difficult to assess in older persons with communication impairment. A recent study (Rapo-Pylkkö *et al.*, 2015) reported that neuropathic pain was diagnosed in 48% of older people living independently, the most common diagnosis being radiculopathy caused by degenerative disease of the spinal cord. Elderly patients are most at risk of neuropathic pain because of the age-related co-morbidities that may be associated: herpes zoster, diabetes, neurodegenerative disorders, stroke, Parkinson's disease, and sequelae of surgery, or oncologic chemotherapy. Neuropathic pain is underdetected, underestimated, and undertreated in elderly patients. A decision-tree was drawn up to help improve pain management in older patients, especially with communication disorders (Pickering *et al.*, 2016). A crucial step is to recognize neuropathic pain before assessing pain and functional limitations.

The challenge of pain treatment in the geriatric context

Older individuals are at increased risk of cardiovascular disease, and renal and hepatic dysfunction naturally increases with age. Ageing is associated with a number of pharmacokinetic and pharmacodynamic changes that affect drug bioavailability (Novotný, 2006; Schuling *et al.*, 2012). These changes, together with the underlying disease, also increase the risk of adverse drug reactions and drug interactions. Patients with several co-morbidities who receive treatment according to professional guidelines for their respective diseases end up using a large number of drugs. Taking multiple medications is predictive of hospital admission and nursing home placement, impaired mobility, and poor drug compliance (Schuling *et al.*, 2012). Guidelines for pain treatment in older people are often extrapolated from guidelines in adults, with the knowledge that drug treatment must 'start low and go slow' in older people, that renal function assessment is mandatory, and that deleterious cognitive effects of drugs, opiates, antidepressants and antiepileptics may be amplified in older people (Novotný, 2006; Pickering *et al.*, 2014; Pickering, 2014; Radat *et al.*, 2013). Guidelines are regularly published by scientific societies and are particularly useful. Monotherapy is frequently advised for elderly persons, because the pharmacology of a drug is well described and/or modelled according to age or renal function. The difficulty arises when the patient takes several drugs for a long time (as is the case in older persons) and the real pharmacokinetics and pharmacodynamics are quickly lost track of when drugs are mixed and given together. There is, at present, no other clinical option, but pharmacologic and geriatric studies are needed to improve advice on drug associations, metabolism (especially hepatic cytochrome inhibition and induction), renal elimination, and dose adaptation.

While acute pain treatment protocols have been standardized successfully, treatments for chronic, and especially neuropathic pain (antiepileptics, antidepressants), give less satisfaction. Insufficient pain relief is reported in 66% of patients in post-herpetic neuralgia (Laurent *et al.*, 2014), as are adverse events such as dizziness, somnolence, or gait disorder leading to falls. Clinical trials including older patients are very few; patients included in phase 3 studies usually being less than 65 years of age. Data on numbers to treat or to harm are still unavailable in the literature for older patients.

The deleterious impact of drugs on cognitive and psychological processes (Pickering *et al.*, 2014) needs particularly to be studied to understand the cognitive impacts of pain (Attridge *et al.*, 2015, 2016) and of several analgesics, benzodiazepines, and even psychotropic drugs (although not officially recommended) in agitated demented patients (Pickering, 2016). Depression and anxiety are common in elderly persons and the depressive state and social situation must be properly assessed. Depression is associated with poor adherence to treatment and possibly poorer outcome, and favours functional decline in chronic patients. Conversely, functional decline is a mode of presentation of depression in older people, emphasizing the need for global evaluation before antidepressant prescription (Clarke and Currie, 2009).

Stepwise pain management approaches have been published to help with drug prescription and titration, but need developing, especially in the situation of cognitive impairment and frailty (McLachlan *et al.*, 2011).

Patient therapeutic education places the patient at the centre of pain management and must be adapted to the medical condition. Its use with elderly patients is not yet well developed in the EU and greatly depends on local facilities, as it is time-consuming and GPs need to be free to care for other aspects of community-living patients' health (Vargas-Schaffer and Cogan, 2014). Therapeutic education has been particularly well developed in rheumatology, and gives good results associated to pharmacological treatment. The long-term effects may be beneficial, as it helps to maintain autonomy and optimize the quality of life of the older patients, especially given the frustrating lack of progress in the development of new treatments for osteoarthritis.

The combination of non-pharmacological and pharmacological treatments is strongly recommended for older persons, especially to maintain mobility (AGS, 2009), despite the lack of evidence-based trials with alternative medicines.

Finally, prevention of pain offers a unique opportunity to improve the quality of life of older patients and significant help in achieving an extended healthy lifespan; however, preventive treatments are rare. Two interventions offer good hope for pain prevention. Prevention of postsurgical neuropathic pain has been shown with memantine, a drug used in moderate to severe Alzheimer's disease (Morel *et al.*, 2016). Herpes zoster vaccine for >60-year-old persons is recommended to diminish the occurrence of post-herpetic neuralgia (Keating, 2016).

Conclusion

Optimization of the development of geriatric pain medicine in Europe targets all aspects of education, research, and clinical practice. For our purposes there are 10 challenges:

1. Building up a multidisciplinary geriatric workforce in Europe;
2. Making geriatric pain medicine attractive to healthcare practitioners: this is linked not only to education facilities, but also to employment opportunities in this field;
3. Specifying indications and limitations for available behavioural scales and promoting their use at national and international levels;
4. Implementing a stepwise approach to detection, evaluation, and pharmacological and non-pharmacological treatment of pain, in combination with focused geriatric assessment;
5. Conducting randomized clinical drug trials in older persons at an international level, to assess the real-life risk/benefit ratio of pain treatments;
6. Enriching the literature and guidelines on geriatric pain medicine with good-quality methodology;
7. Raising awareness of adverse drug events and interactions in the context of multiple medication, comorbidity, cognitive impairment, and frailty;
8. Focusing on the cognitive and emotional aspects of pain, and the cognitive consequences of pain per se and of analgesics and of coping strategies, specifically in older persons;
9. Conducting epidemiological and interventional studies on synergic effects between drugs and non-pharmacological treatment of pain;
10. Preventing pain: a crucial issue for good quality ageing.

References

American Geriatrics Society (AGS) (2009). Panel on the Pharmacological Management of Persistent Pain in Older Persons Pharmacological Management of Persistent Pain in Older Persons. *JAGS*, **57**, 1331–46.

Attridge, N., Crombez, G., Van Ryckeghem, D., Keogh, E., & Eccleston C. (2015). The Experience of Cognitive Intrusion of Pain: scale development and validation. *Pain*, **156**, 1978–90.

Attridge, N., Keogh, E., & Eccleston, C. (2016). The effect of pain on task switching: pain reduces accuracy and increases reaction times across multiple switching paradigms. *Pain*, **157**, 2179–93.

Breivik, H., Eisenberg, E., & O'Brien T. (2013). The individual and societal burden of chronic pain in Europe: the case for strategic prioritisation and action to improve knowledge and availability of appropriate care. *BMC Public Health*, **24**, 1229.

Clarke, D. M. & Currie, K. C. (2009). Depression, anxiety and their relationship with chronic diseases: a review of the epidemiology, risk and treatment evidence. *Med J Aust*, **190**(7 Suppl), S54–S60.

Consortium Herpes Zoster and Functional Decline Consortium (2015). Functional decline and herpes zoster in older people: an interplay of multiple factors. *Aging Clin Exp Res*, **27**, 757–65.

de Tommaso, M., Arendt-Nielsen, L., Defrin, R., Kunz, M., Pickering, G., & Valeriani, M. (2016). Pain Assessment in Neurodegenerative Diseases. *Behav Neurol*, 2949358.

European Commission (EC) (2012). Healthy ageing in relation to chronic pain in the EU. Systematic Literature Report May 2012. Available at: http://ec.europa.eu/eurostat/documents/2995521/7012459/3-29092015-AP-EN.pdf (accessed 6 May 2016) [Online].

Fry, M., Gallagher, R., Chenoweth, L., & Stein-Parbury, J. (2014). Nurses' experiences and expectations of family and carers of older patients in the emergency department. *Int Emerg Nurs*, **22**, 31–6.

Hadjistavropoulos, T., Herr, K., Prkachin, K. M., *et al.* (2014). Pain assessment in elderly adults with dementia. *Lancet Neurol*, **13**, 1216–27.

Kaiser, U., Arnold, B., Pfingsten, M., Nagel, B., Lutz, J., & Sabatowski, R. (2013). Multidisciplinary pain management programs *J Pain Res*, **6**, 355–8.

Keating, G. M. (2016). Shingles (Herpes Zoster) Vaccine (Zostavax(®)): A review in the prevention of herpes zoster and postherpetic neuralgia. *BioDrugs*, **30**, 243–54.

Kung, F. T., Gibson, S. G., & Helme, R. D. (2000). Older people with chronic pain: comparison of pain clinic patients with a community based sample. *The Pain Clinic*, **12**(2), 103–12.

Laurent, B., Vicaut, E., Leplege, A., Bloch, K., & Leutenegger, E. (2014). Prevalence and quality of life impact of postherpetic neuralgia (PHN) in French medical centers specialized in chronic Pain management: the ZOCAD study. *Med Mal Infect*, **44**(11–12), 515–24.

Lazkani, A., Delespierre, T., Bauduceau, B., *et al.* (2015). Healthcare costs associated with elderly chronic pain patients in primary care. *Eur J Clin Pharmacol*, **71**, 939–47.

Lowthian, J. A., Jolley, D. J., Curtis, A. J., *et al.* (2011). The challenges of population ageing: accelerating demand for emergency ambulance services by older patients, 1995–2015. *Med J Aust*, **194**, 574–8.

Manias, E., Gibson, S. J., & Finch, S. (2011). Testing an educational nursing intervention for pain assessment and management in older people. *Pain Med*, **12**, 1199–215.

Martin, E.; Doloplus Collective Team, Pereira, B., & Pickering, G. (2016). Concordance of pain detection using the doloplus and algoplus behavioral scales. *J Am Geriatr Soc*, **64**, e100–2.

McLachlan, A. J., Bath, S., Naganathan, V., *et al.* (2011). Clinical pharmacology of analgesic medicines in older people: impact of frailty and cognitive impairment. *Br J Clin Pharmacol*, **71**, 351–64.

Morel, V., Joly, D., Villatte, C., *et al.* (2016). Memantine before mastectomy prevents post-surgery pain: a randomized, blinded clinical trial in surgical patients. *PLoS One*, **11**, e0152741.

Moustafa, F., Macian, N., Giron, F., Schmidt, J., Pereira, B., & Pickering, G. (2017). Intervention study with Algoplus®, a pain behavioural scale, for older patients in the Emergency Department implementation. *Pain Pract*, **17**, 655–62.

Novotný, J. (2006). Specific issues in pharmacotherapy of the elderly. *Journal of Health Sciences Management and Public Health*, **7**, 81–93.

Parmelee, P. A., Tighe, C. A., & Dautovich, N. D. (2015). Sleep disturbance in osteoarthritis: linkages with pain, disability, and depressive symptoms. *Arthritis Care Res (Hoboken)*, **67**, 358–65.

Pickering, G. (2014). Antiepileptics for post-herpetic neuralgia in the elderly: current and future prospects. *Drugs Aging*, **31**, 653–60.

Pickering, G. (2016). Pharmacological treatment. In: Gibson, S. & Lautenbacher, S. (eds), *Pain and Dementia*. Washington, DC: IASP Press.

Pickering, G., Deteix, A., Eschalier, A., & Dubray, C. (2001). Impact of pain of nursing home residents on their recreational activities. *Aging*, **13**, 44–8.

Pickering, G., Gibson, S. J., Serbouti, S., *et al.* (2010). Reliability study in five languages of the translation of the pain behavioural scale Doloplus. *Eur J Pain*, **14**, 545, e1–10.

Pickering, G., Marcoux, M., Chapiro, S., *et al.* (2016). An algorithm for neuropathic pain management in older people. *Drugs Aging*, **33**, 575–83.

Pickering, G., Pereira, B., Clère, F., *et al.* (2014). Cognitive function in older patients with postherpetic neuralgia. *Pain Pract*, **14**, E1–7

Pickering, M. E., Bunna, P., Rat, P., *et al.* (2013). Acute pain evaluation with Algoplus scale in Cambodian patients. *Pain Med*, **14**, 1971–6.

Platts-Mills, T. F., Esserman, D. A., Brown, L., Bortsov, A. V., Sloane, P. D., & McLean, S. A. (2012). Older US emergency department patients are less likely to receive pain medication than younger patients: results from a national survey. *Ann Emerg Med*, **60**, 199–206.

Radat, F., Margot-Duclot, A., & Attal, N. (2013). Psychiatric co-morbidities in patients with chronic peripheral neuropathic pain: A multicentre cohort study. *Eur J Pain*, **17**, 1547–57.

Rapo-Pylkkö, S., Haanpää, M., & Liira, H. (2015). Neuropathic pain among community-dwelling older people: a clinical study in Finland. *Drugs Aging*, **32**, 737–42.

Roy, R. (2004). *Chronic Pain, Loss and Suffering*. Toronto, Canada: University of Toronto Press; p. 27.

Savvas, S. & Gibson, S. (2015). Pain management in residential aged care facilities. *Aust Fam Physician*, **44**, 198–203.

Savvas, S., Toye, C., Beattie, E., & Gibson, S. J. (2014). Implementation of sustainable evidence-based practice for the assessment and management of pain in residential aged care facilities. *Pain Manag Nurs*, **15**, 819–25.

Schuling, J., Gebben, H., Veehof, L. J., & Haaijer-Ruskamp, F. M. (2012). Deprescribing medication in very elderly patients with multimorbidity: the view of Dutch GPs. A qualitative study. *BMC Fam Pract*, **13**, 56.

Todd, H. K., Ducharme, J., Choiniere, M., *et al.* **for the PEMI Study Group**. (2007). Pain in the emergency department: results of the pain and emergency medicine initiative (PEMI) multicenter study. *J Pain*, **8**, 460–6.

Vargas-Schaffer, G. & Cogan, J. (2014). Patient therapeutic education: Placing the patient at the centre of the WHO analgesic ladder. *Can Fam Physician*, **60**, 235–41.

Chapter 3.2

Pain in children

Julia Wager and Boris Zernikow

Introduction

Pain in children is not only a small piece of a larger puzzle; it is an entirely different entity. Pain aetiology, assessment, and treatment vary at every age from pre-term foetuses at 23 weeks' gestation to adolescents. Every developmental age has its own distinct features and challenges. Furthermore, for many pain conditions, the pathophysiology in children is different from that in adults. For example, with tumour pain, children primarily suffer from painful invasive procedures and side effects of aggressive antineoplastic treatments since the underlying malignant conditions are acute leukaemias, brain tumours, and mesenchymal solid tumours. Because of the aggressive, often painful treatments, the cure rate in children exceeds 80%. Cancer in adults, however, entails epithelial tumours, less aggressive treatments, and pain primarily due to invasive tumour growth. Cancer pain in adults is often neuropathic or mixed. This example shows why children and adolescents need an age-appropriate pain treatment delivered by paediatric experts.

Pain assessment

In *acute pain*, pain-specific behaviour can be observed, including certain verbal, vocal, or facial expressions, certain postures, and movements. These behaviours can be used for pain assessment in children unable to self-report pain (e.g. because of young age, mental impairment, or sedation). In verbal children, acute pain assessment should be conducted with age-appropriate validated tools such as the Faces Pain Scale revised (Hicks *et al.*, 2001). The reliable assessment of pain intensity can be acquired from a child of four years old and upward. The most crucial time point for pain intensity assessment is the postoperative period. Based on this assessment, institutional guidelines for postoperative pain management in children can be carried out to substantially improve postoperative pain treatment.

With *chronic pain*, pain-specific behaviours often cannot be observed. Most likely this effect emerges due to habituation. Instead of pain-specific behaviour, children with chronic pain may exhibit other behaviours that do not specifically suggest the experience of pain. Chronic pain more likely manifests as increased irritability, depressed mood, aggressive behaviour, low or increased appetite, and impaired school functioning. The PedIMMPACT recommendations specify the most relevant factors to be considered when assessing chronic pain in children (McGrath *et al.*, 2008). Importantly, self-reports of more complex concepts require an advanced level of development and therefore can only be obtained from a certain age onwards. For younger children, we rely on parental proxy reports (Chan and von Baeyer, 2016; Jaaniste *et al.*, 2016).

Acute pain

Everyday acute pain

When a child experiences pain in everyday life, this is usually a nociceptive pain either with no or with minor tissue damage. Pain experiences are crucial for healthy child development. In studies with healthy school children utilizing quantitative sensory testing (QST), younger children (6–8 years) were generally less sensitive to all thermal and mechanical detection stimuli but more sensitive to all pain stimuli than older (9–12 years) children, whereas there were little differences between older children and adolescents (13–17 years). In general, girls were more sensitive to thermal detection and thermal pain stimuli, but not to mechanical detection and mechanical pain stimuli (Blankenburg *et al.*, 2010).

Acute pain in the medical context

Although they share the same pathophysiological mechanisms, pain due to medical interventions is not comparable to everyday pains. In the medical context, the experience of pain occurs in an artificial environment that is characterized by other stressful features such as separation from one's parents, uncertainty about the end of the painful experience, or the child's and parents' anxiety. Nociceptive input is accompanied by an overwhelming feeling of anxiety, which intensifies the perception of pain. Therefore, in paediatrics, psychosocial interventions to reduce anxiety are very important and useful; they include education, parental empowerment, and distraction techniques (Uman *et al.*, 2013). They must be accompanied by pharmacological interventions, which range from skin anaesthesia with EMLA (eutectic mixture of local anaesthetics) to reduce needle pain to analgosedation or general anaesthesia for a bone marrow biopsy. If a general anaesthesia cannot be performed due to a lack of resources, often the combination of a central acting analgesic drug like a strong opioid or ketamine together with a sedative medication like a benzodiazepine are admitted by non-anesthesiologists (Tobias, 2015; Leroy *et al.*, 2009). In addition to pain control, patient security during analgosedation is a greater challenge in children than in adults and requires careful attention (Sury *et al.*, 2010).

Prolonged acute pain

Pain management protocols for burn injuries and in intensive care units, particularly in the postoperative setting, reduce the symptom load in children (Messerer *et al.*, 2010). These standard operating procedures should be assertively implemented in every hospital that cares for children. The best way to do this is by committing to pain relief as an institution and by certifying the hospital as a 'comfort place' or 'child-friendly hospital'. These quality management certificates are provided by different organizations worldwide (e.g. CHILDKIND: http://childkindinternational.org/). Benchmarking processes such as PAIN OUT INFANT are an additional helpful step in improving postoperative pain management (http://pain-out.med.uni-jena.de/).

Chronic pain

In what follows, the term '*chronic pain*' will be used for recurrent as well as persistent pain that has lasted for longer than three months. Chronic pain in children is multifaceted. It may arise as a symptom of a chronic condition (e.g. ulcerative colitis), but chronic pain may also become an independent disease. In Europe, at specialized pain clinics, chronic pain disorders without an underlying somatic condition are often classified as somatoform pain disorders (World Health Organization, 1992; Hechler *et al.*, 2014; Zernikow *et al.*, 2012).

Epidemiology of chronic pain

The prevalence rates of chronic pain in children range between 5–54% (King *et al.*, 2011). The differences in prevalence rates can be reduced to variations in the chronic pain definition (e.g. the criterion of time and frequency), variations in the study samples (e.g. age distribution), and variations in the study design (e.g. reference period; interview vs. questionnaire data; self-report vs. proxy report). Additionally, chronic pain has a large economic impact.

For some time, the prevalence of chronic pain in children has clearly increased. The most frequent pain condition in children is headache; it occurs across all ages but increases with age. Musculoskeletal pain, abdominal pain, or back pain also occur in children but are less common. While abdominal pain peaks in early childhood, back pain, and musculoskeletal pain peak in adolescence. Many children with chronic pain experience pain in more than one location. The prevalence of pain is higher in girls compared to boys, and younger children report chronic pain less often compared to adolescents. Recurrent or chronic pain lasts for more than one year in 30–60% of affected children and adolescents. For approximately one-third of children and adolescents with chronic pain, it even continues into adulthood. The risk of pain chronification is particularly high in girls, children with migrant backgrounds, and children with strong emotional distress or frequent pain episodes. One specific external risk factor for chronic pain in children is a chronic pain condition of parents. Approximately 4% of children with chronic pain have a moderate level of pain-related disability, and 1% are severely disabled due to pain.

Multidimensionality of paediatric chronic pain

In children and adolescents, chronic pain is considered a bio-psychosocial phenomenon. Some aspects of this phenomenon may be unique to this age group.

The biological dimension

Various paediatric chronic diseases have pathophysiology that causes repeated nociceptive stimuli. These conditions include genetic disorders (e.g. osteogenesis imperfecta and epidermolysis bullosa), chronic inflammatory diseases (e.g. juvenile idiopathic arthritis, ulcerative colitis, and Crohn's disease), cancer, and degenerative conditions (e.g. arthrosis). However, in children, these defined diseases are rare.

In conditions considered 'functional', physiological features contribute to the development and amplification of chronic pain. For example, in children with functional abdominal pain, the following abnormalities are more common: minor food allergies; slight fructose or lactose malabsorption; altered intestinal microbiomes; increased gastrointestinal permeability; subclinical gut inflammation or subtle variations in local gut immunology with increased mast cell count. '*However, even if minor abnormalities are detected in children with chronic pain, they usually do not explain the severity of the pain problem, such as pain intensity or pain-related disability. Minor abnormalities in common pediatric chronic pain conditions are not specific to children with chronic pain and will not occur in all affected children. Therefore, minor abnormalities cannot be interpreted as the one cause for the pain condition*' (Zernikow and Wager, p. 10).

In children with functional pain disorders, often neurobiological changes can be detected (e.g. central sensitization). '*A recent imaging study shows that the amygdala has more connections with other brain areas in pediatric pain patients with complex regional pain syndrome (CRPS) compared with healthy children (Simons et al., 2014). Specifically, more connectivity was shown for cognitive/emotional (prefrontal, cingulate cortex, basal ganglia), sensorimotor (thalamus, somatosensory cortex) and integrative (cerebellum, parietal lobe, thalamus) processing*' (Zernikow and Wager, p. 13). The excessive connectivity decreases after successful pain treatment. Moreover, not all changes in the CNS resolve along with symptom reduction. This suggests that CNS alterations remain, even in successfully treated patients.

The psychosocial dimension

Mental stress contributes to the development and maintenance of chronic pain in children. Anxious and depressive traits are considered risk factors (Miró *et al.*, 2007). Additionally, childhood sexual and physical abuse and other stressful life events enhance the risk of chronic pain and other somatoform disorders (Lampe *et al.*, 2003, Essau, 2007, Voerman *et al.*, 2015). Compared to healthy children, those with chronic pain spend less time with peers, have fewer friends, and are bullied more often. Taken together, '*the social environment of the child, especially his/her family, peer group and school, may be relevant to the origin and maintenance of pain disorders*' (Zernikow and Wager, p. 22).

Chronic pain treatment

'*Access to pain management is a human right! This has been stated in the Declaration of Montreal by the World Health Organization (WHO) and the IASP (IASP, 2015). However, the subjectivity of pain and the fact that a child with chronic pain is often not taken seriously in his/her report of pain can result in a lack of treatment for these children*' (Zernikow and Wager, p. 11). Today, healthcare providers increasingly recognize that the child's perspective needs to be recorded and respected.

Indications for treatment of chronic pain

'*Chronic pain becomes clinically relevant when it is accompanied by restrictions in everyday life, e.g., school absenteeism, neglecting friends, withdrawal from physical activity or emotional distress. In addition to the parents, the child him-/herself can best judge if a doctor's visit is required [. . .]*' (Zernikow and Wager, p. 15).

The goals of chronic pain treatment are the decrease and/or better handling of pain symptoms; this includes a decrease of functional disability, better psychological well-being, and the reintegration into school or work. A further goal of chronic pain treatment should be the prevention of potentially harmful diagnostic procedures or medical interventions. Reaching these goals also reduces the economic burden on the individual and society.

According to the bio-psychosocial model, often a multimodal treatment is indicated for chronic pain. This multimodal treatment includes the following components: medical interventions to address the modification of biological determinants of pain; psychological interventions to address relevant emotions and cognitions associated with pain; and social interventions to address role functioning in school, family, and with peers. According to the patient's needs, these treatment components need to be combined.

Medical interventions in chronic pain

In many children with diseases associated with chronic pain (e.g. cancer or inflammatory bowel disease), a medical intervention aiming at the primary cause will reduce or eliminate pain. However, some children will still experience pain after the successful treatment of the primary cause (Bromberg *et al.*, 2014). The medical treatment of minor physiological abnormalities in children with chronic pain is not effective in reducing the pain problem in many cases. *'For example, the causative treatments of constipation, lactose intolerance or helicobacter pylori colonization, such as high fiber or lactose free diets or Helicobacter pylori eradication therapy, have in most cases been ineffective in reducing pain and pain-related disability in children with chronic abdominal pain [. . .]'* (Zernikow and Wager, p. 16).

Pharmacological interventions

In children with chronic pain, pharmacological interventions to reduce pain are only indicated when the drug can directly influence nociceptive processing and for causative treatment. Four major groups of drugs are designated for such treatment: triptans, non-opioids, opioids, and adjuvants.

Triptans are effective at treating migraines and cluster headaches in childhood. Non-opioids (e.g. ibuprofen) reduce inflammation in conditions such as migraines, cancer pain, or juvenile idiopathic arthritis. *Opioids* have proven to be effective in postoperative pain, pain associated with burns, and cancer pain. *Adjuvant drugs*, such as antidepressants and anticonvulsants, reduce neuropathic pain which rarely occurs in children. However, adjuvants have not been proven effective in other paediatric chronic pain conditions, such as headaches or abdominal pain. *'On rare occasions and in orphan diseases such as osteogenesis imperfecta, adjuvants may be useful and are sometimes recommended [. . .]'* (Zernikow and Wager, p. 17).

Invasive medical interventions

In chronic pain conditions, evidence on the effectiveness of invasive medical interventions is limited. There might be an indication for the use of regional anaesthesia, or intrathecal medications, such as opioids or baclofen, in cases of localized cancer pain, severe cerebral palsy, or very rare cases of CRPS; however, this therapy should be integrated into a comprehensive multidisciplinary pain treatment. And even in these situations, interventions may only be effective for a very limited number of patients. Generally, the anticipated success of the interventions needs to be carefully balanced against the burden and risk (Zernikow *et al.*, 2015).

Psychological and social interventions in chronic pain

Psychological interventions for paediatric pain patients are versatile. They aim to reduce dysfunctional cognitions, emotions, and behaviour associated with pain and the negative impact of the pain condition. In chronic pain treatment, the most relevant psychological therapies are cognitive behavioural therapy, biofeedback, and hypnotherapy. Psychological interventions are effective in chronic pain patients with underlying physical conditions and functional conditions.

Within paediatric pain treatment, cognitive behavioural therapy can also address parents' cognitions and emotions and other familial factors that contribute to the maintenance of chronic pain. Several studies show the positive effect that psychological therapies involving the parents have on the child's pain symptoms, the parents' behaviour, and their psychological well-being. Additionally, several guidebooks for parents are available that provide detailed descriptions of interventions that parents can use to support their child in the treatment of chronic pain (Palermo and Law, 2015; Coakley, 2016; Dobe *et al.*, 2014).

Health literacy in the context of chronic pain

Psychoeducation is a key element of cognitive behavioural therapy. In chronic pain treatment, it should not only be applied by psychologists, but rather by all professions involved in the treatment. A study on functional abdominal pain shows that six sessions led by a gastroenterologist with a focus on education are as effective as six sessions of comprehensive cognitive behavioural therapy delivered by a psychologist (Van der Veek *et al.*, 2013). The cartoon *'Understanding pain and what's to be done about it . . . In less than 10 minutes'* is one source of education and is available in nearly every European language, please see http://www.deutsches-kinderschmerzzentrum.de/en/about-us/videos/video-understanding-pain/#c2569.

Multidisciplinary treatment of chronic pain

Regular primary care treatment is sufficient for many children with chronic pain. However, others require more intense and specialized treatment (e.g. physiotherapy, comprehensive education, or psychotherapy), or even specialized multidisciplinary pain treatment (Eccleston *et al.*, 2014).

For children severely affected by chronic pain, multidisciplinary, multimodal pain treatment programmes have recently become a standard of care and are offered in inpatient settings (Hechler *et al.*, 2015), day care, and less intensive outpatient settings. Each programme has a different treatment focus, but all are conceptualized as multiprofessional and multidisciplinary offers.

Conclusion

The management of pain in children is a broad domain. Five points summarize the most important aspects:

1. Acute and chronic pain in children should be considered a discrete condition and not be equalized to pain in adults.
2. The treatment of paediatric pain requires paediatric experts.
3. For the assessment of the subjective experience of pain, self-report is the gold standard in children. However, in younger children we rely on parental proxy report.
4. Acute pain in children requires pharmacological treatment. Additionally, psychosocial interventions are very effective.
5. Chronic pain in children is an increasing problem and requires a multidisciplinary treatment approach. Analgesics and co-analgesics are less important than psychosocial interventions and the establishment of a normal life.

Acknowledgements

Text extracts from Zernikow, B. and Wager, J., *The scientific facts and background of the cartoon understanding pain . . . and what's to be done about it in 10 minutes*, German Paediatirc Pain Center, reproduced with permission of the authors. Available from http://www.deutsches-kinderschmerzzentrum.de/fileadmin/media/Inhaltsbilder/Literatur/Cartoon_Scientific_Facts_Zernikow_Wager.pdf

References

Blankenburg, M., Boekens, H., Hechler, T., *et al.* (2010). Reference values for quantitative sensory testing in children and adolescents: Developmental and gender differences of somatosensory perception. *Pain*, **149**, 76–88.

Bromberg, M. H., Schechter, N. L., Nurko, S., Zempsky, W. T., & Schanberg, L. E. (2014). Persistent pain in chronically ill children without detectable disease activity. *Pain Management*, **4**, 211–19.

Chan, J. Y.-C. & von Baeyer, C. L. (2016). Cognitive developmental influences on the ability of preschool-aged children to self-report their pain intensity. *Pain*, **157**, 997–1001.

Coakley, R. (2016). *When Your Child Hurts: Effective Strategies to Increase Comfort, Reduce Stress, and Break the Cycle of Chronic Pain*. London, UK: Yale University Press.

Dobe, M., Zernikow, B., & Stewart, B. (2014). *How to Stop Chronic Panic in Children: A Practical Guide*. Heidelberg, Germany: Carl-Auer-Systeme Verlag und Verlagsbuchhandlung GmbH.

Eccleston, C., Palermo, T. M., Williams, A. C. D. C., *et al.* (2014). Psychological therapies for the management of chronic and recurrent pain in children and adolescents. *Cochrane Database Syst Rev*, **5**, CD003968.

Essau, C. A. (2007). Course and outcome of somatoform disorders in non-referred adolescents. *Psychosomatics*, **48**, 502–9.

Hechler, T., Kanstrup, M., Holley, A. L., *et al.* (2015). Systematic review on intensive interdisciplinary pain treatment of children with chronic pain. *Pediatrics*, **136**, 115–27.

Hechler, T., Ruhe, A., Schmidt, P., *et al.* (2014). Inpatient-based intensive interdisciplinary pain treatment for highly impaired children with severe chronic pain: randomized controlled trial of efficacy and economic effects. *Pain*, **155**, 118–28.

Hicks, C. L., Von Baeyer, C. L., Spafford, P. A., Van Korlaar, I., & Goodenough, B. (2001). The Faces Pain Scale—Revised: Toward a common metric in pediatric pain measurement. *Pain*, **93**, 173–83.

Jaaniste, T., Noel, M. & Von Baeyer, C. L. (2016). Young children's ability to report on past, future, and hypothetical pain states: a cognitive-developmental perspective. *Pain*, **157**, 2399–409.

King, S., Chambers, C. T., Huguet, A., *et al.* (2011). The epidemiology of chronic pain in children and adolescents revisited: A systematic review. *Pain*, **152**, 2729–38.

Lampe, A., Doering, S., Rumpold, G., *et al.* (2003). Chronic pain syndromes and their relation to childhood abuse and stressful life events. *J Psychosom Res*, **54**, 361–7.

Leroy, P., Gorzeman, M. & Sury, M. (2009). Procedural sedation and analgesia in children by non-anesthesiologists in an emergency department. *Minerva Pediatrica*, **61**, 193–215.

McGrath, P. J., Walco, G. A., Turk, D. C., *et al.* (2008). Core outcome domains and measures for pediatric acute and chronic/recurrent pain clinical trials: PedIMMPACT recommendations. *J Pain*, **9**, 771–83.

Messerer, B., Gutmann, A., Weinberg, A., & Sandner-Kiesling, A. (2010). Implementation of a standardized pain management in a pediatric surgery unit. *Pediatr Surg Int*, **26**, 879–89.

Miró, J., Huguet, A., & Nieto, R. (2007). Predictive factors of chronic pediatric pain and disability: A Delphi Poll. *J Pain*, **8**, 774–92.

Palermo, T. M. & Law, E. F. (2015). *Managing Your Child's Chronic Pain*. New York, NY: Oxford University Press

Simons, L. E., Pielech, M., Erpelding, N., *et al.* (2014). The responsive amygdala: treatment-induced alterations in functional connectivity in pediatric complex regional pain syndrome. *Pain*, **155**, 1727–42.

Sury, M., Bullock, I., Rabar, S., Demott, K., & Group, G. D. (2010). Sedation for diagnostic and therapeutic procedures in children and young people: summary of NICE guidance. *BMJ*, **341**, c6819.

Tobias, J. D. (2015). Sedation of infants and children outside of the operating room. *Curr Opin Anesthesiol*, **28**, 478–85.

Uman, L. S., Birnie, K. A., Noel, M., *et al.* (2013). Psychological interventions for needle-related procedural pain and distress in children and adolescents. *Cochrane Database Syst Rev*, **10**, CD005179.

Van der Veek, S. M., Derk, B. H., Benninga, M. A., & de Haan, E. (2013). Cognitive behavior therapy for pediatric functional abdominal pain: A randomized controlled trial. *Pediatrics*, **132**, e1163-e.

Voerman, J., Vogel, I., Waart, F., *et al.* (2015). Bullying, abuse and family conflict as risk factors for chronic pain among Dutch adolescents. *Eur J Pain*, **19**, 1544–51.

World Health Organization (WHO) (1992). *International Classification of diseases*, 10th Revised Edition. Geneva, Switzerland: WHO.

Zernikow, B., Wager, J., Brehmer, H., Hirschfeld, G., & Maier, C. (2015). Invasive treatments for complex regional pain syndrome in children and adolescents: a scoping review. *Anesthesiology*, **122**, 699–707.

Zernikow, B., Wager, J., Hechler, T., *et al.* (2012). Characteristics of highly impaired children with severe chronic pain: A 5-year retrospective study on 2249 pediatric pain patients. *BMC Pediatrics,* **16**, 54–65.

Zernikow, B. & Wager, J. The scientific facts and background of the cartoon Understanding Pain . . . and what's to be done about it in 10 minutes. German Paediatric Pain Center. Available at: http://www.deutsches-kinderschmerzzentrum.de/fileadmin/media/Inhaltsbilder/Literatur/Cartoon_Scientific_Facts_Zernikow_Wager.pdf [Online].

Chapter 3.3

Opioids for pain in Europe: Differing problems and differing solutions

Cathy Stannard

Introduction

The issue of opioid prescribing remains prominent internationally in the medical literature, in the conversations of those responsible for public health, and in written and broadcast media. The harsh lessons learned from the population-based 'experiment' of prescribing opioids for long-term non-cancer pain have been seen most prominently in North America where the prescribing of opioid medicines has led to an undoubted public health crisis of opioid-related harms including addiction, unintentional overdose, and death (CDC, 2016b; Dart *et al.*, 2015; Dunn *et al.*, 2010; Gomes *et al.*, 2011, 2014b; SAMHSA, 2016). Other countries, notably the United Kingdom and elsewhere in Europe have seen similar rises in prescribing of opioids over recent years but we are still getting to grips with whether or not a tide of opioid-related harms is about to engulf us (Häuser *et al.*, 2016; Health and Social Care Information Centre, 2016; Kotecha and Sites, 2013; O'Brien *et al.*, 2017; Stannard, 2013). It is not surprising that the use of opioids for pain management has been brought into sharp focus with critical analysis of the effectiveness or otherwise of opioids for pain, the harms of opioid therapy, and the degree to which these may have been underrecognized. There is thus much clinical, academic, and policy activity to equip prescribers with the information they need to prescribe responsibly and safely (CDC, 2016a; Chou *et al.*, 2015; Faculty of Pain Medicine, 2015; Franklin, 2014; Häuser *et al.*, 2015; NOUGG, 2010; O'Brien *et al.*, 2017; Sullivan and Howe, 2013; Zacny and Lichtor, 2008).

There is a critically important further facet to this debate. Access to opioid medicines varies substantially with North America, Western Europe, and Oceania, which represent 17% of the world's population, consuming 90% of the world's opioid supply (International Narcotics Control Board, 2015; University of Wisconsin, 2016). Throughout a decade or more of efforts to encourage restraint in opioid prescribing, it has been recognized that an unintended consequence may be that access to opioids for those that need them most, notably patients with severe acute pain and cancer sufferers at the end of life, will be restricted further by fears of an opioid addiction epidemic adding to existing regulatory and organizational barriers. The message in any publication calling for increased access to opioids runs the risk of being drowned out by the much-publicized international call to reappraise the role of opioids in the repertoire of pain treatment.

The need to balance appropriate access to essential pain relief and the need to protect individuals and society from harm should not be thought of as two sides of the same coin: improved access with risks of a further opioid epidemic or cautious prescribing with consequent reduced access. Clarity of thinking and a detailed understanding of the antecedents of, and potential solutions for, both of these related, but distinct problems is key. This chapter explores trends in opioid prescribing in Europe, identifying whether there are signals of increasing misuse and mortality relating to prescription opioids, and highlighting the persistent barriers to prescribing in parts of the continent.

Historic perspective: Why we are where we are

In the late twentieth century, there was increasing concern that patients with cancer were dying with avoidable pain because of restricted access to opioids. The World Health Organization analgesic ladder, developed in 1986, espoused a stepwise approach to prescribing for cancer pain based on the reported severity of pain, with non-opioid medicines being first choice for mild pain and strong opioids for severe pain with the recommendation that doses be escalated until pain is controlled (WHO, 1996). This engendered acceptance of the medicinal role of opioids and improved the lives of cancer sufferers. Inevitably however, a moral debate ensued: given the aversive nature of the pain experience, it was argued that access to treatment should be available for patients with pain regardless of the underlying diagnosis and the idea of pain relief as a human right emerged as a prominent influence on prescription of analgesic medicines (Brennan *et al.*, 2007; Cousins *et al.*, 2004). With the support of the pharmaceutical industry, a decade or more of vocal pain advocacy bundled together the themes of increased diagnosis of pain, the right to treatment, and access to opioids with the consequence that free access to opioids was seen as a compassionate and therefore laudable goal of medical practice (Ballantyne *et al.*, 2016; Kotecha and Sites, 2013; Weisberg and Stannard, 2013; Weisberg *et al.*, 2014). The individual and societal burden of undertreated pain was framed as a problem that could be solved by more liberal prescribing of opioids. A rapid and sustained rise in opioid prescribing was then inevitable.

There is no evidence that more liberal use of opioids for non-cancer pain has made any impact on the prevalence of or disabling sequelae of the condition at either a societal or individual level. By contrast, there has emerged a clear association of opioid prescribing and opioid-related harms, particularly prescription opioid deaths, opioid treatment admissions, and addiction and diversion of medicines, most prominently seen in the United States, where between 1999–2015, more than 183,000 people have died from overdoses related to prescription opioids, but also in Canada and Australia (CDC, 2016b; Dart *et al.*, 2015; Dobbin, 2014; Gomes *et al.*, 2011, 2014a, 2014b; National Treatment Agency for Substance Misuse, 2011; Okie, 2010; Rudd *et al.*, 2016; Warner, 2015).

Pain and opioid prescribing in Europe

Prevalence of pain in Europe

Chronic pain of moderate to severe intensity occurs in 19% of adult Europeans. Of this group, one-fifth have a concurrent diagnosis of depression and two-thirds describe being unable to work outside the home (Breivik *et al.*, 2006). A study of disability in relation to a range of physical and medical conditions showed that chronic pain was the single condition that contributed the most to disability measures in all European regions (Barbaglia *et al.*, 2017). This is consistent with the more recent findings of the Global Burden of Disease Study 2013 (Vos *et al.*, 2015). Primary care practitioners in Europe find chronic pain one of the most challenging conditions to treat and patterns of analgesic use vary considerably (Fig. 3.3.1) (Breivik *et al.*, 2006; Castro-Lopes, 2014; Galvez, 2009; Johnson *et al.*, 2013).

Given the uncertain efficacy of many interventions for the treatment of chronic pain (Moore *et al.*, 2013), this sets the scene for resort to opioid prescribing 'when all else fails' in a large, disabled, and distressed population. It is true that pain relief for patients with persistent symptoms is often inadequate. It is also true that prescribing practices in relation to, and cultural acceptability of, use of opioids for chronic pain

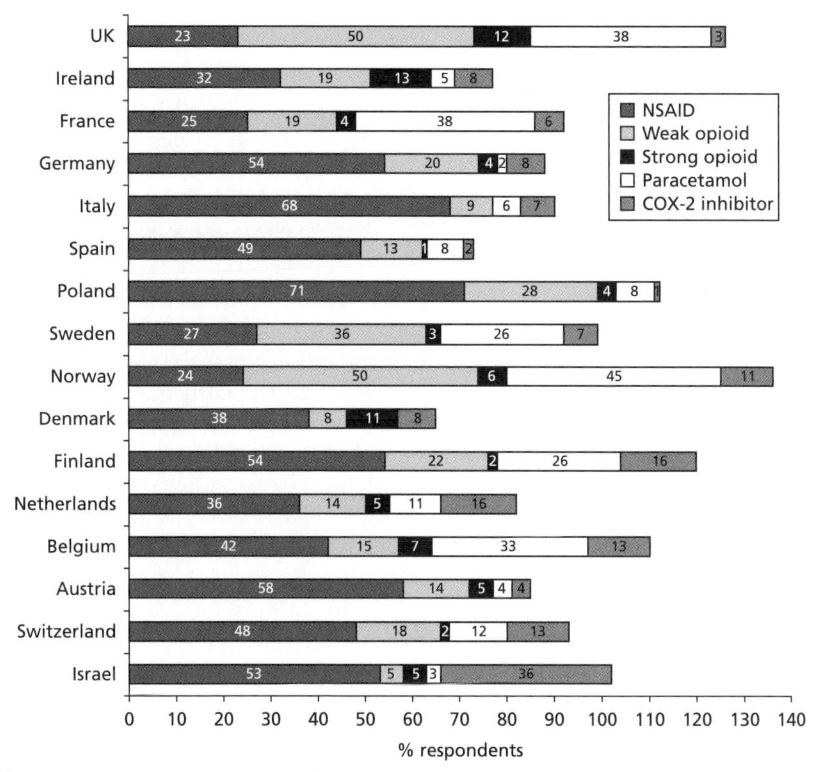

Fig. 3.3.1 European country-specific usages of prescription medications for chronic pain (Breivik *et al* 2006).

Reproduced from Harald Breivik *et al.*, 'Survey of chronic pain in Europe: Prevalence, impact on daily life, and treatment,' *European Journal of Pain*, Volume 10, pp. 287–333, Copyright © 2005 European Federation of Chapters of the International Association for the Study of Pain, with permission from John Wiley and Sons.

vary widely across Europe, but the seemingly refractory problem of making an impact on the societal burden of non-cancer pain cannot be framed scientifically as being causally related to underprescribing of opioids.

Opioid prescribing in Europe

Prescribing of opioids in Europe demonstrates a picture of stark contrasts. This poses challenges in making general comparisons between European and North American prescribing. Although there has been a general picture of increased prescribing in Europe, per capita consumption remains several-fold lower in all European countries compared to the United States and Canada. Estimates of country-specific opioid consumption can be derived from a number of sources. The International Narcotics Control Board gathers data on the amounts of opioid that each country's competent national authority estimates are needed and used annually. The statistical measure of drug consumption used is the defined daily dose (DDD) defined by the World Health Organization (WHO) as 'the assumed average maintenance dose per day for a drug used for its main indication in adults'. Although there is variation in the way different countries report consumption data to the International Narcotics Control Board (INCB), the figures provide a useful broad comparison of opioid use. Table 3.3.1 includes data from a number of European countries and from the United States and Canada for comparison. The table exemplifies the contrasts across Europe and paints a clear picture of less liberal prescribing in Europe compared to North America (regional average DDD/million inhabitants 8,298 and 38,947, respectively—a fourfold difference) (International Narcotics Control Board, 2015).

Opioid use can also be compared by calculating the morphine equivalents in mg per head of population. Figure 3.3.2 shows most recent prescribing data for all European countries using this metric and clearly depicts the extremes of prescribing (University of Wisconsin, n.d.).

The relationship between the rise in prescribing of opioids in the United States and prescription opioid-related harms has generated much discussion as to whether European countries experiencing a similar trajectory in prescribing are likely to be vulnerable to an overwhelming rise in deaths and other prescription opioid-related harms (Stannard, 2013; Weisberg *et al.*, 2014). Examination of trends in opioid prescribing across Europe show more marked and sustained rises in countries with higher morphine equivalences in mg/capita, whereas prescribing has been more static in countries where use has been low (University of Wisconsin, 2016). In the United Kingdom, although there has been a sustained rise in number of prescriptions of opioids and associated costs (23 million opioid prescriptions dispensed in the community in 2015 at a cost of £314 million; see Health and Social Care Information Centre, 2016) there has been a fall in oral morphine equivalents per capita, probably because of increased prescribing of low dose transdermal buprenorphine preparations. This has been confirmed from other data sources (Zin *et al.*, 2014).

Barriers to opioid prescribing in Europe

There are undoubted challenges of managing severe pain, particularly at the end of life, in a number of European countries where cultural beliefs, differing drug policies, poor

Table 3.3.1 Levels of consumption of narcotic drugs in defined daily doses for statistical purposes per million inhabitants per day (excluding preparations in schedule III)

Global ranking	Country	Total DDD
1	United States	50,412
2	Canada	30,540
3	Germany	26,547
4	Denmark	24,460
5	Belgium	21,926
6	Austria	21,376
7	Switzerland	19,297
9	Netherlands	14,344
11	Spain	11,955
13	Norway	11,512
14	United Kingdom	11,418
15	Ireland	11,331
17	Sweden	10,004
20	France	8,706
24	Italy	6,246
27	Greece	5,118
51	Romania	1,323
61	Turkey	757
153	Uzbekistan	10

Source: data from International Narcotics Control Board, *REPORT 2015 Estimated World Requirements for 2016—Statistics for 2014*, Copyright ©1995–2017 International Narcotics Control Board, available from www.incb.org/incb/en/narcotic-drugs/Technical_Reports/2015/narcotic-drugs-technical-report-2015.html.

knowledge, and legal/regulatory controls are interrelated and particularly influential (Cherny *et al.*, 2010). Opioid analgesics remain the mainstay of management of moderate to severe cancer pain and are included in the WHO list of essential medicines (WHO, 1996, 2015).

The single convention on narcotic drugs prohibits production and supply of controlled medicines other than for medical and scientific purposes. In addition, country-specific legislation and regulation, created to prevent misuse and diversion can limit access to opioids and this is the case in many low- and middle-income countries. The seeming tension between the conflicting needs of provision of medicines for those who will benefit and the prevention of diversion and misuse have been addressed in a

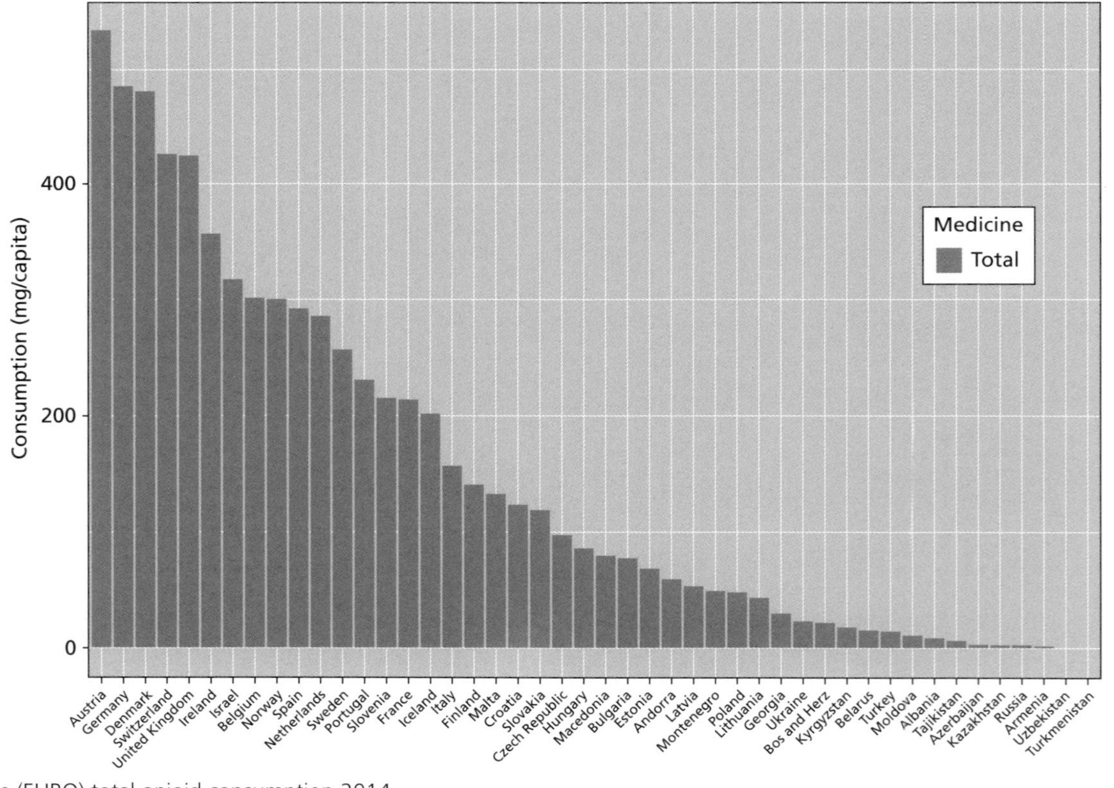

Fig. 3.3.2 Europe (EURO) total opioid consumption 2014.

Generated and reproduced with permission from Pain and Policy Studies Group, *Custom Consumption Graphs for Opioid Medicines*, Copyright © 2016 UW Madison Department of Medicine, https://ppsg-chart.medicine.wisc.edu./. Source: data from International Narcotics Control Board; World Health Organization population data by Pain and Policy Studies Group, University of Wisconsin/WHO Collaborating Center, Copyright © 2016.

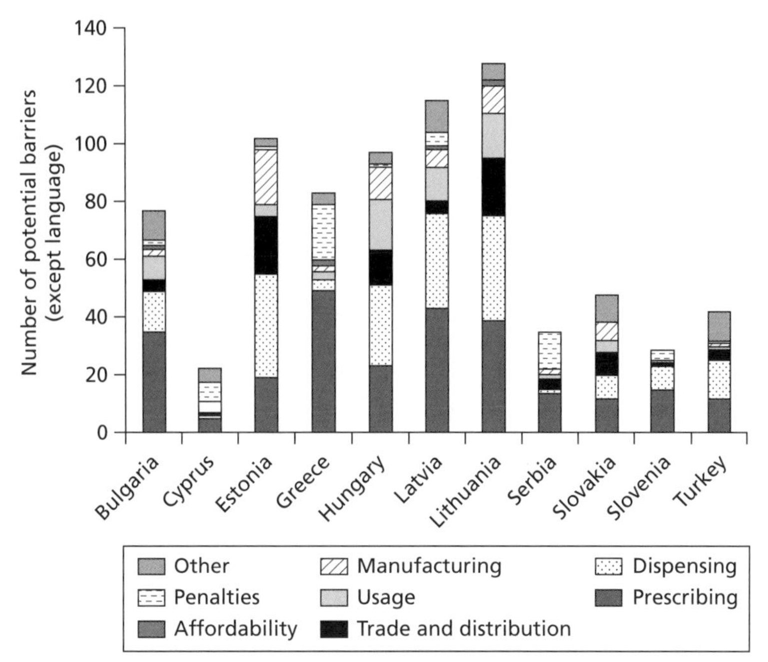

Fig. 3.3.3 Number of potential barriers to appropriate prescriptions of opioids quantitatively identified according to category (except use of stigmatizing language) per country.

Reprinted from *The Lancet Oncology*, Volume 17, Number 1, Vranken MJM *et al.*, 'Barriers to access to opioid medicines: a review of national legislation and regulations of 11 central and eastern European countries,' e13-e22, Copyright © 2016 Elsevier Ltd, with permission from Elsevier, http://www.sciencedirect.com/science/journal/14702045.

WHO guideline, 'Ensuring balance in national policies on controlled substances: guidance for availability and accessibility of controlled substances' (WHO, 2011). This document relates to a European project (ATOME—Access to Opioid Medicines in Europe) to improve access to opioids in 11 European countries (Bulgaria, Cyprus, Estonia, Greece, Hungary, Latvia, Lithuania, Serbia, Slovakia, Slovenia, and Turkey) where data suggest that access to opioids might be problematic. In each country contributing to the project, stakeholder individuals including relevant legal expertise were identified and the teams carried out a systematized review of legal documents using eight of the 21 WHO guidelines referring to legal and regulatory aspects of access to controlled substances encompassing the whole pharmaceutical supply chain (Vranken *et al.*, 2016). Examples of potential barriers to opioid prescribing included:

- **Prescribing** (limited to specific medical discipline, special permit needed, special forms, limited duration of prescription, limited quantity, or dose)
- **Dispensing** (special licences, designated pharmacies, onerous administrative requirements, restrictions on storage)
- **Manufacturing** (onerous administrative and storage requirements)

- **Use** (trade distribution)
- **Affordability**
- **Penalties** (for violation of regulations)
- **Language** (unclear definitions of licit and illicit use, stigmatization of opioid users)

The study found that there were potential barriers to appropriate access to opioid medicines for analgesia in all countries studied ranging from 22 potential barriers (Cyprus) to 128 potential barriers (Lithuania) (Fig. 3.3.3). This analysis has provided a platform for improving access to opioids in the countries studied, but it is not yet possible to evaluate the impact that this has on the important end point of successful pain treatment, particularly for patients with cancer.

Prescription opioid harms in Europe

Prescribing statistics and opioid consumption data tell only part of the story about appropriate use of opioids. Analysis of these statistics should prompt two questions: are we exposing populations to risks of prescription opioid-related deaths and morbidity and are we using opioid drugs, the principal indication for which is pain relief, in an appropriate, effective, and safe way?

There is a relative paucity of studies on misuse, abuse of, and addiction to prescribed opioids in Europe with different countries collecting data in different ways (Casati *et al.*, 2012). Some countries (including the United Kingdom) include over-the-counter opioids in addictions data, whereas the European Monitoring Centre for Drugs and Drug Addiction (ECMDDA) largely focuses on illicit opioid products. The foregoing provides some detail from countries that have specifically studied opioid misuse in relation to increases in prescription opioid prescribing.

Generally, lifetime estimates for non-medical use of prescription psychotherapeutic drugs (e.g. opioids, stimulants, and sedatives) suggests that such use is lower in the EU (7–13%) than in the United States, where the figure is around 20% (Novak *et al.*, 2016; Schubert *et al.*, 2013). A systematic review of studies exploring addiction to prescribed opioids (Vowles *et al.*, 2015) included two non-US studies, a small case notes review and administration of an addiction questionnaire in 104 patients in London, concluding that problematic use was not identified in that cohort (Cowan *et al.*, 2003), and a study comparing utility of different diagnostic criteria in Denmark (Ekholm *et al.*, 2014; Højsted *et al.*, 2010). More recently, a Danish study based on a random sample of 25,000 patients with 13,281 eligible individuals compared addictive behaviours in subjects with and without chronic pain. Individuals with chronic pain were more likely to report addictive behaviours than those without pain and there was a clustering of indicators of addictive behaviours in opioid users with pain, compared to non-opioid users with pain. The study also found a high risk of long-term use of benzodiazepines and hypnotics in long-term opioid users compared to short-term and non-opioid users (Højsted *et al.*, 2013). In Norway, where prescription of weak opioids is prevalent, there are data available from a long-term follow-up of a cohort of opioid-naïve patients initiated on weak opioids for acute pain (Skurtveit *et al.*, 2011). The proportion of patients defined as persistent users of opioids or probable problematic users were 0.3% and 0.08%, respectively. A Norwegian pharmacoepidemiological study concluded that of 14,477 people reporting chronic non-malignant pain, 85% did not use opioids, 3% used them persistently, and 12% occasionally (Fredheim *et al.*, 2010). Three-quarters of those using opioids had severe pain despite their opioid use. The study also concluded that physical inactivity and co-prescription of benzodiazepines were associated with persistent opioid use.

An analysis of drug and alcohol-related deaths in Finland from 2000 to 2008 showed that fatalities in relation to prescription opioids increased as a proportion of all drug-related poisonings from 9.5% (52 cases) to 32.4% (179 cases). Deaths involving weak opioids (codeine and tramadol) were frequently as a result of suicide, but deaths involving buprenorphine and methadone were usually accidental. Consumption of other sedatives and alcohol was a prominent feature of prescription drug-related deaths (Hakkinen *et al.*, 2012; Winstock *et al.*, 2014). More recent data looking at patterns of misuse showed that drug abuse (defined as drug abuse history, drug injecting, or laboratory findings of illicit drugs) was the norm in patients dying in association with buprenorphine and methadone and the exception for tramadol, codeine, fentanyl, and oxycodone deaths, with abuse and fatal poisonings most common in men aged 20–49 (Hakkinen *et al.*, 2014; Winstock *et al.*, 2014).

There was a 37% rise in prescribing of opioids in Germany in the decade 2000–2010, which was mostly a result of increased prescribing for non-cancer pain (77% of all opioid prescribing). Notably, there was a fourfold increase in the use of extended release strong opioid prescriptions, now thought to be a risk factor for sustained high-dose prescribing and associated harms. Trends in strong rather than weak opioid given at initiation of therapy and longer duration of therapy were noted (Schubert *et al.*, 2013). Analysis of a large insured cohort showed that 15.5% of patients on long-term opioid therapy were receiving high doses with a mean morphine equivalent daily (MED) of 173 mg, somewhat lower than populations in United States and Canada (Häuser *et al.*, 2016). Higher dose use was associated with male gender and mental health diagnoses. Of note, the percentage of individuals diagnosed as having an opioid use disorder/addiction was very small at 0.008% and this is in accordance with German data from a tertiary centre (Marschall *et al.*, 2016).

In the United Kingdom, a cross sectional study between 2000 and 2010 showed a sustained increase in strong opioid prescribing with the majority of prescriptions being for non-cancer pain. There was a greater increase in prescriptions than the number of patients exposed to opioids and increasing days of supply were demonstrated (Zin *et al.*, 2014).

UK Data on opioid-related deaths, misuse, and addiction

The National Drug Treatment Monitoring System (NDTMS) is a national database that collects activity data from publicly funded substance use disorder treatment services in England (see Fig. 3.33.4). This includes information on the substances that people present to treatment with including over-the-counter medicines. Analysis of NDTMS data gives a picture of misuse of prescription opioids in patients presenting to drug treatment services. These data are likely to underestimate the prevalence of addiction to medicines, as not all individuals who have developed an addiction to prescribed analgesia will be referred to drug treatment and recovery services.

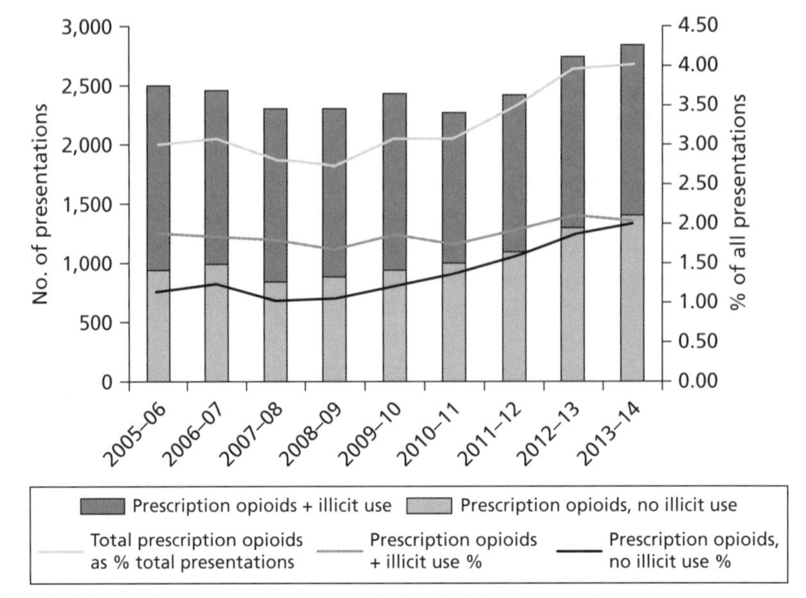

Fig. 3.3.4 Trends in presentation to publicly funded drug dependency and recovery services in England: clients presenting with misuse of prescription opioids with and without additional use of illicit substances.

Source: data from the English National Drug Treatment Monitoring System, 2015.

The data identify two populations presenting to drug services: patients addicted to prescription opioids as their sole drug of dependency and those who use prescription opioids as part of a polysubstance misuse (i.e. in combination with illicit drugs). The number of patients using prescription opioids in conjunction with illicit drugs has remained relatively stable at 2% of the population in treatment. However, the proportion of individuals who use prescription opioids as their sole drug has increased and is also 2% of the treatment population, and this group represents an increasing proportion of presentations to drug dependency and recovery services.

The Crime Survey for England and Wales examines the extent and trends in illicit drug use among a nationally representative sample of 16–59-year-olds resident in households in England and Wales (Home Office, 2016). The most recent data suggest that 7.5% of adults aged 16–59 years had taken a prescription-only painkiller not prescribed to them in the past year:

- 7.4% (around 2.4 million adults) for medical reasons;
- 0.2% (33,000 adults) said it was just for the feeling or experience it gave them;
- Use of non-prescribed prescription-only painkillers for medical reasons decreases as life satisfaction increases: 12.7% of those with low levels of life satisfaction reported use in the last year, compared with 5.7% of those with very high levels of life satisfaction.

The decline in misuse with age is less for prescription painkillers than for other drugs and painkiller misuse is less likely to be associated with misuse of other drugs.

The Office for National Statistics (ONS) publishes annual data on drug poisoning and drug misuse deaths (ONS, 2016). It does not distinguish between prescribed, over-the-counter, and illicitly-obtained medicines. The drug misuse figures only include drugs controlled under the Misuse of Drugs Act. The published data only breaks down poisoning (and not drug misuse) deaths by substance. There is a gradual trend of increasing deaths relating to prescription opioid medicines, particularly tramadol (peaking in 2015 at 240 deaths in which tramadol was mentioned on the death certificate) but the most recent data have shown a small fall in tramadol-related deaths, possibly attributable to scheduling of the drug in 2015. The data report that substances are 'mentioned' on death certificates, so it is not possible to know whether deaths are attributable to that substance, or present but not contributory to death.

Prescription drug misuse: Comparisons between Europe and North America

Although available data are far from conclusive, analysis of prescription opioid-related harms in Europe does not suggest that the problem is of a similar magnitude to that seen in North America. Potential reasons for observed differences have been postulated, some of which are presented in more detail here (Fischer *et al.*, 2013; Häuser *et al.*, 2016; Van Amsterdam and van den Brink, 2015; Weisberg and Stannard, 2013; Weisberg *et al.*, 2014).

Choice and availability of drug

Prescription painkillers are the second most common type of illicit drug used (marijuana being the most common) in the United States (Fig. 3.3.5) (SAMHSA, 2016).

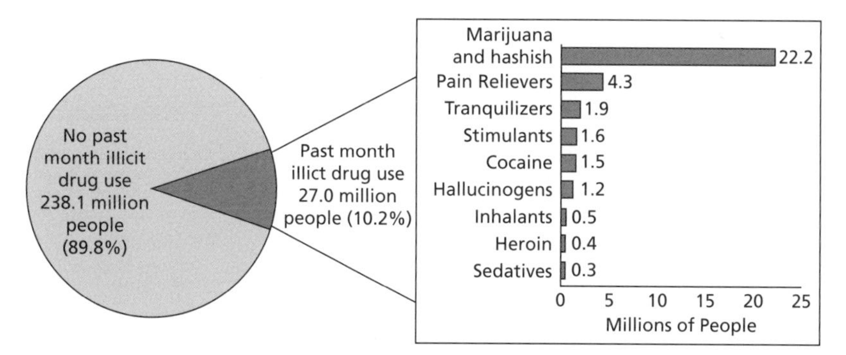

Note: Estimated numbers of people refer to people aged 12 or older in the civilian, non-institutionalized population in the United States. The numbers do not sum to the total population of the United States because the population for NSDUH does not include people aged 11 years old or younger, people with no fixed household address (e.g. homeless or transient people not in shelters), active-duty military personnel, and residents of institutional group quarters, such as correctional facilities, nursing homes, mental institutions, and long-term hospitals.

Note: The estimated numbers current users of different illicit drugs are not mutually exclusive because people could have used more than one type of illicit drug in the past month.

Fig. 3.3.5 Numbers of past month illicit drug users among people aged 12 or older (US): 2014.

Reproduced from Substance Abuse and Mental Health Services Administration (SAMHSA), *National Survey on Drug Use and Health 2014 and 2015*, available from www.samhsa.gov/data/sites/default/files/NSDUH-DetTabs-2015/NSDUH-DetTabs-2015/NSDUH-DetTabs-2015.htm.

Prescription opioids represent two-thirds of non-medical use of psychotherapeutic drugs in the United States. The percentage of users of prescription opioids has been slightly lower in the last two years for which data are available compared to the preceding 10 years. There is likely a shared market for prescription opioids and heroin, with heroin being relatively cheaper and easy to obtain in the United Kingdom and Europe compared to the United States (Weisberg *et al.*, 2014). The data for heroin misuse therefore show a contrasting trend with increase in use in the period during fall in prescription opioid misuse (Banerjee *et al.*, 2016; CDC, 2015a, 2015b; Cicero *et al.*, 2014; Compton *et al.*, 2016; Dasgupta *et al.*, 2014; Hedegaard *et al.*, 2015; Mars *et al.*, 2014; Warner, 2015). As controls on misuse of prescription opioids begin to have an impact, heroin misuse is emerging as a more significant health problem (Kolodny *et al.*, 2015). In Europe, by contrast, opioids (of which heroin is the most commonly misused drug), are less frequently used compared to other illicit substances, but account for the largest proportion of drug-related deaths and drug treatments (ECMDDA, 2016). Misuse of and morbidity relating to buprenorphine and methadone in Europe reflect their predominant use in treatment of heroin addiction (Green *et al.*, 2015). Unlike the United States, methadone use for pain is limited in England, with only 2.6% of methadone prescriptions written for pain (Health and Social Care Information Centre, 2016).

Vertically integrated, publicly funded healthcare systems exemplified by the United Kingdom afford opportunities for close scrutiny of opioid prescribing. Almost all patients are registered with a general practitioner who will be able to see who is being prescribed what, as will other partners in that practice. Prescribing is further scrutinized at practice and local level by medicines management teams, who are empowered (as are dispensing pharmacists) to challenge prescribing outwith the bounds of good practice and can share with prescribers the extent to which their prescribing practices differ from local and regional norms. Increasingly, secondary care specialists do not prescribe for patients but rather ask the patients' general practitioners to prescribe, which further reduces the sources from which prescription opioids can be obtained. The private insurance industry in the United Kingdom is very small and represents only 0.1% of controlled substance prescribing (Care Quality Commission, 2011). This contrasts with decentralized systems—most notably those in the United States—where prescriptions can be obtained from numerous specialist and community practitioners. Direct-to-consumer advertising, notably of potent oxycodone preparations and incentivizing of practitioners to prescribe are not seen in the United Kingdom and largely elsewhere in Europe. Similarly, the impact of patient satisfaction metrics is more potent in a private healthcare system and acquisition of an opioid prescription is associated with increased satisfaction and necessarily influences choice of treatment (Frantsve and Kerns, 2007; Zgierska *et al.*, 2012). Resources are constrained in both private and publicly funded healthcare systems: in the United States prescribing may be more readily reimbursed than more holistic interventions for pain. This desire for and expectation of a 'quick fix' is similarly seen in the United Kingdom and Europe, but there is an emerging understanding of the interplay between emotional and physical well-being and a recognition that detailed assessment and integrated treatment planning is in the best interests of patients and reduces costly and unnecessary, if not harmful, pharmacological and other interventions (The Kings Fund, 2016). These themes are reflected in a wider context of a more general expectation of pharmacotherapeutic solutions to a number of problems in the United States compared to Europe again driven by prominent advertising to patients and prescribers (Flora, 2007; Rose, 2003).

A further influence on prescribing may be the availability of opioid substitution treatment for heroin addiction, which in the more established and decentralized model of community-based provision of methadone and buprenorphine in the United Kingdom and elsewhere in Western Europe is likely better equipped to meet demand for services (Strang *et al.*, 2010).

Motivations for use of non-prescribed prescription painkillers

The inconsistency of data collection particularly in relation to populations studied (age, risk factors for misuse) and drugs used do not allow firm conclusions to be drawn regarding differing motivations for illicit drug use. One United States study of college students identified the three most common motives associated with the non-medical use of prescription opioids were to relieve pain (40%), get high, and to experiment. Use of drugs for pain was less likely to be associated with other substance misuse (McCabe *et al.*, 2007). A UK study of the misuse of tramadol showed that a somewhat higher proportion of non-medical users took the drug for pain relief (nearly 60%) with other motives being to relax, to help sleep, and to relieve boredom (Winstock *et al.*, 2014). The Crime Survey of England and Wales 2015–2016 (see above) suggests that the predominant motive for use of a prescription painkiller not prescribed was for medical reasons, with only 0.2%, (33,000 adults) using prescription medicines for the feeling or experience it gave them (Home Office, 2016).

Conclusion

Any discussion of opioid prescribing is necessarily of its time as patterns of drug use and availability are constantly changing. It is difficult to view opioid prescribing in Europe through a clear global lens as data collection around the world is inconsistent. We must work with the data we have and these indicate that while problematic use of prescription opioids does occur in Europe, the scale of this problem is far from that seen in North America. What is unarguable is that Europe exemplifies a complete spectrum: at one end of poor access to opioids for those with severe pain, particularly at the end of life, who may potentially benefit; and by contrast, a culture of liberal and increasing opioid prescribing. Clinicians and policymakers have acknowledged the problems of widespread opioid prescribing seen in North America and remain alert for emerging problems of opioid use and its related morbidity. Strategies for optimizing use of medicines to retain societal safety also remain an important focus.

The main challenge for clinicians to meet however must always be the patient with enduring and intrusive pain. There are few assurances we can give patients that we have tools to reduce intensity of pain and we must remember that opioids used appropriately may improve the quality of some patients' lives. Our efforts should be directed to identifying and supporting those patients. However, this must not come at the cost of exposing the larger proportion of patients, for whom opioids are unlikely to be a useful adjunct to pain management, to harms unbalanced by analgesic benefit.

References

Ballantyne, J., Kalso, E., & Stannard, C. (2016). The WHO analgesic ladder: a good concept gone astray. *BMJ*, **352**, i20.

Banerjee, G., Edelman, G. J., & Barry, D. T., *et al.* (2016). Non-medical use of prescription opioids is associated with heroin initiation among US veterans: a prospective cohort study. *Addiction*, **111**, 2021–31.

Barbaglia, D., Adroher, N. D., & Vilagut, G. (2017). Health conditions and role limitation in three European Regions: a public-health perspective. *Gac Sanit*, **31**, 2–10.

Breivik, H., Collett, B., Ventafridda, V., Cohen, R., & Gallacher, D. (2006). Survey of chronic pain in Europe: prevalence, impact on daily life, and treatment. *Eur J Pain*, **10**, 287–333.

Brennan, F., Carr, D. B., & Cousins, M. (2007). Pain management: a fundamental human right. *Anesth Analg*, **105**, 205–221.

Care Quality Commission (2011). Annual report and accounts 2010/2011. Available at: https://www.cqc.org.uk (accessed 1 January 2017)[Online].

Casati, A., Sedefov, R., & Pfeiffer-Gerschel, T. (2012). Misuse of medicines in the European Union: a systematic review of the literature. *Eur Addict Res*, **18**, 228–45.

Castro-Lopes, J. (2014). Impact of chronic pain on primary care across Europe. Journal of Pain & Palliative Care Pharmacotherapy, **28**, 158–9.

Centers for Disease Control and Prevention (CDC) (2015a). Drug-poisoning Deaths Involving Heroin: United States, 2000–2013. Available at: https://www.cdc.gov/nchs/products/databriefs/db190.htm (accessed 1 January 2017) [Online].

Centers for Disease Control and Prevention (CDC) (2015b). MMWR 2015. Today's Heroin Epidemic More people at risk, multiple drugs abused. Available at: https://www.cdc.gov/vitalsigns/heroin/index.html (accessed 1 January 2017) [Online].

Centers for Disease Control and Prevention (CDC) (2016a). Draft Guideline for Prescribing Opioids for Chronic Pain CDC. Available at: http://www.cdc.gov/drugoverdose/prescribing/guideline.html (accessed 2 January 2017) [Online].

Centers for Disease Control and Prevention (CDC) (2016b). Prescription Opioid Overdose Data. Available at: https://www.cdc.gov/drugoverdose/data/overdose.html (accessed 1 January 2017) [Online].

Cherny, N. I., Baselga, J., de Conno, F., & Radbruch, L. (2010). Formulary availability and regulatory barriers to accessibility of opioids for cancer pain in Europe: a report from the ESMO/EAPC Opioid Policy Initiative. *Ann Oncol*, **21**, 615–26.

Chou, R., Turner, J., & Devine, E. (2015). The effectiveness and risks of long-term opioid therapy for chronic pain: a systematic review for a National Institutes of Health Pathways to Prevention Workshop. *Ann Intern Med*, **162**, 276–86.

Cicero, T. J., Ellis, M. S., Surratt, H. L., & Kurtz, S. P. (2014). The changing face of heroin use in the United States: a retrospective analysis of the past 50 years. *JAMA Psychiatry*, **71**, 821–6.

Compton, W. M., Jones, C. M., & Baldwin, G. T. (2016). Understanding the relationship between prescription opioid and heroin abuse. *N Engl J Med*, **374**, 1295–6.

Cousins, M., Brennan, F., & Carr, D. (2004). Pain relief: a universal human right? *Pain*, **112**, 1–4.

Cowan, D., Wilson-Barnett, J., Griffiths, P., & Allan, L. (2003). A survey of chronic noncancer pain patients prescribed opioid analgesics. *Pain Med*, **4**, 340–51.

Dart, R. C., Surratt, H. L., Cicero, T. J., *et al.* (2015). Trends in opioid analgesic abuse and mortality in the United States. *N Engl J Med*, **372**, 241–8.

Dasgupta, N., Creppage, K., Austin, A., *et al.*(2014). Observed transition from opioid analgesic deaths toward heroin. *Drug Alcohol Depend*, **145**, 238–41.

Dobbin, M. (2014). Pharmaceutical drug misuse in Australia. *Aust Prescr*, **37**, 79–81

Dunn, A. T., Saunders, K. M., Rutter, K. W., *et al.* (2010). Opioid prescriptions for chronic pain and overdose. *Ann Intern Med*, **152**, 82–5.

Ekholm, O., Kurita, G. P., Højsted, J., Juel, K., & Sjøgren, P. (2014). Chronic pain, opioid prescriptions, and mortality in Denmark: A population-based cohort study. *Pain*, **155**, 2486–90.

European Monitoring Centre for Drugs and Drug Addiction (ECMDDA) (2016). European Drug Report 2016. Available at: http://www.emcdda.europa.eu/edr2016 (accessed 1 January 2017) [Online].

Faculty of Pain Medicine Royal College of Anaesthetists (UK) (2015). Opioids Aware: A resource for patients and healthcare professionals to support opioid prescribing for pain. Available at: https://www.rcoa.ac.uk/faculty-of-pain-medicine/opioids-aware (accessed 2 January 2017) [Online].

Fischer, B., Keates, A., Bühringer, G., Reimer, J., & Rehm, J. (2013). Non-medical use of prescription opioids and prescription opioid-related harms: why so markedly higher in North America compared to the rest of the world? *Addiction*, **109**, 177–81.

Flora, S. R. (2007). *Taking America off Drugs: Why Behavioral Therapy Is More Effective for Treating ADHD, OCD, Depression, and Other Psychological Problems*. New York, NY: State University of New York Press.

Franklin, G. (2014). Opioids for chronic non-cancer pain. A position paper of the American Academy of Neurology. *Neurology*, **83**, 1277–84.

Frantsve, L. M. & Kerns, R. D. (2007). Patient-provider interactions in the management of chronic pain: current findings within the context of shared medical decision making. *Pain Med*, **8**, 25–35.

Fredheim, O. M., Skurtveit, S., Breivik, H., & Borchgrevink, P. C. (2010). Increasing use of opioids from 2004 to 2007: Pharmaco-epidemiological data from a complete national prescription database in Norway. *Eur J Pain*, **14**, 289–94.

Galvez, R. J. (2009). Variable use of opioid pharmacotherapy for chronic noncancer pain in Europe: causes and consequences. *Pain Palliat Care Pharmacother*, **23**, 346–56.

Gomes, T., Mamdani, M., Dhalla, I. *et al.* (2014a). The burden of premature opioid-related mortality. *Addiction*, **109**, 1482–8.

Gomes, T., Mamdani, M. M., Dhalla, I. A., Paterson, J. M., & Juurlink, D. N. (2011). Opioid dose and drug-related mortality in patients with nonmalignant pain. *Arch Intern Med*, **171**, 689–91

Gomes, T., Mamdani, M., Paterson, J. M., Dhalla, I. A., & Juurlink, D. N. (2014b). Trends in highdose opioid prescribing in Canada. *Can Fam Physician*, **60**, 826–32.

Green, J. L., Martinez, E. M., Rosenblum, A., et al (2015). Global impact of prescription opioid misuse: Europe and US. *Drug and Alcohol Dependence*, **146**, 1, e129.

Hakkinen, M., Launiainen, T., Vuori, E., & Ojanpera, I. (2012) Comparison of fatal poisonings by prescription opioids. *Forensic Sci Int*, **222**, 327–31.

Hakkinen, M., Vuori, E., & Ojanpera, I. (2014). Prescription opioid abuse based on representative postmortem toxicology. *Forensic Sci Int*, **245**, 121–5.

Häuser, W., Bock, F., Engeser, P., *et al.* (2015). Recommendations of the updated LONTS guidelines: long-term opioid therapy for chronic noncancer pain. *Schmerz*, **29**, 109–30.

Häuser, W., Petzke, F., Radbruch, K., & Tolle, T. (2016). The opioid epidemic and the long-term opioid therapy for chronic noncancer pain revisited: a transatlantic perspective. *Pain Manag*, **6**, 249–63.

Health and Social Care Information Centre (2016). Prescription Cost Analysis England. Available at: https://www.gov.uk/government/statistics/prescription-cost-analysis-england-2015 (accessed 1 January 2017) [Online].

Hedegaard, H., Chen, L. H., & Warner, M. (2015). Drug-poisoning deaths involving heroin: United States, 2000–2013. NCHS data brief, no 190. Hyattsville, MD: National Center for Health Statistics. Available at: https://www.cdc.gov/nchs/products/databriefs/db190.htm (accessed 1 January 2017) [Online].

Højsted, J., Ekholm, O., Kurita, G. P. Juel, K., & Sjøgren, P. (2013). Addictive behaviors related to opioid use for chronic pain: A population-based study. *Pain*, **154**, 2677–83.

Højsted, J., Nielsen, P. R., Guldstrand, S. K., Frich, L., & Sjøgren, P. (2010). Classification and identification of opioid addiction in chronic pain patients. *Eur J Pain*, **14**, 1014–20.

Home Office (2016). Drug Misuse: Findings from the 2015/16 Crime Survey for England and Wales (Second Edition) Statistical Bulletin 2016. Available at: https://www.gov.uk/government/statistics/drug-misuse-findings-from-the-2015-to-2016-csew (accessed 1 January 2017) [Online].

International Narcotics Control Board Report (2015). Estimated World Requirements for 2016—Statistics for 2014. Available at: https://www.incb.org/incb/en/narcotic-drugs/Technical_Reports/2015/narcotic-drugs-technical-report-2015.html (accessed 1 January 2017) [Online].

Johnson, M., Collett, B., & Catro-Lopes, J. (2013). The challenges of pain management in primary care: a pan-European survey. *J Pain Res*, **6**, 393–401.

Kolodny, A., Courtwright, D. T., Hwang, C. S., *et al* (2015). The prescription opioid and heroin crisis: a public health approach to an epidemic of addiction. *Annu Rev Public Health*, **36**, 559–67.

Kotecha, M. K. & Sites, B. D. (2013). Pain policy and abuse of prescription opioids in the USA. A cautionary tale for Europe. *Anaesthesia*, **68**, 1210–15.

Mars, S. G., Bourgois, P., Karandinos, G., Montero, F., & Ciccarone, D. (2014). 'Every "never" I ever said came true': transitions from opioid pills to heroin injecting. *Int J Drug Policy*, **25**, 257–66.

Marschall, U., L'Hoest, H., Radbruch, L., & Häuser, W. (2016). Long-term opioid therapy for chronic non-cancer pain in Germany. *Eur J Pain*, **20**, 767–76.

McCabe, S. E., Cranford, J. A., Boyd, C. J., & Teter, C. J. (2007). Motives, diversion and routes of administration associated with nonmedical use of prescription opioids. *Addict Behav*, **32**, 562–75.

Moore, A., Derry, S., Eccleston, C., & Kalso, E. (2013). Expect analgesic failure; pursue analgesic success. *BMJ*, **346**, f2690

National Opioid Use Guideline Group (NOUGG) (2010). Canadian guideline for safe and effective use of opioids for chronic noncancer pain. Available at: https://fhs.mcmaster.ca/npc/opioid/ (accessed 1 January 2017) [Online].

National Treatment Agency for Substance Misuse (2011). Addiction to medicine: An investigation into the configuration and commissioning of treatment services to support those who develop problems with prescription-only or over-the-counter medicine. Available at: www.nta.nhs.uk/uploads/addictiontomedicinesmay2011a.pdf (accessed 1 January 2017) [Online].

Novak, S. P., Håkansson, A., & Martinez-Raga, J. (2016). Nonmedical use of prescription drugs in the European Union. *BMC Psychiatry*, **16**, 274.

O'Brien, T., Christrup, L. L., Drewes, A. M., *et al.* (2017). European Pain Federation position paper on appropriate opioid use in chronic pain management. *Eur J Pain*, **21**, 3–19.

Office for National Statistics (ONS) (2016). Deaths related to drug poisoning in England and Wales. Available at: https://www.ons.gov.uk/peoplepopulationandcommunity/birthsdeathsandmarriages/deaths/bulletins/deathsrelatedtodrugpoisoninginenglandandwales/2015registrations (accessed 1 January 2017) [Online].

Okie, S. (2010). A flood of opioids, a rising tide of deaths. *N Engl J Med*, **363**, 1981–5.

Rose, N. (2003). Neurochemical selves. *Society*, **41**, 46–59.

Rudd, R. A., Seth, P., David, F., & Scholl, L. (2016). Increases in drug and opioid-involved overdose deaths—United States, 2010–2015 MMWR Morb Mortal Wkly Rep 2016. Available at: https://www.cdc.gov/mmwr/volumes/65/wr/mm655051e1.htm (accessed 1 January 2017) [Online].

SAMHSA (2016). Center for Behavioral Health Statistics and Quality, National Survey on Drug Use and Health, 2014 and 2015. Available at: https://www.samhsa.gov/data/sites/default/files/NSDUH-DetTabs-2015/NSDUH-DetTabs-2015/NSDUH-DetTabs-2015.htm (accessed 1 January 2017) [Online].

Schubert, I., Ihle, P., & Sabatowski, R. (2013). Increase in opiate prescription in Germany between 2000 and 2010: a study based on insurance data. *Dtsch Arztebl Int*, **110**, 45–51.

Skurtveit, S., Furu, K., & Borchgrevink, P., *et al.* (2011). To what extent does a cohort of new users of weak opioids develop persistent or probable problematic opioid use? *Pain*, **152**, 1555–61.

Stannard, C. F. (2013). Opioids in the UK: what's the problem? *BMJ*, **347**, f5108.

Strang, J., Hall, W., Hickman, M., & Bird, S. M. (2010). Impact of supervision of methadone consumption on deaths related to methadone overdose (1993–2008): analyses using OD4 index in England and Scotland. *BMJ*, **341**, c4851.

Sullivan, M. & Howe, C. (2013). Opioid therapy for chronic pain in the United States: Promises and perils. *Pain*, **154**, 94–S100.

The Kings Fund (2016). Bringing together physical and mental health: A new frontier for integrated care. Available at: https://www.kingsfund.org.uk/publications/physical-and-mental-health (accessed 1 January 2017) [Online].

University of Wisconsin (2016). Pain and Policy Studies Group. Opioid Consumption Data. Available at: http://www.painpolicy.wisc.edu/opioid-consumption-data (accessed 2 January 2017) [Online].

Van Amsterdam, J. & van den Brink, W. (2015). The Misuse of Prescription Opioids: A Threat for Europe? *Curr Drug Abuse Rev*, **8**, 3–14.

Vos, T., Barber, R. M., Bell, B., & Bertozzi-Villa, A. (2015). Global Burden of Disease Study 2013. *Lancet*, **386**(9995), 743–800.

Vowles, K. E., McEntee, M. L., Julnes, P. S., *et al.* (2015). Rates of opioid misuse, abuse, and addiction in chronic pain:a systematic review and data synthesis. *Pain*, **156**, 569–76.

Vranken, M. J. M., Lisman, J. A., Mantel-Teeuwisse, A. K., *et al.* (2016). Barriers to access to opioid medicines: a review of national legislation and regulations of 11 central and eastern European countries. *Lancet Oncol*, **17**, e13–22.

Warner, M. (2015). Trends in Drug-poisoning Deaths Involving Opioid Analgesics and Heroin: United States, 1999–2012. Available at: https://www.cdc.gov/nchs/data/hestat/drug_poisoning/drug_poisoning.htm (accessed 1 January 2017) [Online].

Weisberg, D., Becker, W., Fiellin, D., & Stannard, C. (2014). Prescription opioid misuse in the USA and UK: Cautionary lessons. *Int J Drug Policy*, **25**, 1124–30.

Weisberg, D. & Stannard, C. F. (2013). Lost in translation? Learning from the opioid epidemic in the USA (invited editorial). *Anaesthesia*, **68**, 1207–19.

Winstock, A. R., Borschmann, R., & Bell, J. (2014). The non-medical use of tramadol in the UK: findings from a large community sample. *Int J Clin Pract*, **68**, 1147–51.

World Health Organization (WHO) (1996). Cancer pain relief: with a guide to opioid availability, 2nd Edition. Available at: http://apps.who.int/iris/bitstream/10665/37896/1/9241544821.pdf (accessed 1 January 2017) [Online].

World Health Organization (WHO) (2011). Ensuring Balance in National Policies on Controlled Substances. Guidance for availability and accessibility of controlled medicines. Available at: www.who.int/medicines/areas/quality_safety/guide_nocp_sanend/en/ (accessed 2 January 2017) [Online].

World Health Organization (WHO) (2015). WHO Model List of Essential Medicines, 19th Edition. Geneva, Switzerland: WHO. Available at: http://www.who.int/medicines/publications/essentialmedicines/en/ (accessed 1 January 2017) [Online].

Zacny, J. P. & Lichtor, S. A. (2008). Nonmedical use of prescription opioids: motive and ubiquity issues. *J Pain*, **9**, 473–86.

Zgierska, A., Miller, M., & Rabago, D. (2012). Patient satisfaction, prescription drug abuse, and potential unintended consequences. *JAMA*, **307**, 1377–8.

Zin, C., Chen, L., & Knaggs, R. (2014). Changes in trends and pattern of strong opioid prescribing in primary care. *Eur J Pain*, **18**, 1343–51.

Chapter 3.4

Specialty pain medicine

Andreas Kopf

The rise of specialty pain medicine and implications for education, governance, and professional identity

Chronic pain rehabilitation programmes first appeared in the United States in the 1970s and, by many accounts, are credited to John Bonica, who was one of the first to propose organized pain services as early as in the 1940s. Bonica founded the Department of Anesthesiology at the University of Washington School of Medicine in Seattle, where he established the first multidisciplinary pain centre in the 1960s. In 1974, the International Association for the Study of Pain (IASP) was founded, followed by Chapters in Europe. The German Pain Society was founded as early as 1975. In the past four decades, pain medicine has established itself as an indispensable element of healthcare and has fostered much research and education. The level of pain medicine is, however, very diverse around the world, as we see in section two of this volume. While in the majority of countries pain medicine is still non-existent or represented only be single 'missionary' pioneers, in other countries such as Australia and New Zealand, the United States, and in Western European countries, pain medicine is now a recognized supraspeciality or—as a rare exception in Australia, Ireland, and Israel—a specialty of its own.

Pain medicine as a specialty or as a supraspecialty deals with the management of difficult chronic painful diseases, especially but not exclusively with complex chronic painful states unresponsive to conventional treatment. The very concept of pain medicine is based on the conviction that the effective management of difficult pain conditions is possible only through well-coordinated efforts of a specialist possessing the knowledge and skills to diagnose and treat pain. The clinical advancement were accompanied by an advancement of science and many aspects of pain and its treatment have only been made possible in the last two decades.

Unfortunately, awareness about pain aetiologies and management among medical professionals in general is very limited. Therefore, undertreatment of pain remains a major public health concern. The IASP is advocating for 'Working together for pain relief throughout the world' and it is a sad truth that poor advancement in pain medicine is not a privilege of so-called developing countries, but a reality in most countries worldwide. In Europe this is independent from the gross national product! Advocating therefore needs to include the promotion of pain education to health professionals, patients, communities, and policymakers. Education has to involve the assessment, evaluation, policymaking and research of pain and has to promote the sharing of educational resources within the pain community of all the European Pain Federation Chapters. In 2018, the EFIC in cooperation with the IASP will establish the 'Global Year for Excellence in Pain Education', which will hopefully focus attention on the crucial aspects of education that includes undergraduate and postgraduate education; and especially in the latter, remedying the lack of clarity in methods for continuing professional development. In Europe, this is of utmost importance and should be part of the efforts of the European Union to create cross-European standards. Apart from the contents and structure of education, the aim of this education needs further discussion, with respect to the options of a 'basic competence', a subspecialty, a supraspeciality, or a specialty of pain medicine. This discussion has not been directed so far, and thus European-wide leadership is a priority.

Overview: How pain medicine as a specialty is developing in some countries

In most countries of the world, self-management with little clinician intervention is the first and most widely used approach for the management of pain by patients. A similar approach is taken by primary care providers, in whose practices 'pain' is one of the most frequent causes for a consultation. Certain specialist care providers may also diagnose and treat underlying diseases like rheumatoid arthritis and thereby secondarily treat pain. Only in a few countries do certified pain specialists provide or coordinate a broad range of therapies including interdisciplinary care. Even in countries with 'developed' pain medicine, the supply of pain specialists is exceeded greatly by the demand, causing referrals only after lengthy delay and after visiting a number of other specialists before, thereby allowing the chronification processes to continue. In the United States it has been estimated that only one out of five patients in need of a certified pain specialist will be seen by one (Gatchel *et al.*, 2014). This estimate applies also to European countries with certified pain specialists, meaning that existing pain care is fragmented, inconsistent, and incomplete, with uneven access and disparate quality.

Inadequate education of providers and the lack of a single professional organization to oversee education in, and delivery of, pain care often are the barriers. Regarding education, the insufficient representation of pain medicine starts in undergraduate education, the place where medical students learn about the priorities of healthcare. In the United States, a recent survey identified only four medical schools that require a course on pain. In Europe, the APPEAL-Study has shown that, with the exception of France and Germany, undergraduate education in pain medicine is of variable and mostly insufficient quality and quantity (Briggs *et al.*, 2015). Consequently, the majority of physician respondents in various surveys reported that they lacked adequate training to manage pain. On the postgraduate level there are subspecialty training programmes (for certain specialties only, mostly for anesthesiology) and supraspeciality training programmes (for all clinical specialties), usually in the form of a 'fellowship' after completing the specialty with different requirements regarding practical experience (from unstructured to structured in a certified educational centre) and diplomas (from acceptance of a 'general' certificate to oral and oral/written examinations).

Canada is an example of a unified approach (since 2010) with a required curriculum, objectives of training, standards, and assessment procedures leading to a diploma programme to end fragmentation of care (RCPSC, 2017). The Australian and New Zealand College of Anaesthetists (ANZCA), in 1999, established a separate interdisciplinary Faculty of Pain medicine within the College of Anaesthesists, which was recognized as a medical subspecialty by the federal government of Australia 2006 (FPM, 2015). In Europe, for example in the United Kingdom, advanced training in pain medicine has been regulated by the Royal College of Anaesthesists since 1999 (RCA, 2017), and in Germany by the Federal Medical Chamber since 2003 (FCP, 2008). European countries have a wide variety of programmes. As opposed to palliative care, pain medicine is lacking educational standardization.

There is no European country with a specialty as such, although Israel and Ireland have started specialty-like programmes (but a 'home specialty' is still required before training in pain medicine starts).

Some of the training models are nationally unified, overseen by the Ministry of Health or the Chamber of Medicine (e.g. Germany), or there exist different models in parallel with certification from different medical societies (like in the United States) or individual university bodies (like in Serbia).

Implications for cross-border working

Several professional groups have already identified a core of knowledge and skills basic to pain medicine, generally based on IASP recommendations, encompassing the management of pain such as in the perioperative setting, pain associated with malignancies, pain following peripheral or central nervous system injury, and comprehensive and multimodal treatment of chronic pain. This should be the prerequisite for a united Europe with free transfer of licensing to practice across borders.

Lessons for education and training

The effort of establishing pain medicine in a healthcare system is considerable and therefore takes many years, even decades of work. Since there are some European countries that have already invested a lot of time and effort, it would seem logical to adapt existing common training frameworks including curricula, examination procedures, and education structures in other chapters.

Such a common approach would have also formal advantages within the integration process of the European Union, but also content advantages: after a first phase of establishing courses, treatment centres, and international relations, there cannot be a pain medicine 'light' version anywhere in Europe focusing only on the available human and financial resources. Therefore 'just' some pain management in cancer centres or 'just' some interventional pain management (for private patients) would be a misunderstanding of what is needed. There are a number of curricula of different European countries which are sketchy and are bearing exactly this risk of misunderstanding.

The focus of education has to be a comprehensive approach to pain; comprehensive regarding the syndromes (perioperative, cancer, chronic), and comprehensive regarding the management (according to the bio-psycho-social-spiritual approach of 'total pain'). It has been suggested that we teach the learning objectives of pain medicine therefore in a top-down fashion to allow fellows from the beginning to develop the idea of a multimodal and interdisciplinary approach, which is the philosophy of pain medicine. This approach has been elaborated upon as a 'Flipped Pain Curriculum' by Daniel Carr, from the United States (Carr and Bradshaw, 2014). In this model it would be a prerequisite to establish as early as possible the national recognition necessary to define educational centres for teaching the competency-based curricula. In the absence of a European model by the European Union of Medical Specialists (UEMS), the European Pain Federation has published just such an example.

The above-described diversity and non-structured certifications in pain medicine reflect shortcomings in existing pain education delivery systems. To address these shortcomings, certain medical societies are proposing to recognize pain medicine as its own specialty, which would include creating a single board certification process for pain medicine, developing pain medicine residencies and establishing a unified professional pain medicine organization in each country. The European Pain Federation is prepared to support this process with model curricula, examinations, and teaching guidelines.

A minimum requirement for a pain medicine residency training programme has been proposed by the American Board of Pain Medicine, considering the interdisciplinary character of pain medicine as a cross-sectional field with a four-year residency including pain medicine training, primary care, research training, and physical medicine/rehabilitation, with altogether 70% of the training as residency time (Dubois and Follett, 2014). Interestingly, medical psychology is not included in the defined mandatory rotations.

There should be a dicussion of some of the possible negative aspects of such a residency programme. This should particularly focus on the funding of such training programmes, the funding of reimbursement schemes by the insurance system, the reduction of the diversity of pain specialists by eliminating the different parent fields of expertise, and the possible elimination of the interdisciplinary approach, which would be now represented by one person.

As opposed to the model of a specialty, a supraspeciality model would have some striking advantages: the increased clinical expertise from the parent specialty; the potential triage of complex or rare cases to different subspecialists; improved job satisfaction and work environment (and income security). When staying within a parent specialty, this can enhance the attractiveness of the parent specialty at the same time, promoting better collaboration as an already recognized supraspecialization. But dependence to a parent specialty also carries some risks (e.g. the financial burden to the healthcare systems worldwide could cause a down-stripping of parent specialties of everything that is not their core competencies).

What should happen in the future?

It is a controversial discussion on the pros and cons of establishing a specialty of pain medicine of its own. After many years of pain medicine being a supraspeciality in a number of European countries, it seems logical to move one step forward to make pain medicine an equal discipline within the medical system, especially since a trained pain doctor designation has been developing. Such recognition is needed in order to stimulate the interest of the next—maybe less pioneering—generation to make the otherwise risky decision to decide to go into pain medicine. On the positive side, providing a focus, almost exclusively, on chronic pain disorders brings into focus a unique and very large population of patients with significant healthcare needs. Furthermore, the lack of a specialty status is the reason for a fragmented provision of care to patients. Consider the size of this problem, with 2–3% of the population requiring specialist provision with chronic pain including advanced physical and psychological impairment. Even in 'developed' countries, it is estimated that only around 15% of pain patients will receive management by a pain specialist.

The educational initiative of the European Pain Federation is a sound foundation for the development of different levels of qualifications for pain medicine. The demand for implementation of pain medicine in the undergraduate curriculum in medical faculties as a mandatory cross-sectional field will raise the awareness of patients with pain and encourage new doctors to engage in further specialist training. The postgraduate curriculum of the European Pain Federation will give guidance to medical societies, academic institutions, and healthcare providers about the competences required for specialized pain medicine. And the recently inaugurated European Diploma of Pain Medicine (EDPM) will be another reason to stimulate further individual qualification in pain medicine (for details see https://www.europeanpainfederation.eu/core-curriculum/diploma-in-pain-medicine/).

On the negative side of the discussion, this exclusive focus on the chronic pain patient group is seen by some as a self-amputation of pain medicine. The generalist approach of including acute and cancer pain, for example, within the total pain concept is seen as more valuable and attractive for young doctors, otherwise reducing their professional scope to the chronic pain patient alone. In order for a pain medicine specialist to do multimodal pain management, is more than individual specialism needed? We know that only in a team can one work successfully—for some patients, his/her input may be a minor contribution. Also, pain medicine by definition is a cross-sectional field and therefore the supraspeciality—combining different attitudes and competencies might be better suited to benefit the patient, therefore the supraspeciality's disadvantage of impaired recognition might not be a disadvantage in the end!

A further negative argument is offered in terms of transition to a specialty model. Some have argued that in the period of transition patient care might suffer, while only 'pain specialists' are entitled to treat chronic pain, of which there will inevitably be a shortage. Notwithstanding these reflections, there might be national, regional, or local circumstances regarding legal, administrative, or structural necessities (referral rules, privatization practices, and so on), respectively, making it a reasonable decision to opt for one or the other side. It is unwise at this stage to generalize across Europe.

Conclusion

In past decades, pain medicine was able to demonstrate its ability to improve the care of patients with pain regarding cancer, perioperative pain, and chronic pain. But the improvement is far from adequate. To achieve the goal of adequate care provision for pain patients, a feasible and tempting suggestion would be a multilevel educational initiative with a step-up/step-down approach for patients regarding their management needs:

1. Essential pain medicine to be integrated in all undergraduate education with a level of cognitive, practical, and affective learning objectives orientated at the EFIC Core Curriculum.
2. A general pain medicine competence as a prerequisite in all clinical specialization trainings to enlarge upon the basic pain medicine education.
3. A supraspeciality of pain medicine allowing the education—with the EFIC postgraduate curriculum—in special pain medicine for all clinical specialists to ensure the advancement of multidisciplinary and interdisciplinary pain medicine, which is the prerequisite of the multimodal management approach, providing the graduates to work in hospitals as consultants or in private practices, for example.
4. A specialty of pain medicine on top of the supraspeciality, with a training framework including a multidisciplinary training programme of increased length and more profound insight to ensure adequately trained pain physicians for the academic teaching, research coordination, and as chairmen of pain management referral centres.

References

Briggs, E. V., Battelli, D., Gordon, D., *et al.* (2015). Current pain education within undergraduate medical studies across Europe: Advancing the Provision of Pain Education and Learning (APPEAL) study. *BMJ Open*, **10**, e006984.

Carr, D. B. & Bradshaw, Y. S. (2014). Time to flip the pain curriculum. *Anesthesiology*, **120**, 12–4.

Dubois, M. Y. & Follett, K. A. (2014). Pain medicine: The case for an independent medical specialty and training programs. *Acad Med*, **89**, 863–8.

Faculty of Pain Medicine (FPM) (2015). Australian and New Zealand College of Anaesthetists, 2015 training programme. Available at: http://fpm.anzca.edu.au/training/2015-training-program [Online].

Federal Chamber of Physicians (FCP) in collaboration with the German Society for the Study of Pain (2008). MKB Special Pain Therapy, 2nd Edition. Available at: http://www.bundesaerztekammer.de/fileadmin/user_upload/downloads/MKSpezSchmerz.pdf [Online].

Gatchel, R. J., McGeary, D. D., McGeary, C. A., & Lippe, B. (2014). Interdisciplinary chronic pain management: Past, present, and future. *Am Psychol*, **69**, 119–30.

Royal College of Physicians and Surgeons of Canada (RCPSC) (2017). Eligibility for subspecialists. Available at: http://www.royalcollege.ca/rcsite/credentials-exams/exam-eligibility/practice-eligibility-route-per-sub-subspecialists-e [Online].

The Royal College of Anaesthetists (RCA) (2017). Faculty of Pain Medicine, Training and Assessment. Available at: https://www.rcoa.ac.uk/faculty-of-pain-medicine/training-examination-and-assessment [Online].

Chapter 3.5

Working at the frontiers of pain management in Europe

Nevenka Krčevski-Škvarč

Introduction

Inadequate pain treatment is present worldwide. In Europe it is particularly prominent in Eastern European (EE) countries that are less developed economically than Western European countries. EE countries are commonly grouped into the subregions of Eastern Europe, East Central Europe, the Baltic, and the Balkans. The Eastern Europe subregion includes Russia, Ukraine, Belarus, Romania, and Moldavia. The East Central Europe subregion consists of the Czech Republic, Hungary, Poland, Croatia, Slovenia, and Slovakia. The Baltic subregion comprises Lithuania, Latvia, and Estonia. The Balkans subregion includes the countries of Bulgaria, Serbia, Montenegro, Bosnia and Herzegovina, Albania, Kosovo, and Macedonia.

The majority of EE countries are those which had been cut off by the Iron Curtain or became independent by the separation of former countries in the nineties of last century. Their common characteristics are systems in transition, developing societies, and some of them as lower-resource countries, but are all generally lower-income countries compared to those in Western European. This is the main cause of disparity between the east and west of Europe with regard to the development of pain medicine and the presence of pain management in their healthcare systems. According to the International Monetary Fund, developing countries are in transition from a traditional to modern lifestyle, and could be classified as per the Gross National Index as high-income, middle-income, and low-income countries. Low- and middle-income countries are referred to as developing countries.

Also, among EE countries there are significant differences and disparities in healthcare and pain management. The situation is better in the countries with advanced economies such as Slovakia, Czech Republic, Poland, Slovenia, Croatia, Estonia, and Latvia than in the developing countries such as Albania, Bosnia and Herzegovina, Kosovo, Romania, Turkey, Russia, Ukraine, Serbia, and Moldavia.

Pain management in Eastern European countries

Due to relative poverty, these countries have health priorities in which pain management has no visible place or is neglected. The majority of these countries have no national policies and pain clinics that offer multidisciplinary pain strategies. These countries have relatively few opportunities for education in pain management and palliative care, as well as restrictive regulations on prescribing pain drugs. Some of these countries only recently organized associations for pain management and joined the International Association for the Study of Pain (IASP) and the European Pain Federation (EFIC). These associations are promoting pain medicine in their countries in various manners. With the advocacy of developed pain associations, these countries could improve the situation in their countries and diminish the disparities in pain management. The advocacy can be made through the delivery of grants and financial support, help in education, training, and practice-based learning, and through twinning partnerships.

Palliative care in Eastern European countries

The palliative care situation in Eastern European countries is slightly better in the countries that have joined the European Union (EU), according to the Recommendation of the Committee of Ministers to member states on the organization of palliative care (Rec 24, Council of Europe, 2003). Despite huge variations in the levels of provision across the countries of EE, the development of palliative care in all countries continues to be uneven, uncoordinated, and poorly integrated across wider healthcare systems, mainly as the result of inadequate and limited palliative care capacity.

EFIC councillors' reports on pain management and palliative care in their countries

Two years ago I asked the EFIC Eastern European Chapters' representatives about the situation in their countries regarding the application of pain medicine and palliative care in their healthcare systems. The questions were directed to the existence of facilities for pain management and palliative care; the state of education in pain and palliative care; the existence of national strategies, curricula, and guidelines; and the main obstacles in service development and possible actions for improvement. Acquired data showed that EE countries with a high income and membership of the EU have a slightly better situation than middle- and low-income countries where some do not even have a facility for pain management. The establishers of existing units are generally not governments; they are mainly organized on the hospital level and cover a small percentage of patients who need pain management and acute palliative care (Table 3.5.1). Education for both pain medicine and palliative care at undergraduate level is either not present or is complementary (Table 3.5.2). Postgraduate education and national plans are present in some way in the countries with high income, and more for palliative care than pain management. The same is the case for the existence of curricula (Table 3.5.3). The national pain associations in all countries are active in the production of guidelines predominantly for cancer pain treatment, acute pain treatment, neuropathic pain treatment, and the use of opioids.

In these countries, there is often voiced the opinion that the main obstacles for better implementation of pain medicine and palliative care lies in addressing the problems of lack of money, education, pain specialists and facilities, and in generating more

Table 3.5.1 Facilities for pain management and palliative care in some Eastern European (EE) countries

Country	Facilities	Enough?	% of pain patients	Establisher
Slovenia	4a, 14ch, 1ca, 1po	No	20%	Department
Croatia	2a, 29ch, 8ca, 3m, 1po	No	40%	Ministry, hospital, department
BiH	8	No	–	Hospital
Serbia	M	No	5%	Hospital
Kosovo	Na	No	NA	NA
Estonia	3a, 6m	No	30%	Hospital
Lithuania	/Ch 2 ca	No	10–15%	Hospital
Latvia	1a, 3ch, 6m, 1ca, 5po	No	1–2%	Hospital, department
Slovakia	M44	Yes	–	Ministry
Hungary	–	No	10–20%	–

A = acute pain, CH = chronic pain, CA = cancer pain, PO = palliative care department, M = mixed.

Source: data from Survey on education and certification in pain medicine and implementation of pain management in EE countries, 2014.

interest in healthcare institutions and entire healthcare systems. They see the need for education, national plans, political decisions, and better awareness as main factors for improvement of the situation.

EFIC support of the Eastern European Chapters

The EFIC takes great care to support all its Chapters and their members, especially those from Eastern European countries. EE countries have significant financial and professional support. Federation support is available through grants for their scientific meetings, individual grants for EFIC schools, congresses, and fellowships. Professional support is given with lectures at regional meetings and bidirectional partnerships. The five EFIC schools that cover wide range of pain medicine provide a great opportunity to gain knowledge in the field. The newest school is focuses on research in pain medicine and opens possibilities for cross-border clinical and basic research. Grants for young researchers are also available. Besides, EFIC promotes the implementation of all its initiatives, such as the Societal Impact on Pain (SIP) and the Global Youth Ambassador Project (GYAP) in the member states. It is also working on recommendations and with other scientific contributions which can be used in its Chapters. The newest contribution is the possibility to gain an EFIC Diploma in Pain Medicine,

Table 3.5.2 Undergraduate education in pain medicne and palliative care in some EE countries

Country	Regular/PM	Regular/PC	Complementary/PM	Complementary/PC
Slovenia	No	No	Yes	Yes
Croatia	No	No	Yes	Yes
BiH	No	No	Yes	Yes
Serbia	No	No	No	No
Kosovo	No	No	No	No
Estonia	Yes/No	No	Yes	Yes
Lithuania	Yes	Yes	Yes	No
Latvia	No	No	Yes	Yes
Slovakia	No	No	Yes	Yes
Hungary	No	No	No	No
Romania	Yes	No	Yes	Yes

PM = pain medicine, PC = palliaticve care.

Source: data from Survey on education and certification in pain medicine and implementation of pain management in EE countries, 2014.

Table 3.5.3 Postgraduate education, the existence of national plan and curricula for pain management and palliative care in some EE countries

Country	Postgrad/ PM	Posdtgrad/PC	NP PM	NPPC	Curr PM	Curr PC
Slovenia	Yes	Yes	Yes	No	No	Yes
Croatia	Yes	No	No	Yes	Yes	No
BiH	No	No	No	No	No	No
Serbia	No	No	No	Yes	No	No
Kosovo	No	No	No	No	No	No
Estonia	Yes/No	No	No	No	No	No
Lithuania	No	No	Yes	No	No	No
Latvia	Yes	No	No	Yes	Yes	No
Slovakia	Yes	Yes	No	No	Yes	Yes
Hungary	No	Yes	No	No	No	No
Romania	Yes	Yes	Yes	Yes	Yes	Yes

PM = pain medicine, PC = palliative care, NP = national plan, Curr = curriculum.

Source: data from Survey on education and certification in pain medicine and implementation of pain management in EE countries, 2014.

which is of great value for Chapters of countries that do not offer postgraduate education in the field. All efforts are introduced to diminish disparities among Eastern European and West European countries.

Recently I asked the representatives of EE chapters about the establishment of their Chapters and when they joined EFIC; what they find advantageous about being a Chapter member; what are their expectations of being in EFIC; and what could be improved to meet their expectations.

National pain associations in EE could be divided in two groups; those that were established at the time of the EFIC's founding, and those that have been established with the help of EFIC at the beginning of our century, the youngest being established last year.

Advantages of being a member Chapter in the EFIC are noted as: motivation for progress; sharing experiences; the Federation's support in grants and lecturers; taking part in the Federation's activities; access to the *European Journal of Pain* and other publications. Also ranked as being very important is the building of bridges between the east and west of Europe to approach unique pain medicine education and practice. Financial support is very important to the EE Chapters, especially recently since some bigger pharmaceutical companies are not present in EE countries due to the appearance of generic products.

The EFIC is expected to continue to enlarge support in education and training, and to help in organization and contacts with policymakers. The Federation is viewed as the main scientific and educational body in pain medicine, standardization of education and practice in pain medicine, and that it will continue in efforts to promote pain management as a priority in European healthcare systems.

Improvements for pain medicine are expected, with further empowered activities by the EFIC in EE countries and its engagement in political activities in Chapter states to achieve and introduce national plans for pain management.

Conclusion

The European Pain Foundation (EFIC) has a strong role in supporting the frontiers of pain management, making the work of pain professionals visible, and supporting them in improving pain management in all of its Chapters. Further improvement could be achieved by the continuous presence of EFIC activity in each of the EE chapters with regard to:

- actions for recognition of societal impact of pain;
- actions for the introduction of pain education at all levels of medical schools;
- actions for the establishment of national pain policy;
- actions for gaining skills in pain practice.

As the Eastern European countries differ in their levels of achievement for these aspects, they need to make individual priorities and action plans.

A lot needs to be done to make these dreams come true, to do away with the disparities among Western and Eastern countries, but I am sure the European Pain Foundation could and will do its best to solve this major European problem.

Reference

Council of Europe (2003). Recommendation Rec (2003) 24 of the Committee of Ministers to member states of the organization of palliative care. The Committee of Ministers, 12 November 2003. Available at: http://www.eapcnet.eu/LinkClick.aspx?fileticket=3KJ5U3BQLVY%3d&tabid=1709 [Online].

Chapter 3.6

European pain policy: Challenges and opportunities

Norbert van Rooij, Joop van Griensven, Mariano Votta, and Bart Morlion

Introduction

From cradle to grave, humankind has, to some extent, been faced with pain. Taking its physical and emotional toll, chronic pain can dominate people's lives and those of their families, friends, and caregivers (EFIC, 2001). The prevalence of pain causes a tremendous impact on society in use of healthcare and social resources (Leadley *et al.*, 2012). Given that the costs associated with severe chronic pain are considerable for health systems, individuals, and society, we will need to accept that, from a societal and health policy perspective, pain is a health problem in its own right (EFIC, 2001; Morlion *et al.*, 2012). In the long term, this view will change policies for budgetary and resource allocation in pain care, extending away from a biomedical model dealing with pain as a symptom, to a biopsychosocial model taking into account the biological, psychological, and social factors affecting the societal impact of pain (Behrendt *et al.*, 2016; Vandenbroeck *et al.*, 2016).

Prioritizing pain in policies calls for a whole systems perspective (Phillips *et al.*, 2008). This will to jointly address the societal impact of pain with policymakers sparked the initiation of the platform 'Societal Impact of Pain' (SIP) in 2009. The SIP platform is driven by the continuous advocacy of the European Pain Federation (EFIC), supported by Grünenthal and, since 2016, joined by Pain Alliance Europe (PAE), and Active Citizenship Network (ACN) as active partners. Since the start of the platform, over 300 international and national pain advocacy groups, scientific organizations, and authorities have endorsed the objectives of the SIP meetings (SIP, 2016b). The Societal Impact of Pain platform aims to address access to pain treatment in policies, through raising awareness of the relevance of the impact that pain has on our societies, health, and economic systems, by exchanging information and sharing best practices across all member states of the European Union, and by developing and fostering European-wide policy strategies and activities for improved pain care in Europe. The platform provides opportunities for discussion for healthcare professionals, pain advocacy groups, politicians, insurances, representatives of health authorities, regulators, and budget holders.

Pain: An increasing problem for individuals

Being a major symptom in many medical conditions, pain can interfere with a person's quality of life and general functioning. People in pain can experience impairments in attention, control, working memory, mental flexibility, problem-solving, and information processing speed (Hart *et al.*, 2003). Pain is associated with increased depression, anxiety, fear, and anger (Bruehl *et al.*, 2009). In the presence of chronic pain, other dimensions of health (physical, psychological, social) are severely reduced (Elliott *et al.*, 1999; Smith *et al.*, 2001). Chronic pain is related to low self-rated health in the general population (Mäntyselkä *et al.*, 2003). On top of all this, severe chronic pain is associated with an increased risk of 10-year mortality, independent of sociodemographic factors (Torrance *et al.*, 2010). In daily life, risk factors associated with chronic pain include sociodemographic, clinical, psychological, and biological factors. Pain also increases the risk of other social problems, including social exclusion, loss of income, and can even result in poverty (Pain Concern, 2016; Phillips *et al.*, 2008; van Hecke *et al.*, 2013).

Pain is commonly connected with numerous chronic health conditions, such as cancer and musculoskeletal diseases (IASP, 2009; Majithia *et al.*, 2016; Mieritz *et al.*, 2016; Roberto *et al.*, 2016). Indeed, chronic pain is one of the most common co-morbidities of other long-term illnesses (Barnett *et al.*, 2012). Therefore it is of no surprise that a large proportion of physician visits are caused by pain complaints (Gureje *et al.*, 2001; Mäntyselkä *et al.*, 2001; Koleva, 2005). Additional to pain being a frequent complaint, people with chronic pain consult their general practitioner five times more frequently than those without chronic pain complaints (Von Korff *et al.*, 1990). Overall, individuals reporting chronic pain have a significantly higher healthcare system utilization than individuals without chronic pain complaints (Eriksen *et al.*, 2004).

During the SIP symposium in 2011, the European Commissioner for Health and Consumer Policy, John Dalli, stated: '*We should also realise that as the demographic profile of Europe changes and as the population becomes older, pain will become an increasingly important issue in the future*' (SIP, 2011b). The ageing society addressed by the European Commissioner is a serious challenge for Europe. It is estimated that the European population aged ≥ 65 will increase from 18.5% in 2014 to 28% in 2050 (Eurostat, 2015). This will come at a high price, as the prevalence of health states related to age will also increase (König *et al.*, 2010). Many chronic conditions especially prevalent among the ageing population, such as diabetes and arthritis, are often linked to chronic pain (Haanpää and Hietaharju, 2015; Neogi, 2013). The elderly population shows a higher incidence of chronic and neuropathic pain conditions (Molton and Terill, 2014). In some indications, older people get less access to pain treatment than the general population as chronic pain is often overlooked by health professionals (Booker *et al.*, 2016; WHO, 2015).

Negative impact on work-related outcomes

Pain disorders are among the most prevalent, costly, disabling, and commonly researched conditions in the workplace (Schultz *et al.*, 2007). Several literature reviews and database analyses indicate that chronic pain has a considerable negative impact on work-related outcomes (Patel *et al.*, 2012). While including 46,934 respondents in the United Kingdom (UK), France, Spain, Germany and Italy researchers analysed population, prevalence, and attributes of pain experience utilizing a large-scale Internet-based study (Langley, 2011). As they focused on the impact of pain on labour force participation, the analysis demonstrated that the experience of pain—severe daily pain in particular—had a substantial negative association with ability to work, as well as reported absence from work (absenteeism), and attending work while sick (Langley *et al.*, 2010). As a health status measure, severe daily pain outweighed many other health status measures (Langley *et al.*, 2011; Sternbach *et al.*, 2013).

Due to the effects of pain on rates of absenteeism, reduced productivity, and even the risk of employees leaving the labour market, social protection systems spend a large budget on pain-related complaints (Barmer GEK, 2016). Nearly half of all absences from work, lasting more than three days, are caused in Europe by musculoskeletal disorders (Bevan, 2013). Data from the Labour Force Survey show that over 2.3 million people in the UK report conditions or disabilities related to their back or neck as their main health problem (UK, 2016). In the UK in 2014, more days were lost to back, neck, and muscle pain than any other cause (Jenkins, 2014). In England in 2013, low back pain was ranked highest of all injury-related disabilities and yielded the largest total number of 'years lived with disability' (England, 2015). Longitudinal data from Finland show that physically heavy work at a young age can have a long-lasting effect on the risk of low back pain (Lallukka *et al.*, 2017). Worldwide chronic pain conditions (in particular back pain) are by far the greatest cause of disability (Newton *et al.*, 2015; Vos *et al.*, 2016). Unsurprisingly, chronic pain is one of the major reasons why people exit the labour market prematurely and it contributes significantly to disability retirement (Saastamoinen *et al.*, 2012).

A growing problem for society

In 2015 the Swedish Minister for Social Security, Annika Strandhäll, set a pain policy benchmark when she proposed a seven-point action programme for improved health and reduced sick leave including support for people with chronic pain (Gov. Offices of Sweden, 2015; Gustafsson, 2016). Taking into account these aspects, it becomes obvious that chronic pain in the working population poses a substantial burden on individuals, employers, healthcare systems, and society.

Affecting between one-third and one-half of the population pain, in particular chronic pain, is one of the major health problems in Europe (Fayaz *et al.*, 2016; Goldberg and Summer, 2011; Harstall and Ospina, 2003). The impact of pain represents a huge burden to society associated with enormous costs; financial and in terms of degraded quality of life for the persons involved, their family, and those immediately around them. Rough estimates place the cost of chronic pain, as a disease state, in similar cost categories as heart disease, cancer, and diabetes (Gaskin and Richard, 2012).

One of the biggest challenges for policymakers is that pain needs to be addressed in policies for both primary and secondary care. In secondary care, pain is highly correlated with trauma and postoperative (acute) pain (Estebe, 2016; Schug and Pogatzki-Zahn, 2011). At the same time, a great deal of the costs caused by chronic pain are dealt with in primary care (Andersson *et al.*, 1999; Grobe *et al.*, 2016; Smith *et al.*, 1999). Given the frequency of chronic pain as a presentation in primary care, one would expect general practitioners to have adequate evidence, training, and resources to assess and manage chronic pain. This is not the case, and often clear guidance on to how to refer pain patients is absent or insufficient. The process of trial and error of different specialties and treatment possibilities often results in a long and costly treatment pathway (Itz *et al.*, 2016). Besides the lack of dedicated policies and budgets, one of the factors contributing to inadequate pain treatment for persons in pain is the often inadequate medical training in pain management (Pergolizzi *et al.*, 2013). In most European member states, high-quality primary-care-focused education and research in chronic pain is not integrated in the healthcare system (Mills *et al.*, 2016; Treede and van Rooij, 2011).

Recently, French patient associations and health professionals urged for the urgency of new concrete measures in an open letter to the President of the French Republic. They stressed the undertreatment of acute pain in the emergency department and the need to expand medical undergraduate education in the management of acute and chronic pain (Bouhassira *et al.*, 2016).

The prevalence of pain in the general public has been confirmed by the EU Directorate General SANCO in 2007 (DG SANCO, 2007). According to the Eurobarometer Survey related to activity restriction due to health problems and specifically to musculoskeletal pain, 32% of all respondents experienced muscle, joint, neck, or back pain which affected their daily activities in the week leading up to them being interviewed for the survey, while 25% experienced pain in their muscles, joints, neck, or back lasting three months or more, affecting their ability to carry out the activities of daily living. These findings were confirmed in 2014 when the Austrian national health survey identified chronic low back pain and other chronic pain problems as the most commonly named illnesses (Statistik Austria, 2014).

Although the overarching economic impact of chronic pain in Europe has not been quantified, data from different countries give a good idea. In the UK, back pain alone is estimated to cost the economy £12.3 billion per year (Maniadakis and Gray, 2000). The direct costs caused by back pain are modest compared to the cost of informal care and the production losses related to it. In Sweden, the socioeconomic burden of patients with a diagnosis related to chronic pain was estimated to amount to €32 billion per year, which equals a fifth of the total Swedish tax burden or about a tenth of Swedish GDP in 2007 (Gustavsson *et al.*, 2012).

Unfortunately throughout the EU, chronic pain patients report insufficient pain control and dissatisfaction with treatment (Breivik *et al.*, 2006). Chronic pain is often not only underdiagnosed but also under-, over- or just wrongly-treated (Dietl and Korczak, 2011). In this light it does not come as a surprise that international experts call for strategic prioritization and coordinated actions to address the unacceptable and unnecessary burden of uncontrolled chronic pain that plagues European communities and economies (Breivik *et al.*, 2013).

The SIP approach to improve pain policies in Europe

The United Nations (UN) Universal Declaration of Human Rights (Art. 5) states: 'No one shall be subjected to torture or to cruel, inhuman or degrading treatment or punishment'

(United Nations, 1948). As most countries have no national policy at all or very inadequate policies regarding the management of pain, representatives from Chapters of the International Association for the Study of Pain (IASP) in 64 countries, plus IASP members in 129 countries agreed to declare that 'pain management is a fundamental human right' (Declaration of Montreal, 2010). Although the agreement on the Montreal declaration was a major achievement, the next step—inserting pain in health policies—is a big challenge.

National pain strategies

In 2011 IASP published its 'Desirable Characteristics of National Pain Strategies' (IASP, 2014). This comprehensive document contains guidance for governmental and non-governmental organizations that seek to improve pain care.

Key recommendations by IASP are:

- Access to pain education for health professionals and the general population
- Coordination of the care system to ensure timely access to the right support
- A quality improvement programme to address access and standards of care
- A reasonable proportion of direct and dedicated funding for pain research

Critical factors for success identified by IASP are:

- Gathering of evidence on the burden of pain to the nation
- Gathering of information on access to care
- Development of government policy on pain services
- Formation of a broad coalition of stakeholders
- A clear plan with timescales to achieve strategic actions

From International Association for the Study of Pain® (IASP), *Desirable Characteristics of National Pain Strategies: Recommendations by the International Association for the Study of Pain*, Copyright © 2014 IASP, www.iasp-pain.org/DCNPS?navItemNumber=655. This text has been reproduced with permission of the International Association for the Study of Pain® (IASP).

In some countries, the call for a national strategy for chronic pain management has become louder (Fullen *et al.*, 2006). In Belgium, the authorities recognized 35 pain centres (Belgian Pain Society, 2013). In Scotland, the conclusions of the report 'Getting Relevant Information on Pain Services' (GRIPS) were endorsed by the Scottish Government resulting in a National Lead Clinician for Chronic Pain (IASP, 2015; NHS Quality Improvement Scotland, 2008).

While it has been argued that recognition of pain medicine as an independent medical specialty would generate credibility for the specialty and its providers among medical peers, payers, regulatory and legislative agencies, and the public at large, in Germany pain medicine has been included as a mandatory subject in undergraduate medical studies (Drießen, 2012; Dubois and Follett, 2014; Kopf *et al.*, 2014). As with the EU Directive 2011/24/EU in Italy, in France, Slovenia, and Ireland pain has been included in the national implementation of the cross-border health directive (European Parliament and the Council, 2011; Presidente della Repubblica, 2014; LegiFrance, 2002; Predsednik Republike Slovenije, 2008; Ireland; Stationery Office, 2014).

At the EU level the societal impact of pain was highlighted under the Italian presidency of the council of the European Union, when ministers from 28 EU member states agreed on the need to create a European network for pain therapy, ensuring training of professionals in the sector, and the exchange of information on the effectiveness of therapies for the most vulnerable population groups (Italian Presidency of the Council of the EU, 2014). Unfortunately, despite these positive trends, in some EU member states pain centres are hardly available, or are even being closed (Szilagyi *et al.*, 2015).

The roadmap: Seven practical steps to move forward in pain policy

As policymakers are seldom pain specialists, a clear path is required. One of the key documents developed by the SIP platform is the 'SIP Road Map for Action'. This instrument outlines seven steps for policymakers and health institutions to effectively address the societal impact of pain at EU and national level (SIP, 2011a; Varrassi, 2011).

1. Acknowledge that pain is an important factor limiting the quality of life and should be a top priority of the national healthcare system.
2. Activate patients, their families, relatives, and caregivers through the availability of information and access to pain diagnosis and management.
3. Raise awareness of the medical, financial, and social impact that pain and its management has on the patients, their families, caregivers, employers, and the healthcare system.
4. Raise awareness of the importance of the prevention, diagnosis, and management of pain amongst all healthcare professionals, notably through further education.
5. Strengthen pain research (basic science, clinical, epidemiological) as a priority in EU framework programmes and in equivalent research road maps at national and EU level, addressing the societal impact of pain and the burden of chronic pain on the health, social, and employment sectors.
6. Establish an EU platform for the exchange, comparison, and benchmarking of best practices between member states on pain management and its impact on society.
7. Use the EU platform to monitor trends in pain management, services and outcomes, and provide guidelines to harmonize effective levels of pain management to improve the quality of life of European Citizens.

In order to qualify the progress of the roadmap implementation, EFIC installed the roadmap monitor (Treede and van Rooij, 2011). The results show that adequate pain therapy is still not accessible for all European citizens, nor is a sufficient policy framework in place to prevent the negative impact of pain on society (Wells, 2016).

The Societal Impact of Pain's 'Time for Action'

With the intention to discuss policy issues related to the societal impact of pain, the SIP 2016 symposium hosted delegates representing European institutions, policymakers, pain specialists, scientific researchers, patient representatives, and other stakeholders. Under the scientific auspices of EFIC and guided by the SIP cooperation partners PAE and ACN, the following eight overarching policy recommendations were formulated (SIP, 2016a):

1. Implementation of Article 8.5 of Directive 2011/24/EU (the Cross-border Healthcare Directive)
2. Establish an EU platform on the societal impact of pain
3. Integrate chronic pain within EU policies on chronic diseases
4. Ensure that pain care is a part of policies and strategies on cancer
5. Initiate policies addressing the impact of pain on employment
6. Implement workplace adjustments for people with chronic pain
7. Increase investment in pain research
8. Prioritize pain within education for healthcare professionals, patients, and the general public

These recommendations form a comprehensive base for future policy development addressing the societal impact of pain at the institutional levels of the European Union and national governments.

Addressing pain in future healthcare policies

As aforementioned, pain is a major healthcare problem in Europe. The enormous burden and costs society has to bear, caused by pain, calls for policymakers and decision-makers to adopt effective policies and strategies addressing healthcare service provision and resource allocation. In order for healthcare systems to remain sustainable, we need to accept that, from a societal and health policy perspective, pain is a health problem in its own right. Addressing pain in healthcare policies will be a challenge, but the implementation of the 'SIP Roadmap for Action' and the 'SIP policy recommendations' may be regarded as concrete opportunities to put pain at the top of political and health policy agendas (SIP, 2011b; SIP, 2016c).

References

Andersson, H. I., Ejlertsson, G., Leden, I., & Scherstén, B. (1999). Impact of chronic pain on health care seeking, self care, and medication. Results from a population-based Swedish study. *J Epidemiol Community Health*, **53**, 503–9.

Barmer GEK (2016). *Press: Barmer GEK Arztreport 2016; Über drei Millionen Patienten mit chronischem Schmerz.* Available at: https://presse.barmer-gek.de/barmer/web/Portale/Presseportal/Subportal/Infothek/Studien-und-Reports/Arztreport/Arztreport-2016/BARMER-GEK-Arztreport-2016.html (accessed 26 July 2016) [Online].

Barnett, K., Mercer, S. W., Norbury, M., Watt, G., Wyke, S., & Guthrie, B. (2012). Epidemiology of multimorbidity and implications for health care, research, and medical education: a cross-sectional study. *Lancet*, **380**(9836), 37–43.

Behrendt, S., Kulas, H., Marschall, U., Steffens, M., Schiffhorst, G., & Bleß, H.-H. (2016). Which back pain patients benefit from multidisciplinary pain management? A comparative cost analysis using claims data of statutory health insurance. *Gesundheitswesen*, **78**(S 01), e120–7.

Belgian Pain Society (2013). *Pain centers*. Available at: http://www.belgianpainsociety.org/information-patient/pain-centers (accessed 28 July 2016) [Online].

Bevan, S. (2013). *Reducing Temporary Work Absence Through Early Intervention: The case of MSDs in the EU*. Lancashire, UK: The Work Foundation.

Booker, S., Bartoszczyk, D., & Herr, K. (2016). Managing pain in frail elders. *American Nurse Today*, **11**(4). Available at: https://www.americannursetoday.com/managing-pain-frail-elders/ [Online].

Bouhassira, D., Chauvin, M., Perrot, S., & Robert, C. (2016). Il faut écrire un nouveau chapitre de la lutte contre la douleur. *Le Monde*, 31 Oct.

Breivik, H., Collett, R., Ventafridda, V., Cohen, R., & Gallacher, D. (2006). Survey of chronic pain in Europe: prevalence, impact on daily life, and treatment. *Eur J Pain*, **10**, 287–333.

Breivik, H., Eisenberg, E., & O'Brien, T. (2013). The individual and societal burden of chronic pain in Europe: the case for strategic prioritisation and action to improve knowledge and availability of appropriate care. *BMC Public Health*, **13**, 1229.

Bruehl, S., Burns, J. W., Chung, O. Y., & Chont, M. (2009). Pain-related effects of trait anger expression: neural substrates and the role of endogenous opioid mechanisms. *Neurosci Biobehav Rev*, **33**(3), 475–91.

Declaration of Montreal (2010). *Declaration of Montreal*. Available at: http://www.iasp-pain.org/files/Content/NavigationMenu/Advocacy/DeclarationOfMontreal.pdf (accessed 29 July 2016) [Online].

DG SANCO (2007). *Special Eurobarometer 272e, Health in the European Union*. Brussels, Belgium: Directorate General SANCO and coordinated by Directorate General Communication.

Dietl, M. & Korczak, D. (2011). Over-, under- and misuse of pain treatment in Germany. *GMS Health Technol Assess*, **19**, 7, Doc03.

Drießen, M. (2012). *Endlich: Schmerzmedizin wird Pflichtfach*. Available at: http://idw-online.de/de/news477678 (accessed 28 July 2016) [Online].

Dubois, M. Y. & Follett, K. A. (2014). Pain medicine: The case for an independent medical specialty and training programs. *Acad Med*, **89**, 863–8.

Elliott, A. M., Smith, B. H., Penny, K. I., Smith, W. C., & Chambers, W. A. (1999). The epidemiology of chronic pain in the community. *Lancet*, **354**(9186), 1248–52.

England, P. H. (2015). *Burden of Disease Study for England*. Available at: https://www.gov.uk/government/uploads/system/uploads/attachment_data/file/460518/Global_Burden_of_Disease_England_infographics.pptx (accessed 13 November 2016) [Online].

Eriksen, J., Sjøgren, P., Ekholm, O., & Rasmussen, N. (2004). Health care utilisation among individuals reporting long-term pain: an epidemiological study based on Danish National Health Surveys. *Eur J Pain*, **8**, 517–23.

Estebe, J. P. (2016). A plea for acute pain service: Is it time to move forward towards perioperative pain service?. *ESA Newsletter online*, Summer, Issue 65.

European Pain Federation (EFIC) (2001). EFIC's Declaration on Pain: Pain is as a major health problem, a disease in its own right. In: **EFIC** (ed.) *EFIC-Europe Against Pain*. Brussels, Belgium: EFIC.

European Parliament and the Council (2011). *Directive 2011/24/EU of the European parliament and of the council on the application of patients' rights in cross-border healthcare*. Available at: http://eur-lex.europa.eu/LexUriServ/LexUriServ.do?uri=OJ:L:2011:088:0045:0065:en:PDF (accessed 26 July 2016) [Online].

Eurostat (2015). *Population structure and ageing; Eurostat Statiscis explained.* [Online] Available at: http://ec.europa.eu/eurostat/statistics-explained/index.php/Population_structure_and_ageing (accessed 26 June 2016) [Online].

Fayaz, A., Croft, P., Langford, R. M., Donaldson, L. J., & Jones, G. T. (2016). Prevalence of chronic pain in the UK: a systematic review and meta-analysis of population studies. *BMJ Open*, **6**, e010364.

Fullen, B., Hurley, D. A., Power, C., O'Keeffe, L. D. (2006). The need for a national strategy for chronic pain management in Ireland. *Irish Journal of Medical Science*, **175**, 68–73.

Gaskin, D. J. & Richard, P. (2012). The economic costs of pain in the United States. *J Pain*, **13**, 715–24.

Goldberg, D. S. & Summer, J. M. (2011). Pain as a global public health priority. *BMC Public Health*, **11**, 770.

Gov. Offices of Sweden (2015). Åtgärdsprogram för ökad hälsa och minskad sjukfrånvaro. *Bilaga till protokoll vid regeringssammanträde*, **249**, 1–9.

Grobe, T. G., Steinmann, S., & Szecsenyi, J. (2016). *Barmer GEK Arztreport 2016: Schwerpunkt: Alter und Schmerz.* 37th Edition. Berlin, Germany: Barmer GEK.

Gureje, O., Simon, G. E., & Von Korff, M. (2001). A cross-national study of the course of persistent pain in primary care. *Pain*, **92**, 195–200.

Gustafsson, A.-K. (2016). *Sweden: Combating rise in sick leave and investing in work environment training.* Available at: http://www.eurofound.europa.eu/observatories/eurwork/articles/working-conditions-social-policies/sweden-combating-rise-in-sick-leave-and-investing-in-work-environment-training (accessed 28 July 2016) [Online].

Gustavsson, A., Bjorkman, J., Ljungcrantz, C., *et al.* (2012). Socio-economic burden of patients with a diagnosis related to chronic pain—Register data of 840.000 Swedish patients. *Eur J Pain*, **16**, 289–99.

Haanpää, M. & Hietaharju, A. (2015). Halting the march of painful diabetic neuropathy. *IASP PAIN: Clinical Updates*, **April, XXIII**(2). Available at: http://iasp.files.cms-plus.com/Content/ContentFolders/Publications2/PainClinicalUpdates/Archives/pcu_vol23_no2_april2015_1428006215952_2.pdf [Online].

Harstall, C. & Ospina, M. (2003). How prevalent is chronic pain? *IASP PAIN: Clinical Updates*, **June, XI**(2). Available at: https://www.iasp-pain.org/files/Content/ContentFolders/Publications2/PainClinicalUpdates/Archives/PCU03-2_1390265045864_38.pdf [Online].

Hart, R. P., Wade, J. B., & Martelli, M. F. (2003). Cognitive impairment in patients with chronic pain: the significance of stress. *Curr Pain Headache Rep*, **7**, 116–26.

International Association for the Study of Pain (IASP) (2009). *Musculoskeletal Pain Fact Sheet*, s.l. Available at: https://www.iasp-pain.org/Advocacy/Content.aspx?ItemNumber=1101 [Online].

International Association for the Study of Pain (IASP) (2014). *Desirable Characteristics of National Pain Strategies: Recommendations by the International Association for the Study of Pain.* Available at: https://www.iasp-pain.org/DCNPS?navItemNumber=655 (accessed 26 July 2016) [Online].

International Association for the Study of Pain (IASP) (2015). *Scotland Makes Systematic Improvements in Treatment of Chronic Pain.* Available at: https://www.iasp-pain.org/PublicationsNews/NewsDetail.aspx?ItemNumber=4538&navItemNumber=645 (accessed 28 July 2016) [Online].

Ireland Stationery Office (2014). *S.I. No. 203 of 2014; European Union (Application of Patients' Rights in Cross-Border Healthcare) Regulations.* Available at: https://www.hse.ie/eng/services/list/1/schemes/cbd/Stutory_Instrument.pdf (accessed 26 July 2016) [Online].

Italian Presidency of the Council of the EU (2014). *Summary of the conclusions of EU Health Ministers meeting in Milan*. Available at: http://italia2014.eu/en/news/post/conclusioni-informale-salute (accessed 26 July 2016) [Online].

Itz, C., Huygen, F., & Kleef, M. (2016). A proposal for the organization of the referral of patients with chronicnon-specific low back pain. *Curr Med Res Opinion*, **32**, 1903–9.

Jenkins, J. (2014). *UK Office for National Statistics. Full Report: Sickness Absence in the Labour Market*. Available at: http://www.ons.gov.uk/employmentandlabourmarket/peopleinwork/labourproductivity/articles/sicknessabsenceinthelabourmarket/2014-02-25 (accessed 26 07 2016) [Online].

Koleva, D. (2005). Pain in primary care: an Italian survey. *Eur J Public Health*, **15**, 475–9.

König, H.-H., Heider, D., Lehnert, T., *et al.* (2010). Health status of the advanced elderly in six European countries: results from a representative survey using EQ-5D and SF-12; Health Qual Life Outcomes. *Health and Quality of Life Outcomes*, **8**, 143.

Kopf, A., Dusch, M., Alt-Epping, B., & Treede, R. D. (2014). Das Querschnittsfach „Schmerzmedizin". *Der Schmerz*, **28**, 405–13.

Lallukka, T., Viikari-Juntura, E., Viikari, J., *et al.* (2017). Early work-related physical exposures and low back pain in midlife: the Cardiovascular Risk in Young Finns Study. *Occup Environ Med*, **74**, 163–8.

Langley, P. C. (2011). The prevalence, correlates and treatment of pain in the European Union. *Curr Med Res Opin*, **27**, 463–80.

Langley, P. C., Molina, J. T., Cesar, M., & Ruiz-Ibán, M. (2011). The association of pain with labor force participation, absenteeism, and presenteeism in Spain. *Journal of Medical Economics*, **14**, 835–45.

Langley, P. C., Müller-Schwefe, G., Nicolaou, A., Liedgens, H., Pergolizzi, J., & Varrassi, G. (2010). The impact of pain on labor force participation, absenteeism and presenteeism in the European Union. *Journal of Medical Economics*, **13**, 662–72.

Leadley, R., Armstrong, N., Lee, Y. C., Allen, A., & Kleijnen, J. (2012). Chronic diseases in the European Union: the prevalence and health cost implications of chronic pain. *Journal of Pain & Palliative Care Pharmacotherapy*, **26**, 310–25.

LegiFrance (2002). *Loi n°2002-303 du 4 mars 2002—art. 3 JORF 5 mars 2002—Article L1110-5—Chapitre préliminaire: Droits de la personne*. Available at: https://www.legifrance.gouv.fr/affichCode.do;jsessionid=CD09FBD4D4356479A6B6BA73CE3C1223.tpdila16v_2?idSectionTA=LEGISCTA000006170991andcidTexte=LEGITEXT000006072665anddateTexte=20090722 (accessed 26 July 2016) [Online].

Majithia, N., Loprinzi, C., & Smith, T. (2016). New practical approaches to chemotherapy-induced neuropathic pain: prevention, assessment, and treatment. *Oncology (Williston Park)*, **30**, 1020–9.

Maniadakis, N. & Gray, A. (2000). The economic burden of back pain in the UK. *Pain*, **84**, 95–103.

Mäntyselkä, P., Kumpusalo, E., Ahonen, R., *et al.* (2001). Pain as a reason to visit the doctor:a study in Finnish primary health care. *Pain*, **89**, 175–80.

Mäntyselkä, P., Turunen, J., Ahonen, R., & Kumpusalo, E. (2003). Chronic pain and poor self-rated health. *JAMA*, **290**, 2435–42.

Mieritz, R. M., Thorhauge, K., Forman, A., Mieritz, H. B., Hartvigsen, J., Christensen, H. W. (2016). *Musculoskeletal Dysfunctions in Patients With Chronic Pelvic Pain: A Preliminary Descriptive Survey*. Available at: http://www.jmptonline.org/article/S0161-4754(16)30213-5/abstract (accessed 18 Nov 2016) [Online].

Mills, S., Torrance, N., & Smith, B. H. (2016). Identification and management of chronic pain in primary care: a review. *Curr Psychiatry Rep*, **18**, 22.

Molton, I. R. & Terill, A. L. (2014). Overview of persistent pain in older adults. *Am Psychol*, **69**, 197–207.

Morlion, B., Pergolizzi, J., & Huygen, F. (2012). *Towards a multidisciplinary team approach in chronic pain management*. Available at: http://www.pae-eu.eu/wp-content/uploads/2013/12/Multidisciplinary-approach-in-chronic-pain-management.pdf (accessed 29 July 2016) [Online].

Neogi, T. (2013). The epidemiology and impact of pain in osteoarthritis. *Osteoarthritis Cartilage*, **21**, 1145–53.

Newton, J. N., Briggs, A. D. M., Murray, C. J. L., *et al.* (2015). Changes in health in England, with analysis by English regions and areas of deprivation, 1990–2013: a systematic analysis for the Global Burden of Disease Study 2013. *Lancet*, **386**, 2257–74.

NHS Quality Improvement Scotland (2008). *Getting to GRIPS with Chronic Pain in Scotland*. Edinburgh, UK: NHS Quality Improvement Scotland.

Pain Concern (2016). *Transcript—Programme 76: Pain, poverty and employment*. Available at: http://painconcern.org.uk/transcript-programme-76-pain-poverty-employment/ (accessed 26 July 2016) [Online].

Patel, A. S., Farquharson, R., Carroll, D., *et al.* (2012). The impact and burden of chronic pain in the workplace: a qualitative systematic review. *Pain Pract*, **12**, 578–89.

Pergolizzi, J., Ahlbeck, K., Aldington, D., *et al.* (2013). The development of chronic pain: physiological CHANGE necessitates a multidisciplinary approach to treatment. *Curr Med Res Opin*, **29**, 1127–35.

Phillips, C., Main, C., Buck, R., Aylward, M., Wynne-Jones, G., & Farr, A. (2008). Prioritising pain in policy making: The need for a whole systems perspective. *Health Policy*, **88**, 166–75.

Predsednik Republike Slovenije (2008). *455. Patients' Rights Act (PACPA) Page 1045th; Art. 17*. Available at: https://www.uradni-list.si/1/content?id=84936 (accessed 26 July 2016) [Online].

Presidente della Repubblica (2014). *Decreto legislativo, n°38, art.9.5*. Available at: http://www.gazzettaufficiale.it/eli/id/2014/03/21/14G00050/sg (accessed 26 July 2016) [Online].

Roberto, A., Deandrea, S., Greco, M. T., *et al.* (2016). Prevalence of neuropathic pain in cancer patients: pooled estimates from a systematic review of published literature and results from a survey conducted in 50 italian palliative care centers. *J Pain Symptom Manage*, **51**, 1091–102.e4.

Saastamoinen, P., Laaksonen, M., Kääriä, S. M., et al. (2012). Pain and disability retirement: a prospective cohort study. *Pain*, **153**, 526–31.

Schug, S. A. & Pogatzki-Zahn, E. M. (2011). Chronic pain after surgery or injury. *IASP Clinical Updates*, Jan., **XIX**(1). Available at: https://www.iasp-pain.org/files/Content/ContentFolders/Publications2/PainClinicalUpdates/Archives/PCU_19-1_for_web_1390260524448_6.pdf [Online].

Schultz, I., Stowell, A., Feuerstein, M., & Gatchel, R. (2007). Models of Return to Work for Musculoskeletal Disorders. *Journal Occupational Rehabilitation*, **17**, 327–52.

Smith, B. H., Elliott, A. M., Chambers, W. A., Smith, W. C., Hannaford, P. C., & Penny K. (2001). The impact of chronic pain in the community. *Fam Pract*, **18**, 292–9.

Smith, B. H., Hoptona, J. L., & Chambers, W. A. (1999). Chronic pain in primary care. *Fam Pract*, **16**, 475–82.

Societal Impact on Pain (SIP) Roadmap (2011a). *The Societal Impact of Pain—A Road Map for Action*. Available at: https://www.sip-platform.eu/events/sip-2011/materials.html (accessed 26 July 2016) [Online].

Societal Impact on Pain (SIP) (2011b). *Welcome by John Dalli, European Commissioner, Health and Consumer Policy*. Available at: https://www.sip-platform.eu/events/sip-2011/programme/plenary-3-may.html (accessed 26 June 2016) [Online].

Societal Impact on Pain (SIP) (2016a). *SIP 2016 builds a strong legacy*. Available at: https://www.sip-platform.eu/events/sip-2016/materials.html (accessed 26 July 2016) [Online].

Societal Impact on Pain (SIP) (2016b). *SIP events*. Available at: https://www.sip-platform.eu/endorsers.html (accessed 16 July 2016) [Online].

Societal Impact on Pain (SIP) (2016c). *Societal Impact of Pain 2016, 8 policy recommendations: Time for Action*. Available at: https://www.sip-platform.eu/events/sip-2016/materials.html (accessed 28 July 2016) [Online].

Statistik Austria (2014). *Österreichische Gesundheitsbefragung 2014 (ATHIS)*, Vienna, Austria: Statistik Austria.

Sternbach, N., Annunziata, K., & Isherwood, G. (2013). Profile of Back Pain Sufferers Across 5EU Countries. *Poster Presented at the ISPOR 16th Annual European Congress, Health Outcomes Practice*, November.

Szilagyi, I.-S., Bornemann-Cimenti, H., Messerer, B., Vittinghoff, M., Sandner-Kiesling, A. (2015). Schmerztherapeutische Versorgung österreichischer Gesundheitszentren. Fragebogenstudie zum Istzustand österreichischer Schmerzambulanzen. *Der Schmerz*, **29**, 616–24.

Torrance, N., Elliott, A. M., Lee, A. J., & Smith, B. H. (2010). Severe chronic pain is associated with increased 10 year mortality. A cohort record linkage study. *Eur J Pain*, **14**, 380–6.

Treede, R. & van Rooij, N. (2011). *The Societal Impact of Pain—A Road Map for Action European Road Map Monitor*, Brussels, Belgium: EFIC®.

UK, D. f. W. a. P. D. o. H. (2016). *Work, Health and Disability Green Paper Data Pack*. London, UK: Government Digital Service.

United Nations (UN) (1948). *The Universal Declaration of Human Rights*. Available at: http://www.un.org/en/universal-declaration-human-rights/ (accessed 29 July 2016) [Online].

van Hecke, O., Torrance, N., & Smith, B. H. (2013). Chronic pain epidemiology and its clinical relevance. *Br J Anaesth*, **111**, 13–18.

Vandenbroeck, S., Verjans, M., Lambreghts, C. & Godderis, L. (2016). *Research review on rehabilitation and return to work*. Luxembourg City, Luxembourg: Office of the European Union.

Varrassi, G. (2011). Conference Scene: Symposium on the Societal Impact of Pain (SIP). *Pain Manage*, **1**, 405–8.

Von Korff, M., Dworkin, S. F., & Le Resche, L. (1990). Graded chronic pain status: an epidemiologic evaluation. *Pain*, **40**, 279–91.

Vos, T., Allen, C., Arora, M., et al. (2016). Global, regional, and national incidence, prevalence, and years lived with disability for 310 diseases and injuries, 1990–2015: a systematic analysis for the Global Burden of Disease Study 2015. *Lancet*, **388**, 1545–602.

Wells, C. (2016). *Roadmap to action*. Available at: https://www.sip-platform.eu/events/sip-2016/program/plenary-24-may.html (accessed 16 July 2016) [Online].

World Health Organization (WHO) (2015). *Draft global strategy and plan of action on ageing and health*. Available at: http://www.who.int/ageing/ageing-global-strategy-revised-draft-for-who-eb.pdf (accessed 26 June 2016) [Online].

Chapter 3.7

European pain management: Future directions

Christopher Eccleston, Christopher Wells, and Bart Morlion

Introduction

Pain and suffering respect no borders. In the 37 countries who are members of the European Pain Federation (EFIC), there are approximately 740 million people, all of whom have pain management needs: at birth, throughout life, and on dying. Conservatively, we expect 20%, or almost 150 million of them to have chronic pain (i.e. intermittent, episodic, or persistent pain), fluctuating over an adult lifetime. This personal, societal, and economic burden of pain might appear overwhelming—so much suffering—but the humanitarian and scientific response to pain has been to organize: to develop a skills base, facilitate learning, nurture talent, and to innovate.

What we have gathered here is in part a taking stock, and in part an exploration. We asked leaders from each country to educate us about the size of their nation, its people, the structure of its health system, and how the pain societies are responding to the need within those structures. We were also interested in their challenges. Some of the challenges are specific, defined by geography, history, finance, or culture. But some of the challenges are common across European nations. We asked leaders from Europe to give their perspective on how those challenges affect them in their home nations.

In this final chapter we take the opportunity to discuss three common issues that face us as a European pain community, specifically: (i) the peculiar demands of working as a specialist healthcare professional in the face of overwhelming population need; (ii) the role of science in innovating and translating research into practice; and (iii) the task to develop multidisciplinary, multimodal, multisite delivery to meet the demands of a changing population. We end with an invitation, an invitation to build on the strong foundation of European pain medicine, an invitation to imagine and construct a stronger future together. Before discussing our common issues, we first offer a summary of the current state of practice, difficulties, and innovations across our 37 countries.

Taking a European view

'Underserved' is the dominant view that emerges when considering the population who could benefit from pain management. There were no countries who could confidently claim that they had sufficient resource, technology, skill, or organization to deliver optimal evidence-based treatment to those presenting with pain management needs. Even in the Western economies such as France or Germany, in which significant investments have been made over a sustained period, the organization and delivery was considered still suboptimal. In the Eastern countries, the picture is varied. In Estonia, Latvia, and Lithuania, there is a strong tradition of pain services, often with a history in neurology or anaesthesia. Sole working is common, and there is recognition that dealing with change in the health system is a feature of everyday work. Russia deserves special attention. It is a massive country of 143 million people for whom there are 465 people who identify enough as pain-interested professionals to join the Russian Association for the Study of Pain. Some countries focus heavily on primary care provision, for example the Ukraine. Some are focused on building better links with universities, such as Norway, and others on population planning for pain in the future, such as Italy.

Although there is tradition and precedent of pain management service in all countries, it is clear that the task of building stronger foundations can be difficult. For example, some countries are still operating in the shadow of current or recent military conflict, or of revolution and the establishment of new government. In Slovakia, the history of pain services is long, but the national history dates only to the early 1990s. In Bosnia and Herzegovina, the health services were rebuilt after almost complete depletion after the end of the Bosnian war in 1995. In this region, Kosovo, which joined the European Pain Federation in 2012, offers interesting insight. Nevenka Krčevski-Škvarč provides an informed analysis, in Chapter 3.5, of the challenges facing the Eastern European nations. Without falling into a trap of overgeneralizing across diverse nations with diverse histories, she draws our attention to the demands of practising and growing pain management in lower-resource nations, or in nations who have recently emerged as independent states, with all of the systems development that creates.

However, even in those countries with long-established governmental systems, including medical systems, change can still be difficult to engineer. In Switzerland, for example, pain medicine is still, along with the majority of other countries, not recognized as a specialty. In Portugal the concentration of expertise in secondary and tertiary care is proving difficult to disperse into primary care, and in Denmark the challenge is education, at all levels of the system. A priority for the European Pain Federation is to promote education, training, mentoring, and certification, at all levels, and in all countries. There is now an extensive curriculum, including supporting materials available with a focus on medical training (see https://www.europeanpainfederation.eu/core-curriculum/core-curriculum-for-european-pain-diploma-in-pain-medicine/). There are now plans for further diploma training and certification for other healthcare professionals. In nearly all of the EFIC Chapters, there was discussion of the challenges of working with or without medicines. Most classes of analgesic medication are widely available, including non-steroidal anti-inflammatory drugs (NSAIDs), paracetamol, antidepressant, and anticonvulsant medicines. However, more variety, and greater social concern was evident in most countries, particularly around the use of opioid and cannabinoid medicines, and the use of cannabis for pain relief.

Despite the concerns around opioid use, discussed in some detail by Cathy Stannard in Chapter 3.3 and put in historical context by Harold Breivik in Chapter 1.2, most people are struggling to explain the medicinal benefits of opioids, and to educate government to innovate legislation that discriminates between the medical and non-medical use, or to control for abuse, diversion, and other social problems. There have been successes, as in Estonia, but in most cases, and Greece was a good example of this, even with the recognition that opioids have a role to play in pain management (particularly in palliative care), the bureaucracy associated with social protection of opioid misuse is experienced as a major barrier to effective medical use. In some places, as in Moldova, that barrier is supported by a dominant cultural view of pain as something to be borne unaided, meaning that the use of opioids for pain is rare.

The use of cannabis medicinally is also cited as a cause of current concern and debate for many countries. Israel is a good example. There are advocates who see the addition of cannabis as a positive move, and the Israeli Ministry of Health has approved its use in certain conditions such as cancer pain. But there are also strong concerns against its use, concerns for social and medical harms. Improving the supply, access, and control of analgesic medicines remains a challenge in many countries. The safe and reasonable access to and use of medicines for pain management is a policy focus of the European Pain Federation, which has established a task force to review the evidence for safe use and provide policy support to our members.

Pain management is, of course, more than just the use of drugs. Many countries are keen to develop their national capacity in neuromodulation. The Czech Republic, for example, is investing in non-invasive techniques of electrical stimulation. And many countries, including Belgium, France, Germany, Ireland, and the United Kingdom, are increasingly interventionist, which requires an investment often in new skills, supporting procedures, and education. Lithuania, for example, has successfully invested in specialized day care facilities for pain surgery, and there is an increasing demand, as shown by Andreas Kopf in Chapter 3.4, for specialty interventional pain training across Europe.

Chronic pain is now being recognized as a long-term condition, a consequence perhaps of lives lived longer, and so increasingly each clinical presentation can be complicated enormously by patient behaviour (Treede *et al.*, 2015). How one acts in the context of pain, the decisions one makes, the mental health impact of persistent pain, the effects upon family, occupation, and expectations of the future, all influence suffering. So much so that it is sometimes hard to unpick what is treatable as pain management, and what is a life lived and defined by pain. In many of the chapter contributions there is a recognition that ageing populations, and in some cases shrinking and ageing populations, bring into sharp focus the importance of patient pain behaviour. Focusing on behaviour and how to improve it is arguably the job of all clinical pain professionals. However, psychologists have long been identified as central to the pain management multiprofessional team, and are expert at promoting the self-management of long-term conditions, at empowering individuals to learn how to pursue meaningful goals in the context of pain. Despite this recognition, experts in behaviour change are still a rarity. In some countries the poor supply of psychologists was recognized and discussed as a problem, for example Ireland. In others there have been explicit attempts to improve the supply through education, training, and professionalization. In Finland there is a specific course for psychologists, and 70 have already completed the 800 hours of intensive study in pain psychology. For the majority of countries, however, the reality of pain medicine is one of individual medical practice, with some opportunities for consulting other specialists when available—access to specialized pain psychology remains in most European countries largely an aspiration.

By the same reasoning, there is a multitude of other professionals who can contribute to behaviour change. With a shift in focus from the reduction of pain experience to the engagement of meaningful activity, there is a great opportunity to expand and broaden the pain workforce. In some countries, chronic pain is managed by healthcare professionals including physiotherapists, occupational therapists, specialized nurses, and social workers. We recognize that the reporting of activities in many countries has focused on medical training and medical interventions. To an extent, this reflects the historical and current investments. However, there is recognition that this is a starting point. The European Pain Federation has the ambition to broaden its membership, as individual Chapters expand their multidisciplinary base. We plan to establish specific curricula and dedicated certification processes for all these different groups of clinical pain professionals.

Common issues for the European pain community

A picture is developing of 37 countries, with different histories, cultures, and societies, who all share a common goal: to relieve the suffering of those in pain. Despite the variety in practice, in investment, and in possibilities, there is a shared motivation. Looking across Europe, we see three specific issues that deserve further discussion, both here and beyond these pages. The first concerns the daily life and professional practice, ambitions, and futures, of the people involved: what future is there for the pain management specialist, and how do we protect that future? The second is about science: in the pursuit of clinical progress, what guidance is there from European pain science? And the third is about aspiration: if the optimal model of service remains the full multidisciplinary and multiagency pain unit, how can we accelerate progress? Or, more critically, is that the only model of care to aspire to?

Investing in individuals

Of course, attempts to manage pain are made by individuals, patients, and doctors alike, at all levels of care. But the role of the pain specialist is still only emerging. The dominant model of European specialty pain management is of a physician-led consulting service. In many cases the services are new, innovated by current staff, or individuals are working in the presence, or the historical shadow, of a pioneer who established the clinic, its practices, and the standards. In Chapter 3.4 Andreas Kopf gives a good historical summary of the emergence of the medical discipline, and attempts made internationally to establish education, skills, and licencing, and neatly draws attention to the dilemma at the heart of specialty pain medicine. Untreated pain is common, the norm in fact. Part of the reason for poor pain management is the lack of knowledge and skills in the general community. In specializing, one provides a resource for that knowledge and skill, but then risks creating a barrier of access to both patients and experts. Kopf warns that it is dangerous to generalize. But, paradoxically perhaps, it will be important to understand that as we become more specialized, so there is a responsibility to share skills. As the workforce becomes more multidisciplinary and varied, we need to move to a focus on behaviour change. As we learn more, we need to teach more. In this area the European Pain Federation can play a crucial supporting role. There are mechanisms for providing that support. For example, the biannual congress remains an important place for scientific communication, but critically also for the sharing of models of practice, and the sharing of experiences in training. Regional meetings are encouraged and could be expanded, such as the meetings in Scandinavia, or the Baltics. Curricula development, training, and examinations are expanding. And the policy initiative, spearheaded by the work of the Societal Impact on Pain (SIP), expanded upon in Chapter 3.6, is a crucial part of our strategy. Collective, collaborative, European policy leadership, hand in hand with the patient organizations, is perhaps the most important of investments.

Despite these current investments, more work is needed now on the professional protection and support of the members at an individual level. In particular, working with distressed pain patients, often with minimal treatment options, and no team support, can significantly increase the risk of clinician burnout, and of system failure. As we emerge out of a model of individual treatment and responsibility to shared responsibility and multiple working, we should be mindful to provide, at the very least, adequate clinician management and support.

Science research and development

At the heart of clinical progress is scientific advancement. There is a need for strategic direction and further investment in defining the agenda for pain research in Europe. There are examples from elsewhere. For example, the American Pain Society published its pain research agenda in 2014 (Gereau *et al.*, 2014). See also http://americanpainsociety.org/about-us/press-room/aps-research-agenda-21st-century. Pain research has been chronically underfunded in the United States, as in the rest of world. In comparison with all other common long-term conditions, it is the most economically burdensome problem, and received the least amount of research funding from national agencies. They suggest an agenda that focuses on improving 'clinically meaningful' outcomes, from cure to improved function, mental health outcomes, and the management of the adverse effects of treatment. But also important in this agenda is the recognition that existing treatments which are effective can be optimized, that access to existing treatments is a major problem in most states, and that efforts on treatment should be matched with equal efforts on prevention. This work supported the US National Pain Strategy, published in 2016, that reinforced this agenda, and called also for population-based work to be developed in addition to individual treatment and prevention. There are other, older examples, in and outside of Europe. There has been European Union Funding for pain research. As of 2015, €46 million had been invested over eight programmes: six in neuropathic pain, one in low back pain, and one in headache. Germany and the United Kingdom were the most research-intensive recipients (Kringel and

Lötsch, 2015). There have been further investments. For example, the Relief project is a collaboration between Spain, France, and Sweden, with a focus on procuring digital solutions from innovative companies and supporting them into practice (http://relief-chronicpain.eu/). The 'selfback' project is focused on developing one of these solutions (http://selfback.eu/) in low back pain. And, a recent success is 'Dolorisk', a €6 million-funded project with nine countries involved in determining the risk factors for chronic neuropathic pain (http://dolorisk.eu/). These projects show what is possible when European experts focus on European solutions to European problems.

Despite these successes, there is a need for a new 'pain research strategy' to raise awareness of the mismatch between clinical need and research investment in most of our countries, and to support the policy roadmaps. Currently, there is no strategy for focus or development on pain. Such a strategy could involve the European Research Council, the World Health Organization (WHO), national research funders, and significant charities. A critical task is to determine a pathway for the basic science study of pain pathology, prevention, treatment and management of pain conditions, and to establish effective mechanisms for knowledge translation and implementation.

Innovating in service delivery

Finally, and arising from the focus on current practice models and research investments, is the need to develop novel methods of service delivery, to capitalize on what is known, to prepare for future treatment developments, and ultimately to invest in scalable, effective, modern working practices. This enterprise will require discussion, debate, and sensitive deliberation. It is foolish to confidently predict the future, but irresponsible not to plan for inevitable change. This debate, we suggest, could usefully consider two key components to inform the plan: models of working and the use of technology.

IASP discussed the desirable characteristics of a pain clinic in 2007 (http://www.iasp-pain.org/Education/Content.aspx?ItemNumber=1471), and sought to differentiate between single modality clinics, pain clinics, and fully staffed multidisciplinary pain centres. The questions for debate are whether it is realistic or even appropriate any more, in the European context, to promote the idea of full multidisciplinary pain centres. For some countries, the IASP standard of a full centre is a motivational aspiration. Belgium, for example, has officially implemented this standard in 35 centres over the last decade. For others it can be the opposite of aspirational, an unrealistic model from another place and time. What are needed are novel methods of clinical organization. For example, one could consider integrated networks of pain clinicians operating geographically, but linked for diagnostic, treatment, and case management support over larger networks, with subspecialization delivered at different sites. Central to this is the idea of specialization to a curriculum that is shared between countries, and licencing that crosses traditional borders. Other systems may already be in place that could be used to drive innovation and creativity.

A key component to future working will be the widespread adoption of modern communication technology. As computing power increases and becomes pervasive, integrated, and linked, so one's expectations of delivery and support of all services, including healthcare, change. Modern computing will change pain practice at all levels. At the basic level there is the opportunity in electronic health recording to better monitor patient presentation at healthcare settings, improved prediction of future pain episodes, using big data to identify classes of responding, and the determination of risk factors for chronic pain. Although this has been achieved in small-scale epidemiological research, it could be possible as a feature of everyday clinical practice. More advanced will be the use of shared decision-making platforms supported by diagnostics, and access to expert systems, both automated machine learning, and expert specialists working remotely in real time. The frontier of e-health developments, however, is the attempt to promote behavioural self-management remotely from a therapist using self-determined coping strategies. It is not yet successful. But it will come. In a patient-centred, patient-driven, electronically mediated lifetime pain management system, the specialist could evolve into a health systems architect and operator role, managing the expertise in a whole system, rather than delivering direct care to a list of individual patients.

Future directions

There is a wealth of talent, skill, and expertise in the 37 countries of the European Pain Federation. From individuals working to build whole systems and establish new clinics in adverse social and economic climates, to highly integrated, fully multidisciplinary, university-based pain centres, driving forwards internationally competitive research and clinical innovation. European pain has much to celebrate.

Despite this asset infrastructure, the future direction of European pain management is uncertain; it is unclear how it should develop. Populations are changing, migrating, blending, and ageing. Expectations of both quality of life and quality of healthcare are changing as the opportunities from pervasive computing technology increase. And what it means to be a pain doctor, or a specialist in pain, is also changing. How far can one balance the technical skills of the increasingly complex interventions needed for the individual in one's office, with the social, political, and public health skills needed to respond to a population in need? Such uncertainty, however, brings opportunity. We know that people will continue to need pain management. The demand is not going away. The opportunity we have is to re-vision, re-imagine, what a modern twenty-first-century system for delivering pain management should look like. Such a creative re-crafting will take energy and collaboration, and local leadership, but it will be worth the enterprise. We invite your participation. Such an evolution will only come from the ground, from those working to deliver the highest quality pain management wherever it is needed, from the dedicated experts who make up the invaluable human resource essential to the future of European pain management.

References

Gereau, R. W., Sluka, K. A., Maixner, W., *et al.* (2014). A pain research agenda for the 21st Century. *J Pain*, **15**, 1203–14.

Kringel, D. & Lötsch, J. (2015). Pain research funding by the European Union Seventh Framework Programme. *Eur J Pain*, **19**, 595–600.

Treede, R.-D., Rief, W., Qasim, A., & Bennet, M. I. (2015). A classification of chronic pain in ICD-11. *Pain*, **156**, 1003–7.

Index

abdominal pain, paediatric 218, 219, 220, 221
absenteeism 52, 53, 257
Access to Opioid Medication in Europe (ATOME) project 157, 231
Active Citizenship Network (ACN) 255, 261
acute pain 4, 8
- Austria 25
- children 216, 217–18
- Germany 75, 78
- Moldova 123
- older people 208
- risk factors for persistence 9–11
- Romania 145
- San Marino 153
- *see also* postoperative pain

acute postoperative pain outpatient clinic (APS-OPC) 65–6
adjuvant analgesics (co-analgesics) 158, 220
adverse drug reactions 211
Albania 19–21
Albanian Pain Association 21
algology 29, 113, 192–3
Algoplus scale 210
American Pain Society 271
analgesia *see* treatment, pain
Analgesic Guidelines (Analgetikai útmutató) 88
analgesic ladder, WHO 226
analgesics
- access to 228–32, 268–9
- children 217, 220
- Moldova 124–5
- older people 210–12
- policies 231, 269
- Serbia 158
- usage in Europe 227
- *see also* opioids

analgosedation 217
Anastasiou, Emmanouil 82
anxiety 10, 217
APPEAL-Study 244
Arias, Madrid 169
ARSD *see* Romanian Association for the Study of Pain
assessment, pain
- children 216–17
- Kosovo 109–10
- Moldova 126
- older people 209–10
- Romania 145

Association for Pain Therapy-Bosnia Herzegovina (APT-B&H) 34, 35
Associazione Italiana per lo Studio del Dolore (AISD) 103, 104
ATOME *see* Access to Opioid Medication in Europe
attitudes to pain, patients 109, 123–4, 208
Australian and New Zealand College of Anaesthetists 245
Austria 22–6
Austrian Pain Society (ÖSG) 22–3, 25–6

back pain 24, 114, 183, 257, 258
behaviour change 269–70
Belgian Pain Society (BPS) 28, 29, 30
Belgium 27–30
Berzins, Juris 111
Besson, J.M. 162
Bevan, Aneurin 199
biopsychosocial model 187, 218–19, 220
Birkhan, Jesmond 98
Blake, Catherine 95–6
Bonica, John 162, 186, 243
Bosnia and Herzegovina 31–5, 251, 252
Bosnian war (1992–1995) 31, 32–3
BPS *see* Belgian Pain Society; British Pain Society
Brill, Siviu 100–1
British Pain Society (BPS) 93, 201, 203
Bulgaria 37–40
Bulgarian Association for the Study and Treatment of Pain (BASTP) 38–40
buprenorphine 233, 236
Bytyqi, Adem 107
Bytyqi, Agron 107

Canada 228, 229, 245
cancer pain 5
- Bulgaria 39
- children 216
- Estonia 60
- Finland 64, 65
- Greece 80–1
- opioid use 11, 226, 229
- Serbia 158
- Slovenia 167
- United Kingdom 203

cannabis/cannabinoids 50, 101, 269
capsaicin 89
Carr, Daniel 246
Casale, Roberto 144

Chayen, Mark 98
childhood experiences, traumatic 10–11, 219
children 216–22
  acute pain 217–18
  chronic pain 9, 218–19
  chronic pain treatment 219–21
  pain assessment 216–17
  Spanish initiative 173
Chimonitsy-Cypriou, Vassiliki 82
chronic disease 256
chronic pain 4, 8
  Austria 24
  children 216–17, 218–19
  definition 4
  Denmark 52
  as disease entity 89, 105
  Finland 64, 65–6
  France 67
  individual burden 11–12, 256
  Ireland 93–5
  Latvia 114
  Lithuania 119
  older people 210
  Poland 134
  Portugal 138–9
  prevalence 8–9, 227, 258
  risk factors 9–11
  societal burden 11–12, 257–8
  United Kingdom 202
  work-related outcomes 256–7
chronic pain management
  Belgium 29
  Bulgaria 39
  children 219–21
  Estonia 60
  France 73
  future directions 12, 13, 269–70
  Germany 75
  Greece 83
  Ireland 93–5
  Israel 101
  Kosovo 109
  Latvia 114
  Moldova 123
  Netherlands 186, 187, 188, 189
  older people 208, 211
  opioid use 11, 233
  Poland 132, 134
  Romania 141–2, 144
  Russia 150
  San Marino 153
  Serbia 156, 157, 158–9
  Slovenia 166, 167
  speciality pain medicine 247
  Sweden 175–6, 178
clinical trials 13, 211
co-analgesics (adjuvant analgesics) 158, 220
codeine 233
cognitive behavioural therapy 221
cognitive effects of pain 211
cognitive impairment (dementia) 208–9, 211
communication impairments 210
complex regional pain syndrome (CRPS) 9, 219
computer-based systems 272–3
congenital insensitivity to pain 8
Continuing Education in Algology 82, 83
COST programme 209
costs, chronic pain 12, 258
CPS *see* Czech Pain Society
Crime Survey for England and Wales 234, 237
Croatia 41–5, 251, 252
Croatian Pain Society 41, 43, 44
cross-border working 245
Crul, Ben 187
cultural attitudes to pain 109, 123–4, 269
Czech Pain Society (CPS) 48–9, 50, 162
Czech Republic 46–50, 269

Dalli, John 256
Danish Pain Society 52–4, 56
day care units 120, 269
Declaration of Montreal (2010) 3, 219, 259
defined daily dose (DDD) 228
dementia (cognitive impairment) 208–9, 211
demographic trends 207
Denmark 12, 52–6, 232
depression 10, 211
development, economic 249
diclofenac 157
disability 227, 257
disparities, among European countries
    249–51, 253
Dolorisk 272
Doody, Catherine 95–6
drug misuse, prescription 11, 232–7
drug use, illicit 234–5
Dutch Pain Society (DPS) 187, 188, 189–90

Eastern European (EE) countries 249–53, 268
  country reports 250–1, 252
  EFIC support for 251–3
  pain management 249–51
  palliative care 250–1
economic costs, chronic pain 12, 258
education 243–4
  pain medicine *see* training and education
  patient 211–12, 221
EFIC *see* European Pain Federation
Eisenberg, Elon 100–1
elderly *see* older people
electronic health systems 272–3
emergency departments 208–9
EMLA (eutectic mixture of local
    anaesthetics) 217
employment 10
end-of-life care *see* palliative care
Engel, G. 187
England 200, 202

English Pain Summit 203
e-PAIN 203
epidemiology 8–13
Estonia 57–61, 251, 252
Estonian Headache Society 60
Estonian Pain Society 59, 60, 61
Europe 3–6
  barriers to opioid prescribing 228–32
  chronic pain prevalence 8–9, 227, 258
  cross-border working 245
  disparites within 249–51, 253
  future of pain management 267–73
  older people 207–12
  opioid prescribing 227–8, 229, 230
  paediatric patients 216–22
  pain policy 255–61
  population ageing 207, 256
  prescription opioid harms 232–7
  speciality pain medicine 244, 245–7
European Association for Palliative Care 65
European Diploma of Pain Medicine 173, 247, 251–3
European Journal of Pain 5
European Observatory on Health Systems 79
European Pain Federation (EFIC) 3, 5–6
  Eastern European chapters and 38, 39, 48, 144, 251–3
  foundation 5, 103
  future directions 12, 268, 271
  Israel and 100–1
  Societal Impact of Pain platform *see* Societal Impact of Pain platform
  Spain and 171
  training and education 244, 246, 247, 248
European Society for Rehabilitation (ESPRM) 144
European Union (EU) 78–9, 244, 250, 259–61, 271
European Union of Medical Specialists (UEMS) 105, 246
evidence-based care 189, 190

Fabuš, Stanislav 162
Faculty of Pain Medicine (FPM) 201, 203, 245
FASP *see* Finnish Association for the Study of Pain
FEDELAT 171–2, 173
fentanyl 124, 233
Finland 10, 62–6, 233, 270
Finn, David 95
Finnish Association for the Study of Pain (FASP) 62, 64, 65, 66
Finnish Medical Society Duodecim 65
Flipped Pain Curriculum 246
FPM *see* Faculty of Pain Medicine
France 67–73, 258
functional pain disorders 219

Gabovich, Boris 59
Garstka, Jerzy 130
gate control theory of pain 187
general anaesthesia 217
genetics 9
geriatric patients *see* older people
German Interdisciplinary Pain Association (DIVS) 75–6
German Pain Society 75–8, 243
German-speaking pain societies 22, 25
Germany 75–9, 233, 245
Global Year Against Pain 54, 88, 119
Global Year for Excellence in Pain Education (2018) 244
governance 243–4
Greece 80–4, 269
Groupe Régional Interdisciplinaire Douleur (GRID) 28
Gudelj, Marijana Persoli 41
guidelines, clinical
  Croatia 43
  Denmark 55
  Estonia 60
  Finland 65
  Hungary 88
  Latvia 111
  Poland 133
  Serbia 157
  Slovenia 167
  United Kingdom 202

harms, opioid-related 11, 225, 226, 232–7
headache 114, 218, 220
health, impact of pain 256
healthcare system
  Albania 19–20
  Austria 23–4
  Belgium 27–8
  Bosnia and Herzegovina 31–3
  Bulgaria 37
  Croatia 42–3
  Czech Republic 46–8
  Denmark 52
  Estonia 57–8
  Finland 62–3
  France 67–8
  Germany 75
  Greece 80–1
  Hungary 85–7
  Ireland 91–3
  Israel 98
  Italy 103–4
  Kosovo 107–8
  Latvia 111–13
  Lithuania 117–19
  Moldova 121–2
  Netherlands 185–6, 187
  Norway 127
  Poland 130–1

healthcare system (*cont.*)
Portugal 136–8
Romania 141–2
Russia 147–8
San Marino 152
Serbia 155–7
Slovakia 161
Slovenia 165
Spain 169
Sweden 174–5
Switzerland 181–3
Turkey 191–2
Ukraine 195–6
United Kingdom 199–201
health literacy 221
Hellenic Pain Society (HPS) 82, 83
Hellenic Society of Algology (HSA) 82, 83
heroin misuse 236
herpes zoster vaccine 212
home care services 154
hospices 105
hospitalized patients 208
human right, to pain management 3, 71, 82, 101, 219, 259
Hungarian Pain Society 87–8, 89, 90
Hungary 85–90, 251, 252

IASP *see* International Association for the Study of Pain
illicit drug use 234–5
individual burden of pain 11–12, 256
innovations
Albania 21
Austria 25–6
Belgium 29–30
Bosnia and Herzegovina 35
Bulgaria 39–40
Croatia 44–5
Czech Republic 50
Denmark 56
Estonia 60–1
Finland 65–6
France 71–3
Germany 78–9
Greece 83–4
Hungary 89–90
Ireland 95–6
Israel 102
Italy 105–6
Kosovo 109–10
Latvia 115
Lithuania 120
Moldova 125–6
Netherlands 189–90
Norway 129
Poland 134
Portugal 139–40
Romania 145–6
Russia 150–1
San Marino 154
Serbia 158–9
service delivery 272–3
Slovakia 163–4
Slovenia 167–8
Spain 173
Sweden 178–9
Switzerland 183–4
Turkey 193
Ukraine 197
United Kingdom 202–3
International Association for the Study of Pain (IASP) 5, 243–4
first Congress (1975) 103, 104
national pain strategies 259
pain centres/clinics 272
Spain and 171
International Narcotics Control Board 102, 228, 229
interventional pain therapies 269
children 220–1
Czech Republic 49, 50
Latvia 114
Spain 170
Ireland 12, 91–6
Irish Pain Research Network (IPRN) 95–6
Irish Pain Society 91, 93, 95, 96
Ischia, Stefano 104
Israel 98–102, 269
Israeli Medical Association (IMA) 99, 100
Israeli Pain Association (IPA) 99–100
Israeli Pain Nursing Forum 102
Italian Agency for Drugs (AIFA) 103–4
Italian Association for the Study of Pain (AISD) 103
Italy 103–6

Jagiellonian University, Krakow 132–3, 134

Kolesnikov, Yuri Alex 59
Koorits, Ursula 59
Kosovo 107–10, 251, 252
Kress, Hans G. 144
Kryeziu, Fadil 107
Kulichová, Marta 162

later life *see* older people
Latvia 111–15, 251, 252
Latvian Association for the Study of Pain (LASP) 111, 115
Lindblom, Ulf 5, 52, 103
Lithuania 117–20, 232, 251, 252, 269
Lithuanian Pain Society 117, 119–20
Loeser, John 143
Logina, Inara 111
low- and middle-income countries 249

Macfarlane, Gary 12
Magora, Florella 98

Májek, Milan 163
Malina, M. 115
Melzack, Ronald 187
memantine 212
methadone 124, 233, 236
migraine 220
Mission d'Intérêt Général et d'Aide à la Contractualisation (MIGAC) 70
Missions d'Intérêt Général (MIG) 70
mobile pain management teams 208
Mocavero, Guiseppe 104
Moldova 121–6, 269
Moldovan Society for the Study and Management of Pain 123, 125–6
morphine 11, 81, 124, 157, 158
multidisciplinary pain management 270
  Belgium 29
  Bosnia and Herzegovina 34
  Bulgaria 39
  children 221
  Croatia 44–5
  France 68
  Greece 83
  Hungary 88
  Latvia 114–15
  Netherlands 188, 189–90
  Norway 128–9
  older people 209
  Switzerland 184
  see also pain centres; pain clinics
musculoskeletal pain 96, 114, 257, 258

narcotic analgesics *see* opioids
National Clinical Care Programme, Ireland 96
National Drug Treatment Monitoring System (NDTMS) 233–4
National Institute for Health and Care Excellence (NICE) 202
national pain strategies 259–60
neck pain 24, 257, 258
Netherlands, the 185–90
Netherlands Organization for Health Research and Development (ZonMw) 187
neurologists 123, 157
neuromodulation 49, 50, 269
neuropathic pain 158, 210, 211
Nica, Sarah Adriana 144
Niv, David 38, 99, 100
non-pharmacological management 212, 217
non-steroidal anti-inflammatory drugs (NSAIDs) 124, 157, 158
Noordenbos, William 186–7
North America, opioid misuse 225, 228, 235–7
Northern Ireland 200–1, 202
Norway 127–9, 232–3
Norwegian Pain Society (NPS) 127, 128–9
NSAIDs *see* non-steroidal anti-inflammatory drugs
nurses, pain 29, 59, 64, 93, 94, 102

Office for National Statistics (ONS) 235
older people 5, 207–12, 256
  back pain 183
  pain evaluation 209–10
  pain management 207–9
  pain medicine education 207
  pain treatment 210–12
omnopon 124
opioids 11, 225–38, 269
  Austria 25
  barriers to access 228–32, 269
  Bulgaria 39
  children 220
  Estonia 60
  Europe vs North America 235–7
  Greece 81
  harms related to 11, 225, 226, 232–7
  historic perspective 11, 226
  Israel 102
  Moldova 124–5
  prescribing in Europe 227–8, 229, 230
  Romania 141–2
  Russia 150
  San Marino 154
  Serbia 157, 158
  Ukraine 197
  United Kingdom 203, 228
organisation of care 272–3
  see also pain services
Organization of Danish Medical Societies 56
orofacial pain 176, 177, 179
orthopaedic surgery 9
osteoarthritis 24, 210
osteogenesis imperfecta 220
Österreichische Schmerzgesellschaft *see* Austrian Pain Society
Österreichische Schmerzwochen 26
oxycodone 233

paediatric patients *see* children
pain
  congenital insensitivity 8
  impact on work-related outcomes 256–7
  individual burden 11–12, 256
  patients' attitudes to 109, 123–4, 208
  societal burden 12, 257–8
  see also acute pain; cancer pain; chronic pain
PAiN *see* Pijn Alliantie in Nederland
Pain Alliance Europe (PAE) 187, 255, 260–1
pain assessment *see* assessment, pain
pain behaviour 269–70
pain centres 272
  Belgium 29
  Bulgaria 39–40
  Czech Republic 48–9, 50
  Denmark 52
  France 69–71, 73
  Ireland 93
  Norway 128–9
  Romania 143

pain clinics 272
Croatia 43
Denmark 52
Estonia 59–60
Finland 63–4
France 68–9
Greece 80, 81, 83
Hungary 88
Israel 98, 101, 102
Lithuania 120
older people 209
Poland 132
Slovakia 162
Sweden 176, 177, 179
Switzerland 182–3, 184
Turkey 193
Pain-Free Hospitals 105, 125, 132, 133
pain management 4–5, 268
children 217–18, 219–22
chronic pain *see* chronic pain management
Eastern Europe 249–51
future directions 267–73
human right to 3, 71, 82, 101, 219, 259
multidisciplinary *see* multidisciplinary pain management
older people 207–9
policy 255–61
postoperative 10, 65–6, 78, 142, 145
services *see* pain services
workforce *see* pain workforce
see also treatment, pain
pain medicine
as a speciality *see* speciality pain medicine
as a subspeciality 157, 244–5
as a supraspeciality 243, 246–7, 248
training and education *see* training and education
PAIN OUT project 102, 126, 218
pain services
Albania 21
Austria 25
Belgium 29
Bosnia and Herzegovina 34–5
Bulgaria 39
Croatia 44
Czech Republic 50
Denmark 55–6
Estonia 60
Finland 64–5
France 70–1
future directions 272–3
Germany 77–8
Greece 83
Hungary 89
Ireland 93–5
Israel 101
Italy 105
Kosovo 109
Lithuania 119–20
Moldova 123–5
Netherlands 188–9
Norway 128–9
Poland 133–4
Portugal 139
Romania 144–5
Russia 150
San Marino 153–4
Serbia 158
Slovakia 162–3
Slovenia 167
Spain 170–3
Sweden 177–8
Switzerland 183
Turkey 193
Ukraine 197
United Kingdom 202–3
pain specialists 244, 270–1
Albania 21
Czech Republic 49, 50
Estonia 59
Finland 64
Germany 76
Latvia 111, 113
Netherlands 188
Sweden 176, 177, 179
Turkey 192–3
United Kingdom 201, 202
see also speciality pain medicine
pain units
Bosnia and Herzegovina 34
Latvia 114–15
San Marino 152–3
Slovenia 165, 167
Spain 169–70
Switzerland 182, 184
pain workforce 270
Albania 21
Austria 24–5
Belgium 28–9
Bosnia and Herzegovina 34
Bulgaria 38–9
Croatia 43–4
Czech Republic 48–9
Denmark 52–4
Estonia 59–60
Finland 63–4
France 68–70
Germany 75–7
Greece 82
Hungary 87–8
Ireland 93, 94
Israel 98–101
Italy 104–5
Kosovo 108–9
Latvia 113
Lithuania 119
Moldova 122–3
Netherlands 186–8
Norway 128
Poland 131–3

Portugal 138–9
Romania 142–4
Russia 148–50
San Marino 152–3
Serbia 157–8
Slovakia 162
Slovenia 166–7
Spain 169–70
Sweden 175–7
Switzerland 183
Turkey 192–3
Ukraine 196–7
United Kingdom 201–2
palliative care 5, 48, 105
barriers to opioids 228–9
Eastern Europe 250–1
Finland 65
Greece 81
older people 208
Serbia 155–6
Slovenia 167
United Kingdom 203
paracetamol 124
patient-centred care 187, 273
patient education 211–12, 221
phantom pain 21
photoplethysmography 115
physiotherapists 64, 93, 94, 176
Pijn Alliantie in Nederland (PAiN) 188, 189, 190
Pjevic, Miroslava 157
Plesia, Helen 82
Poland 130–4
policy, pain 255–61, 271
access to analgesics 231, 269
national pain strategies 259–60
rationale 256–8
SIP approach *see* Societal Impact of Pain (SIP) platform
Polish Association for the Study of Pain (PASP) 130, 132–4
population ageing 207
Portugal 136–40, 268
Portuguese Association for the Study of Pain (APED) 136, 139
post-herpetic neuralgia 211, 212
postoperative pain
chronic 10, 126, 212
management 10, 65–6, 78, 142, 145
post-traumatic stress disorder (PTSD) 32–3
prevalence, chronic pain 8–9, 227, 258
prevention, pain 212
primary care 257–8
Professional Health Association (PHA) (Kosovo) 107, 109
professional identity 243–4
promedol 124
Przewlocka, Barbara 133
psychological impact of pain 211, 269–70
psychologists 64, 93, 94, 269–70
psychosocial factors, chronic pain 9, 10–11, 219
psychosocial interventions, children 217, 221
Pud, Dorit 100–1

quality criteria, Austrian pain institutions 26
quality indicators, pain 77–8

Raftery, Hugh 91
RASP *see* Russian Association for the Study of Pain
Rawal, Narinder 4
registers, pain patients 177, 178
rehabilitation
Bosnia and Herzegovina 35
Bulgaria 39
Romania 144
Sweden 177, 178–9
Relief project 272
research, pain 13, 260, 271–2
Albania 21
Belgium 30
Czech Republic 50
Estonia 60
Finland 66
Hungary 89
Ireland 95–6
Israel 102
Latvia 115
Romania 142, 145
Switzerland 183–4
residency training programmes 246
Israel 100
Italy 104, 105
Latvia 113, 115
residential care facilities, elderly 209
rheumatologic disease 210
risk factors, chronic pain 9–11
Rokyta, Richard 50
Romanenko, Igor 195
Romania 141–6, 252
Romanian Association for the Study of Pain (ARSD) 141–4, 145
Russia 147–51, 268
Russian Association for the Study of Pain (RASP) 148–50, 268

Sandu, Lucian 142, 143
San Marino 152–4
San Marino Pain Society 152
Santayana, George 11
SASP *see* Scandinavian Association for the Study of Pain; Swiss Association for the Study of Pain
Scandinavian Association for the Study of Pain (SASP) 52, 62, 127
Scandinavian Society of Anaesthesiology and Intensive Care (SSAI) 179
Schmerznachrichten 26
scientific research *see* research, pain
Scotland 201, 202, 259
selfback project 272

Semmelweis Plan 87
Serbia 155–9, 251, 252
Serbian Association of Pain Research and Treatment (SAPRT) 157–8
services, pain management *see* pain services
sexual abuse, childhood 10–11
SIP *see* Societal Impact of Pain
Škvarč, Nevenka Krčevski 165
Slovakia 50, 160–4, 251, 252
Slovak Society for the Study and Treatment of Pain (SSSTP) 50, 162, 163–4
Slovenia 165–8, 251, 252
Slovenian Association for Pain Management (SZZB) 165, 166–7
Sluijter, Menno 187
Smilov, Ivan 38, 39
societal burden of chronic pain 12, 257–8
Societal Impact of Pain (SIP) platform 255, 258–61, 271
  individual chapters 35, 79, 144, 158, 167, 187
  national pain strategies 259–60
  population ageing and 256
  roadmap 260
  Time for Action 260–1
somatoform pain disorders 218
Spain 169–73
Spanish Pain Foundation (FED) 171
Spanish Pain Society (SED) 170–3
speciality pain medicine 243–8, 270–1
  cross-border working 245
  education and training 245–6
  future prospects 245–6
  international comparisons 244–5
  Ireland 93, 95
  Israel 100, 101
  Italy 104–5
  Latvia 113
  Sweden 176
  see also pain specialists
Společnost pro studium a léčbu bolesti ČLS JEP *see* Czech Pain Society
SSSTP *see* Slovak Society for the Study and Treatment of Pain
stomatognathic physiology 176
Strandhäll, Annika 257
subspeciality
  algology as 192
  pain medicine as 157, 244–5
  pain therapy as 163
supraspeciality, pain medicine as 243, 246–7, 248
Suru, Virgil 143
Sweden 12, 174–9, 258
Swedish Agency for Health Technology Assessment and Assessment of Social Services (SBU) 176–7
Swedish College for Pain Medicine 179
Swedish Pain Society (SPS) 176, 179
Swedish Quality Registry for Pain Rehabilitation (SQRP) 178–9
Swiss Association for the Study of Pain (SASP) 181, 182, 183
Switzerland 181–4, 268
Sylaj, Bashkim 107

Temelkov, Atanas 39
Tiengo, Mario 104
total pain concept 246
training and education (pain medicine) 245–7, 248, 268
  Austria 26
  Belgium 29
  Bosnia and Herzegovina 34
  Bulgaria 39
  Croatia 44
  current developments 244–5
  Czech Republic 49, 50
  Denmark 55–6
  Eastern Europe 250, 252
  Estonia 60
  Finland 64
  Germany 75
  Greece 82, 83
  Hungary 89–90
  Ireland 93, 96
  Israel 100, 101, 102
  Italy 104–5
  Kosovo 109
  Latvia 113, 115
  Moldova 123–4, 125–6
  Norway 128
  older people 207
  Poland 131–3, 134
  Portugal 138, 139
  Romania 143–4, 145
  Russia 150, 151
  San Marino 152
  Serbia 157
  Slovakia 163
  Slovenia 167
  Spain 170, 172, 173
  Sweden 176, 177–8, 179
  Switzerland 183
  Turkey 192–3
  Ukraine 196–7
  United Kingdom 201, 203, 245
tramadol 124–5, 233, 235, 237
treatment, pain
  children 217–18, 220–1
  inadequate 258, 260
  non-pharmacological 212, 217
  older people 210–12
  research needs 13
  see also analgesics; interventional pain therapies; pain management
Treede, Rolf-Detlef 96

trimeperidine 124
triptans 220
Turkey 191–3
Turkish Society of Algology 191, 192–3

UEMS *see* European Union of Medical Specialists
Ukraine 195–7
Ukrainian Association for the Study of Pain (UASP) 195, 196–7
United Kingdom 199–203, 258
  opioid use 203, 228, 233, 236–7
  training in pain medicine 201, 203, 245
United States
  costs of chronic pain 12
  opioid use 11, 228, 229, 232–5, 235–7
  pain research 271
  training and education 246
Universal Declaration of Human Rights 258–9

Vasili, Petrit 21
Vlaamse Anesthesiologische Vereniging voor Pijnbestrijding (VAVP) 28

Wales 201, 202
Wall, Patrick 187
Wells, Chris 82, 163
White Book project, Belgium 29
workforce, pain management *see* pain workforce
work-related outcomes 256–7
World Health Organization (WHO)
  access to opioids guideline 231
  analgesic ladder 226
  defined daily dose 228

Xanti, Michaelis 144

Zimmermann, M. 162
Zupping, Rein 59
Zuurmond, Wouter 187

SAM.KYNMAN@EFIC.ORG